THE PRETERM BABY
and other babies with low birth weight

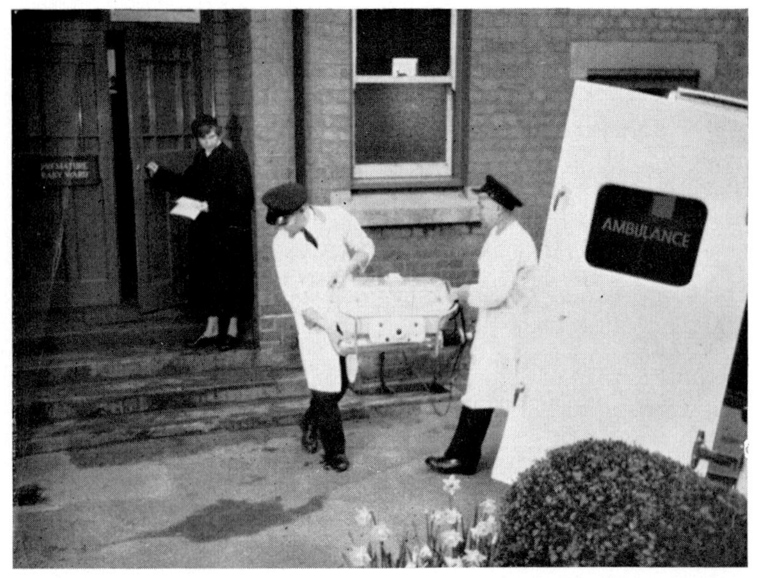

(Photo by Camera Talks)

A baby arrives at the Special Care Baby Unit, Sorrento Maternity Hospital

THE PRETERM BABY

and other Babies with Low Birth Weight

By

V. MARY CROSSE, O.B.E.

M.D. (Lond.), D.P.H., M.M.S.A., D.(Obstet.)R.C.O.G.

Hon. Consultant Paediatrician East Birmingham General Hospital, Solihull Hospital, Sorrento Maternity Hospital, Marston Green Maternity Hospital. Past Lecturer in Paediatrics and Child Health, University of Birmingham. Past Lecturer in Paediatrics, Central Midwives Board. Member of Expert Advisory Panel on Maternal and Child Health (with special relation to Prematurity), World Health Organization, 1950–1970.

SEVENTH EDITION

With 50 Illustrations

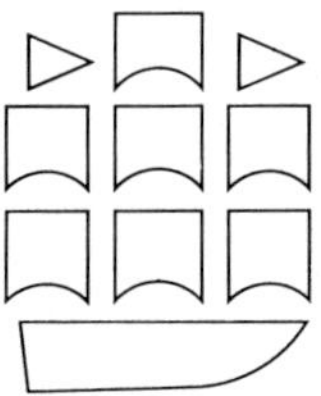

CHURCHILL LIVINGSTONE

Edinburgh and London

1971

First Edition	1945
First Edition reprinted	1946
Second Edition	1949
Third Edition	1952
Fourth Edition	1957
Fifth Edition	1961
Japanese translation	1963
Sinhala translation	1965
Sixth Edition	1966
Spanish translation	1967
Seventh Edition	1971

International Standard Book Number
0 7000 1526 4

All correspondence relating to this volume should be directed to the publishers at 104 Gloucester Place, London, W1H 4AE

Printed in Great Britain at the Pitman Press, Bath

PREFACE

In this edition the recommendations of the Second European Congress of Perinatal Medicine (held in London in 1970) have been followed, and low-weight infants (2500 g and less at birth) are divided into (1) pre-term infants (those born before 37 completed weeks gestation) and (2) light-for-dates term infants (born after 37 weeks). The light-for-dates infants are subdivided into the two generally accepted groups, i.e. malnourished and hypoplastic.

The recent concept of perinatal care (rather than neonatal care) has necessitated the inclusion of a section on the management of pregnancy and the enlargement of the section on care during and immediately after delivery. These sections include new techniques for assessing the gestational age of the foetus, and for monitoring its condition during pregnancy and labour.

The necessity for more intensive neonatal care for a minority of low-weight infants is now generally recognized, and such care is included, e.g. the use of respirators, monitoring equipment, etc.

All chapters have been brought up to date, especially the chapter on complications which has again been almost completely re-written. New sections are included on hypomagnesaemia, idiopathic neonatal diabetes, infants of mothers addicted to narcotics, neonatal necrotizing enterocolitis, and the Wilson-Mikity Syndrome.

Now that statistics for pre-term and low-weight babies are available on a country-wide basis (British Perinatal Mortality Survey 1958), figures from this survey are used instead of those from the City of Birmingham.

Acknowledgements are due to many people who have helped me in the preparation of this edition. I particularly want to thank Dr. Eileen Hill (Consultant Paediatrician) for reading the typescript and making valuable suggestions; and also for reading proofs. I am indebted to Miss S. T. Davy, S.R.N., S.C.M., M.T.D., for once again reading proofs; and to Dr. E. L. M. Miller (Medical Officer of Health, Birmingham) for permission to use some of the Birmingham statistics. I wish also to thank my publishers for their continued help and advice.

V. Mary Crosse.

Birmingham 1971.

CONTENTS

INTRODUCTION

In 1948 the first World Health Assembly recognized the importance of prematurity as a world-wide cause of infant deaths and adopted an international definition of prematurity, i.e. a baby whose birth weight is 2,500 g. ($5\frac{1}{2}$ lb.) or less. The W H O Expert Group on Prematurity (W H O Technical Report Series No. 27, 1950) endorsed this international definition but realized that it would not be applicable in all countries. In many parts of the world the international definition has proved useful for separating off babies which require some special care, but in other countries the use of this standard has resulted in unusually high proportions of premature babies, many of whom were not born prematurely and did not seem to require any special care. This led to the local adoption of various lower birth weight levels, which has created confusion and prevented comparisons.

The time for re-assessment had arrived and a W H O study on birth weight was carried out in 18 countries (countries at different stages of socio-economic development). A study of these birth weights showed that any unduly increased proportion of babies weighing 2,500 g. and less at birth was not due to an increased proportion born prematurely (before 37 completed weeks of gestation) but due to a general reduction of birth weight at all stages of maturity. Many of the babies weighing 2,500 g. and less at birth were born after 37 weeks gestation but with a low birth weight. In view of the convincing evidence that many of the babies included in the international definition were not born prematurely, an Expert Committee on Maternal and Child Health (W H O 1961) recommended that the concept of "prematurity" should give way to that of "low birth weight".

To conform with this recommendation the term low-weight baby is used throughout this book when referring to a baby weighing 2,500 g. or less at birth. A pre-term infant is one born before 37 complete weeks of pregnancy.

As other causes of infant mortality are reduced, low birth weight becomes an increasingly important factor. In England and Wales, between 1928 and 1968, the death rate between the ages of 1 week and 1 year fell from 45·8 to 7·7 per 1,000 live births, while the perinatal death rate (stillbirths plus deaths during the first week of life per 1,000 total births) only fell from 61·1 to 24·7. In England and Wales low-weight babies form 7% of all births and 61% of all perinatal deaths.

The reduction of deaths due to low birth weight can be divided into two distinct parts: firstly, the prevention of a curtailed pregnancy and other causes of low birth weight; and secondly, the care of the low-weight baby before, during and after labour. The first of these problems is an extremely important one and is discussed in Chapter 8; the major portion of this book deals with the second problem.

A complete service for the care of low-weight babies has been in existence in Birmingham for many years. In 1931, the first English unit for the care of low-weight babies was built in the grounds of Sorrento Maternity Hospital. Shortly after the opening of this unit the necessity for suitable transport and for a follow-up service by the health visitors was recognized, and these services were implemented; and in 1933 a home-care service was set up to deal with the larger low-weight babies born in their own homes.

Sorrento Maternity Hospital is a training centre for Parts I & II of the C.M.B. Certificate, and pupil midwives spend a short period of their training working in the special unit. In addition, the unit is recognized by the Ministry of Health for the training of doctors, midwives, nurses and health visitors in the care of the low-weight baby. Some of these people are being trained for the domiciliary care of low-weight babies, and for this reason a special feature has been the teaching of simple methods of care for larger babies which can be used in the babies' own homes.

In 1961, the Ministry of Health Central Health Services Council (Report of the Sub-committee on the Prevention of Prematurity and the Care of Premature Infants) drew attention to the advantages of combining the hospital care of pre-term babies with that of mature sick newborn infants who require similar care and supervision. They suggested the setting up of special baby care units in large and medium sized maternity departments to which mature infants suffering from intracranial birth injury, asphyxia, haemolytic disease of the newborn, babies of diabetic mothers, etc., would be admitted, as well as low-weight babies. A small number of such babies have always been treated in the Sorrento Unit, but they have only been included in the statistics if they weighed 2,500 g. and less at birth.

CHAPTER I

DEFINITION OF LOW BIRTH WEIGHT AND CHARACTERISTICS OF PRE-TERM BABIES AND LOW-WEIGHT TERM BABIES

Definition of Low Birth Weight

THE definition "premature baby" recommended by the World Health Assembly 1948 and the Expert Group on Prematurity (W H O 1950) has now been replaced by that of "low birth weight baby" (W H O 1961). Thus, any infant weighing 5½ lb. (2,500 g.) or less at birth is now regarded as a low-weight baby.

At the Second European Congress of Perinatal Medicine held in London (April 8–10, 1970) it was decided that the birthweight should be related to the gestational age; and that infants born before 37 completed weeks gestation should be called pre-term infants while those born after 37 weeks should be called term infants (this is in agreement with the W H O recommendation of 1950). This decision divides low-weight infants into two groups (1) pre-term infants and (2) term infants who are light for dates (light-for-dates infants).

In well developed countries (with a high mean birth weight and a relatively small proportion of low-weight babies) between 30–40% of all babies weighing 2,500 g. and less are born after 37 completed weeks gestation, and many of these require special care. In less well developed countries (which have a low mean birth weight and a high proportion of low-weight babies) the percentage of light-for-dates babies born after 37 weeks is very much higher, and this accounts for most of the increased proportion of low-weight babies (W H O 1961). Obviously all these term babies do not require special care, and there would still appear to be a place for local adoption of a suitably lower birth weight level solely as an indication for greater care.

Characteristics of Pre-Term Babies

The characteristics of a pre-term baby vary with the gestational age. They are most marked in the babies with the shortest gestational age and become less distinctive as the gestational age increases. The presence or absence of pathological conditions in the baby, or its mother, has a definite effect on the development of the baby, but in the following account it is assumed that the baby is healthy and has the normal characteristics of the gestational age at which it is born.

Length. Measurement of the length of the infant from vertex to heel is the most reliable single method of estimating the gestational age of a healthy pre-term baby because it bears a remarkably constant relationship to it and is little affected by biological factors, such as sex, multiple birth, age of mother, birth order, etc. After the 28th week, the infant measures approximately $\frac{1}{2}$ × weeks of gestational age in inches ($1\frac{1}{4}$ × weeks of gestational age in cm.) i.e. 14 inches (35 cm.) at 28 weeks, 16 inches (40 cm.) at 32 weeks, etc. The length must, however, be measured accurately: if the infant is placed on its back, with both legs straight (knees pressed on to the mattress and feet dorsiflexed), the measurement can be taken from the top of the head to the heels in one straight line.

Weight. The mean birth weight at different gestational ages varies in different countries, and even in different districts, because the birth weight is influenced by many factors (see p. 244). The mean birth weight at 28, 32, 36 and 40 weeks gestation is given below for all single-born babies (male and female) born in England, Scotland and Wales during 1 week in 1958 (Butler and Alberman, 1969).

Maturity	Mean birth weight	
	Grammes	Pounds
28 weeks	1,130	2 lb. 8 oz.
32 ,,	1,890	4 lb. 3 oz.
36 ,,	2,790	6 lb. 2 oz.
40 ,,	3,415	7 lb. 8 oz.

These figures are higher than those used by the author in Birmingham (see p. 95). They are also higher than those reported by Harper (1962), Lubchenco *et al.* (1963), Kitchen (1968) and Usher and McLean (1969). In these five investigations the mean birth weight has ranged between 1020–1236 g. at 28 weeks; 1590–1890 at 32 weeks; 2350–2790 at 36 weeks; and 3226–3500 at 40 weeks.

The loss of weight during the first few days of life is relatively greater in the pre-term baby than in the term baby, the percentage of weight lost increasing as the birth weight decreases. This initial loss of weight is regained more slowly, the birth weight sometimes not being reached until the third week in the case of the smallest infants. But after regaining the birth weight, pre-term babies gain relatively more rapidly than term babies; for example, a baby weighing only 2 lb. will double this weight in a further 6–8 weeks, and at the age of 1 year may weigh more than nine times the birth weight. This relatively rapid growth of the pre-term baby explains its increased requirement of calories, protein, vitamins and mineral salts, these needs being greatest for the infants with the smallest birth weights.

The ratio of the weight of the infant to the weight of the placenta increases as the gestational age increases. Hendricks (1964) gives the following ratios from 28–40 weeks; 3½ at 28 weeks, 4 at 32 weeks, 5 at 36 weeks and 5¾ at 40 weeks.

General proportions. The pre-term infant has a large head in proportion to the size of its body. This is, however, only a stage in development; the foetal head is as long as the rest of the foetus at two months' gestation, while at the fifth month it is about one-third of the total length, and at term it is only one-quarter of the total length. The average circumference of the head (from analysis of the author's cases) at the various gestational ages is given below. These figures are practically the same as those given by Usher and McLean (1969).

Gestational age	Average circumference of head	
	Inches	Centimetres
28 weeks	10	25
32 "	11½	29
36 "	12¾	32
40 "	14	35

The chest is relatively small in the pre-term infant, while the abdomen is relatively large; the head circumference usually exceeds the circumference of the chest (nipple line) by 1½ inches (3·75 cm.) or more. The shorter the gestational age of the infant, the nearer is the umbilicus to the symphysis pubis. The limbs are thin in comparison with the rest of the body.

Activity. The lower the gestational age of the infant, the less is its activity, but even the smallest infants show periods of muscular activity if the general condition is good and if they are not restricted by clothing. The shorter the gestational age of the infant, the weaker and less frequent the cry.

Temperature control. The body temperature tends to be subnormal because of the poor heat production and increased heat loss. Less heat is produced because of the sluggish circulation, feeble respiration with poor oxygen combustion, muscular inactivity and poor intake of food. Loss of heat is increased because of the relatively greater body surface and the lack of subcutaneous fat, particularly brown fat. Brown fat cells begin to differentiate from reticular cells at 26–30 weeks gestational age and their development continues for some weeks after birth. Brown fat is found round the neck, between the scapulae, in the axillae, in the mediastinum and round the kidneys and adrenals (Aherne and Hull, 1964) and there is evidence that brown fat plays a role in the response of human babies to cold (Silverman *et al.*, 1964; Dawkins and Scopes, 1965).

Unless artificial heat is supplied, the temperature of a pre-term infant falls, but care must be taken to control the amount of heat supplied, as the child is also easily overheated. This lack of ability to regulate the body temperature is partly due to the poor development of the heat regulating centre and partly due to the failure of the peripheral responses to heat and cold, i.e. sweating and shivering (Day *et al.*, 1943; Young, 1962).

Respiratory system. The development of the lungs depends on the length of gestation. The lung of an infant weighing 2 lb. (900 g.) or less at birth shows small alveoli lined with low cubical epithelium and surrounded by a cellular stroma with few blood vessels; whereas the lung of an infant weighing 6 lb. (2,730 g.) at birth shows large alveoli, the walls of which are virtually formed by bare capillaries. There is a great increase in the capillary network between the 26th and 36th weeks of intra-uterine life and for this reason the ability of the lungs to sustain extra-uterine life increases with each week that the foetus remains *in utero* during this period. The lower the gestational age the less blood flows through the lungs; the remainder being shunted through the ductus arteriosus (Potter, 1953).

Primary atelectasis (lack of complete lung expansion) is common in the smaller pre-term babies, not only because of the poor development of the lung tissues but also because of the weak respiratory muscles, yielding thoracic cage and poorly developed respiratory centre. Secondary atelectasis (idiopathic respiratory distress of the newborn, see p. 129) is also common, pre-term babies being particularly prone to this condition by reason of a decreased pulmonary lipoprotein, i.e. a surfactant which reduces surface tension in the lungs (see p. 131). Respiration is largely diaphragmatic, and if much atelectasis is present the thoracic cage is dragged down with each inspiration. In the worst cases, the sternum is sucked back towards the spine with inspiration, and expiration is accompanied by a short feeble grunt.

Respiration tends to be irregular in rhythm and depth: there are often periods of apnoea, during which cyanosis may develop. Respirations must be counted for at least one minute if the respiration rate is to be estimated at all accurately.

The cough reflex is absent in the smallest pre-term infants, making the danger of inhalation of regurgitated fluids a very real one.

The nasal passages are extremely narrow, and the mucous membrane is easily injured. Great care must be taken where passing catheters and endotracheal tubes through the nose.

Circulatory system. The heart is relatively large at birth. In some cases its action is slow and feeble: extrasystoles occur and murmurs may be present at or shortly after birth which disappear later as the foetal openings gradually close; or murmurs may appear for the first time several days after birth and these may or may not disappear later. The peripheral circulation is often poor. The walls of the blood vessels are weak, especially those of the intracranial vessels, and this probably accounts for the special tendency to intracranial haemorrhage which is shown by the pre-term infant.

The systolic *blood pressure* at birth is lower than that of term infants and the level decreases with the birth weight. Thus infants weighing 2–5 lb. (900–2,270 g.) at birth have a systolic blood pressure of 45–60 mm. of mercury compared with a pressure of 80 mm. in a term child. The level rises with the age of the child, the rise being approximately 20 mm. by the end of the second week, and another 5 mm. by the age of 2 months. The diastolic level is proportionately low, varying from 30–45 mm.

The *pulse rate* varies between 100 and 160 per minute for some time after birth, the average being 140. Because of a tendency to arrhythmia the pulse rate of a pre-term baby is most accurately obtained by counting the pulse (or preferably the apex beat with a stethoscope) for a whole minute.

As regards the *blood* of the pre-term baby, both the haemoglobin and the red cell count rise as gestation advances until about the 30th week, after which they remain stationary. The usual concentration of blood occurs during the first few hours of life (Gairdner *et al.*, 1958) but the subsequent fall in both the red cell count and the haemoglobin level is greater and the final rise is slower than usual, especially in regard to the haemoglobin level. The pre-term baby has a relatively higher proportion of foetal haemoglobin than the term infant and the foetal haemoglobin disappears more slowly. Schulman *et al.* (1954) and Schulman (1959) demonstrated a steady decrease in the body haemoglobin content (both foetal and adult) in pre-term babies during the first few weeks of life. After this, the body content of adult haemoglobin began to rise (coinciding with an increase in reticulocytes) while that of foetal haemoglobin continued to fall; and it took some weeks for the infant to regain the haemoglobin mass with which it started life. These workers also showed a decreased survival time for the initial red cell population in pre-term babies, i.e. 77 days instead of 100–120 days. More immature cells are present in the blood at birth and throughout the first weeks of life.

The white cell count is high at birth but it is lower than that usually found in the term child. The same predominance of polymorphonuclear cells is found and the same fall in the total white cell count occurs during the first week of life, but the change over to a lymphocytic predominance develops more slowly than in the term infant.

Medoff (1964) found platelet counts of 31,000–197,000/cmm. in pre-term babies during the first five days of life. In babies weighing less than 1,700 g. the count fell to 50,000 by 10–20 days, but in babies weighing more than 1,700 g. the count rose until the 10th day.

An early diminution of blood formation combined with a shortened life span of the red blood cells (Foconi and Sjölin, 1959; Schulman, 1959) leads to the development of anaemia in pre-term babies. The more rapid destruction of the immature cells contributes to the development of neonatal jaundice; this jaundice can be severe and prolonged.

There is a deficiency of several clotting factors in the blood and this, combined with the increased fragility of the capillary walls, contributes to the increased liability of the pre-term infant to haemorrhagic disease of the new-born (see p. 181).

The serum total protein, albumin and globulin levels are all lower in pre-term babies than in babies born at term; the lower the gestational age, the lower the levels. Serum albumin levels fall for a few weeks instead of rising after the first week of life as in term babies. Pre-term babies have relatively lower gamma globulin levels than term babies (but still often higher than adult levels): these decrease rapidly during the first 4–6 weeks of life and then remain low for some time (Crosse *et al.*, 1954 and 1960); and this low gamma globulin level probably contributes to the poor response of the pre-term baby to infection.

In pre-term infants the blood glucose falls to a lower level after birth than in term infants. The normal fall in the blood calcium level and normal rise in the potassium level after birth occur, but the pre-term infants tend to have lower blood calcium levels than term infants (Smith 1959).

Digestive system. The larger infants have good powers of suction and swallowing. As the gestational age decreases, these reflexes become progressively more feeble and the smallest infants are unable to feed effectually. Owing to the poorly developed mechanism for closure of the cardia and the relatively strong pyloric sphincter, regurgitation is common.

The powers of digestion depend on the gestational age, being rudimentary in infants born at 26–28 weeks' gestation, but becoming rapidly less defective as the gestational age increases. The stomach of a baby weighing approximately 2 lb. (900 g.) at birth shows little folding of the mucosal surface and poor development of the secretory glands and muscle fibres, as compared with the stomach of a term baby, with its deeply folded mucosal layer and well-developed glands and muscle tissue. The birth weight bears a close relationship to the development of the gastric mucosa (Miller, 1941). Pre-term infants digest and absorb proteins and carbohydrates easily but they absorb fats badly, even though fat-splitting enzymes are present at birth. As soon as a newborn pre-term baby has used its glycogen stores it depends as usual on its body fat for energy; but when food becomes available, a pre-term baby uses less calories from fat and more from carbohydrates than a term baby. In this way a pre-term baby resembles the foetus which apparently depends on carbohydrates for its main source of energy.

The musculature of the bowel wall is weak and easily distended so that there is a tendency to constipation. Owing to the thin abdominal wall, normal gastric peristalsis is easily seen; and if slight distension is present, intestinal peristalsis also becomes visible.

The liver is relatively large but its function is poorly developed in the smaller infants. This immaturity of the liver predisposes to jaundice by reason of the inability of the liver to conjugate and excrete bilirubin (see p. 231). It has also been suggested that the low blood glucose level found in pre-term babies is hepatogenic, due to small liver glycogen stores (Van Creveld, 1929). The lower serum protein levels, the deficiency of certain blood clotting factors, and the deficient conjugation and detoxication of certain drugs are all due to liver immaturity.

The tip of the spleen is usually palpable.

Urinary system. Urination is scanty and infrequent for a few days after birth, due to the small amount of fluid taken. Urates are commonly present in some excess, giving a false positive for albumin by the heat, acetic acid or trichloracetic acid tests (Doxiadis, 1952).

Pre-term infants have relatively more extracellular fluid than term infants. They also have less ability to concentrate urine and this is important when they suffer from conditions involving an excessive loss of water, e.g. diarrhoea or vomiting.

Pre-term infants show a tendency to become oedematous shortly after birth and this is partly due to poor development of the kidneys (which are markedly immature until 35 weeks gestation, and tubules continue to be formed until term; Smith, 1959) with their inability to excrete sodium and chloride and the consequent retention of water (see p. 228). Potter and Thierstein in 1943 reported a relationship between glomerular development and the weight of the foetus; the smaller the infant the more defective the renal function.

The tendency to a more marked and more prolonged acidosis in newborn pre-term babies is probably also due to the relatively poor development of their kidneys. Since low pH levels are regularly found in apparently healthy pre-term babies there is no proof that this is harmful unless it is increased by respiratory distress, diarrhoea, etc.

Due to renal immaturity, the excretion of many drugs is deficient.

The kidneys may be easily palpable, being relatively lower during foetal life.

Genital system. In the female, the labia minora are not covered by the labia majora until almost at term. In the male, the testicles may be in the abdomen, inguinal canal or scrotum, according to the gestational age, but they may be found in the scrotum as early as 28 weeks' gestation. There is a special tendency to inguinal hernia.

Nervous system. The development of the nervous system depends on the length of gestation. Those with the shortest gestational age tend to lie quietly unless disturbed, only waking at intervals for feeding. External stimulation results in weak purposeless jerky movements and perhaps a feeble cry. At first these infants may lie on the side in the foetal position but they gradually uncurl until, after a few days, they lie on the back with the head rolled over to one side, the hips flexed and abducted, and the knees and ankles flexed ("frog position"). The shorter the gestational age the less good is the muscle tone.

The centres controlling the vital functions, e.g. respiration, control of body temperature, are poorly developed, and so also are the centres controlling the vital reflexes, e.g. coughing, swallowing and sucking.

The Moro and tonic neck reflexes are present in normal pre-term infants; so also are the Chvostek and Babinski signs. Tendon reflexes are variable.

Eyes. By 24 weeks gestational age, the retinal vessels have grown about 6 mm. from the optic nerve. Between 24 and 30 weeks no further growth occurs ("immature fundus") but after this time growth re-commences ("transitional fundus") and by about 34 weeks (weight 4 lb. 6 oz. or 2,000 g.) the fundus is usually mature.

During the "immature" and "transitional" developmental stages of the fundus, infants are liable to become blind if oxygen is given in excess of requirements (see Retrolental fibroplasia, p. 206).

The presence of hyaloid remnants is frequently seen in the eyes of pre-term infants. Roper-Hall (1960), working in two of the units under the author's care, reported these as an almost constant finding among babies weighing less than 3 lb. at birth. They were also found in 58·2% of babies weighing 3–4 lb. at birth, 36·4% of babies weighing 4–5 lb. and 13% of babies weighing 5–6 lb. at birth. These remnants regress and disappear in most cases in a few weeks.

Presence of the pupillary membrane is also a feature of the pre-term baby during the first few days of life (Schmöger, 1955; Gans, 1959). The frequency of persistent pupillary membrane also varies directly with the gestational age.

Skeletal system. Unfortunately, centres of ossification do not appear at sufficiently constant ages to be of value in determining the gestational age. Practical difficulties, moreover, exclude this observation from the routine examination of the pre-term baby.

Skin, hair and nails. The skin is red and wrinkled, and little subcutaneous fat is present in infants up to 28 weeks' gestation; but after this the skin becomes paler and subcutaneous fat begins to appear. In the smallest infants, the nipples are flat pigmented areas and it is only after 36 weeks gestation that they rise above the surrounding skin. Engorgement of the breast is rare in pre-term babies.

Lanugo is plentiful up to 28 weeks, then becomes less in amount; the back, the face and extensor surfaces of the limbs being most commonly affected. Hair is short and scanty and eyebrows are often absent.

The nails are softer than at term. They may even project beyond the finger tips; and contrary to general belief, they reach almost to the tips as early as 28 weeks' gestation.

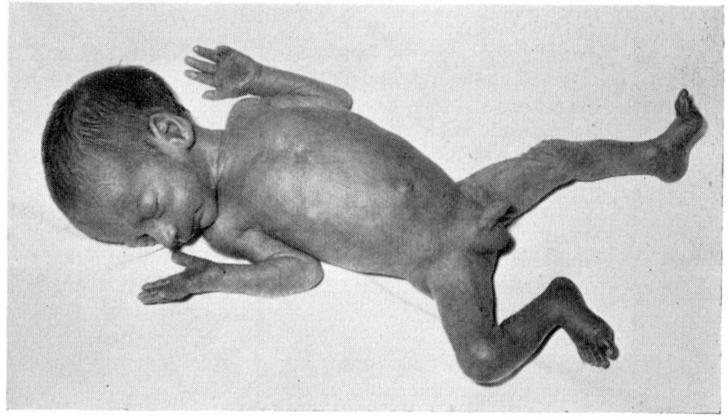

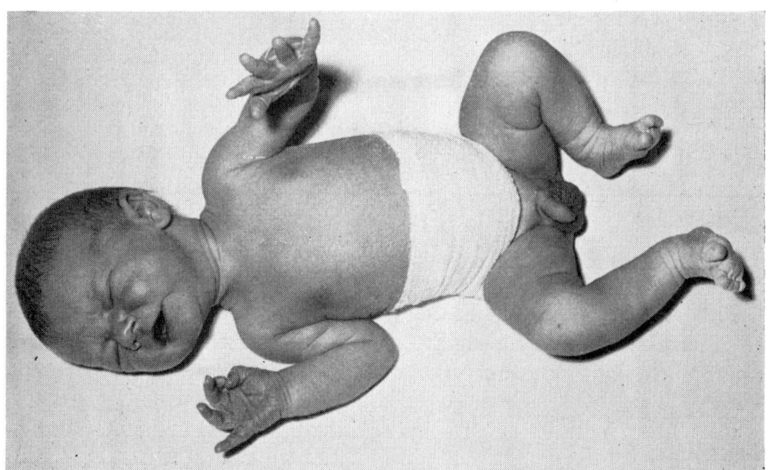

FIGS. 1 and 2. These photographs illustrate some of the difference between the pre-term and term baby, as listed on p. 10.

Comparison between Term and Pre-term Infants

The following table sets out the chief differences which can be observed on examination:

	Term infants	Pre-term infants
Length	20 in. (50 cm.)	Less than 18½ in. (47 cm.).
Weight	7–8 lb. (3,180–3,640 g.)	5½ lb. (2,500 g.) or less.
Proportion	Circumference of head 14 in. (35·5 cm.) Circumference of chest 13 in. (33 cm.) Umbilicus midway between symphysis pubis and xiphisternum.	Less than 13 in. (33 cm.) Less than 11½ in. (29 cm.) Umbilicus nearer symphysis
Vitality	Strong and active Wakes for feeds Lusty cry Normal temperature Suction strong	Weak and sluggish Drowsy Weak mewing cry Subnormal temperature Suction feeble or absent
Skin	Pink and smooth Subcutaneous fat present Nipples raised	Red and wrinkled Little fat present Nipples flat
Hair	Silky strands	Short and fuzzy
Ears	Ears firm and stand out	Ears soft and flat
Soles of feet	Complex series of criss-crossed creases cover soles of feet	One or two transverse creases
Nails	Hard Project beyond finger tips	Soft Just to finger tips or not quite to finger tips
Genitals	Testicles in scrotum Labia minora covered by labia majora	Testicles in abdomen, inguinal canal or scrotum Labia minora not covered by labia majora

Estimation of Gestational Age

If there is any doubt about the gestational age of any infant, this can be determined by a neurological examination of the reflexes (André-Thomas *et al.*, 1960; Prechtl and Beintema, 1964; Robinson, 1966; Amiel-Tison, 1968; Graziani *et al.*, 1968; Saint-Anne Dargassies, 1970). Other methods are to use specified external characteristics to judge the gestational age (Usher *et al.*, 1966; Farr and Mitchell, 1969); or to measure nerve conduction velocity, which increases as the gestational age increases (Ruppert and Johnson, 1968).

Light-for-dates Babies

Low-weight term babies are the result of intra-uterine growth retardation. They are referred to in this book as light-for-dates babies. About 35–40% of all low-weight babies in this country are light-for-dates babies (Butler and Bonham, 1963).

Growth retardation can only be recognized in relation to gestational age. For statistical purposes various standards have been suggested, i.e. the tenth percentile (Lubchenco *et al.*, 1963), or two standard deviations below the mean birthweight (Gruenwald, 1963) which corresponds approximately to the third percentile. For practical purposes one can get a good idea of the degree of growth retardation if the infant's birth weight is plotted against both weight and gestational age (see growth chart on p. 95).

If growth retardation occurs in an infant born before 37 weeks gestation the infant will have the handicaps of a pre-term baby as well as those of a growth-retarded baby.

Light-for-dates babies are not a homogeneous group, and it is usual to divide them into two main groups according to the cause of growth retardation:

(1) **Malnourished group.** This group includes the majority of light-for-dates babies, i.e. multiple-born babies; babies born to mothers with severe toxaemia of pregnancy, hypertension, placental insufficiency, poor socio-economic conditions, etc.; and to mothers who smoke excessively (see causes of low birth weight, p. 244).

These infants have a more alert facies, a stronger cry and more hair than expected for their birth weight. The head and chest measurements are greater than expected and there is less difference between these two measurements than is usual for their birth weight. The skin is pale or meconium-stained, and the backs of the hands and dorsa of the feet may be dry and scaling. There is little subcutaneous fat. The abdomen may be scaphoid and the cord is withered and often meconium-stained.

If the malnutrition has lasted for a period of weeks, the length of the infant corresponds to the weight; but if it has lasted only for days, the body length is more in proportion to the gestational age than the body weight because malnutrition has a more immediate effect on weight increase than on linear growth. The neurological reflexes are in accordance with the gestational age.

Compared with a normal pre-term infant of the same birth weight, the liver, lungs and thymus are relatively smaller in the light-for-dates baby while the heart and brain are relatively larger (Gruenwald, 1963; Butler and Alberman, 1969), especially the brain (Dawkins, 1965). The liver glycogen store is inadequate (Shelly, 1964) and the brown fat is often depleted (Aherne and Hull, 1964). Histological examination shows that maturation of the pulmonary alveolar structure and of the renal glomeruli are in accordance with gestational age. Reduction in the size of the various organs is due to a reduction in the size of the cells rather than in the number of cells (Naeye, 1965a).

Like pre-term babies, the light-for-dates babies tend to develop hypothermia (due to lack of subcutaneous fat), skin and other infections, jaundice (due to depressed liver function and high haemocrit), and late anaemia (from rapid neonatal growth). In addition they are more liable, than pre-term babies, to develop respiratory distress from meconium aspiration or massive pulmonary haemorrhage, hypoglycaemia, and neonatal tetany. They also have a greater risk of intra-uterine anoxia and birth asphyxia.

(2) **Hypoplastic group.** This smaller group includes a variety of syndromes, i.e. genetically small infants (dwarfs); infants with chromosomal abnormalities, and with congenital malformations such as congenital heart disease, anencephaly, etc.; infants born after transplacental infections (see p. 173), etc.

The genetically small infants are well proportioned but small for their gestational age and they behave in accordance with their gestational age. The remainder of this group show signs of the cause of their retarded growth.

In these babies there is a marked reduction in the weight of all organs and histological examination shows a reduction in cell population of all organs (Naeye, 1965b).

It is mainly this group that increases the incidence of physical and mental defects among light-for-dates babies. This group also has a high mortality rate.

Considering all these facts, it is reasonable to presume that low-weight term babies (light-for-dates babies) require as much special care as pre-term babies.

REFERENCES

AHERNE, N. and HULL, D. (1964). *Proc. roy. Soc. Med.*, **57**, 1172.

AMIEL-TISON, C. (1968). *Arch. Dis. Childh.*, **43**, 89.

ANDRÉ-THOMAS, CHESNI, Y. and SAINT-ANNE DARGASSIES, S. (1960). *Cerebral Palsy Bulletin.* Suppl. 1.

BUTLER, N. R. and ALBERMAN, E. D. (1969). *Perinatal Problems.* E. & S. Livingstone, Edinburgh.

BUTLER, N. R. and BONHAM, D. G. (1963). *Perinatal Mortality.* E. & S. Livingstone, Edinburgh.

CROSSE, V. M., HICKMANS, E. M., HOWARTH, B. E. and AUBREY, J. (1954). *Arch. Dis. Childh.*, **29**, 178.

CROSSE, V. M., WALLIS, P. G., LOW, A. and HENLEY, A. A. (1960). *Nutrition*, **14**, 65.

DAWKINS, M. (1965). *Develop. Med. Child. Neurol.*, **7**, 74.

DAWKINS, M. R. and SCOPES, J. W. (1965). *Nature*, **206**, 201.

DAY, R., CURTIS, J. and KELLY, M. (1943). *Amer. J. Dis. Child.*, **65**, 376.

DOXIADIS, F. A. (1952), *Lancet*, **2**, 1242.

FARR, V. and MITCHELL, R. G. (1969). *Amer. J. Obstet. Gynec.*, **103**, 380.

FOCONI, S. and SJÖLIN, S. (1959). *Acta Paediat. Uppsala*, **48**, 18.

GAIRDNER, D., MARKS, J., ROSCOE, J. D., and BRETTELL, R. O. (1958). *Arch. Dis. Childh.*, **33**, 489.

GANS, B. (1959). *Arch. Dis. Childh.*, **34**, 292.

GRAZIANI, L. T., WEITZMAN, E. D., and VELASCO, M. S. A. (1968). *Pediatrics*, **41**, 483.

GRUENWALD, P. (1963). *Biol. Neonat.*, **5**, 215.

HARPER, P. A. (1962). "Preventive Pediatrics". *Child Health and Development.* Century Crofts, New York.

HENDRICKS, C. H. (1964). *Obstet. and Gynec.*, **24**, 357.

HUGGETT, A. St. G. (1946). *Brit. med. Bull.*, **4**, 196.

KITCHEN, W. H. (1968). *Aust. paediat. J.*, **4**, 29.

LUBCHENCO, L. O., HANSMAN, C., DRESSLER, M. and BOYD, E. (1963). *Pediatrics*, **32**, 793.

MEDOFF, H. S. (1964). *J. Pediat.*, **64**, 287.

MILLER, R. A. (1941). *Arch. Dis. Childh.*, **16**, 22.

NAEYE, R. L. (1965a). *Arch. Path.*, **79**, 284.

NAEYE, R. L. (1965b). *Amer. J. Path.*, **47**, 905.

POTTER, E. L. (1953). "Advances in Pediatrics", Vol. 6, Interscience Publishers Ltd., New York and London.

POTTER, E. L. and THIERSTEIN, S. T. (1943). *J. Pediat.*, **22**, 695.

PRECHTL, H. F. R. and BEINTEMA, D. (1964). *Little Club Clin. develop. Med.*, **12.**

ROBINSON, R. J. (1966). *Arch. Dis. Childh.*, **41**, 437.

ROPER-HALL, M. J. (1960). *Brit. med. J.*, **2**, 231.

RUPPERT, E. S. and JOHNSON, E. W. (1968). *Pediatrics*, **42**, 255.

SAINT-ANNE DARGASSIES, S. (1970). *Journées Parisiennes de Pédiatrie*, **1**, 310, Flammarion, Paris.

SCHMÖGER, R. (1955). *Kinderarztl. Prax.*, **23**, 433.

SCHULMAN, I. (1959). *J. Pediat.*, **54**, 663.

SHELLY, H. J. (1964). *Brit. med. J.*, **1**, 273.

SHULMAN, I., SMITH, C. H. and STERN, G. S. (1954). *Amer. J. Dis. Child.*, **88**, 567.

SILVERMAN, W. A., ZAMELIS, A., SINCLAIR, J. C. and AGATE, F. J. Jr. (1964). *Pediatrics*, **33**, 984.

SMITH, C. A. (1959). "The Physiology of the Newborn", 3rd ed. Blackwell, Oxford.

USHER, R., MCLEAN, F. and SCOTT, K. E. (1966). *Pediat. Clin. N. Amer.*, **13**, 835.

USHER, R. and MCLEAN, F. (1969). *J. Pediat.*, **74**, 901.

VAN CREVELD, S. (1929). *Amer. J. Dis. Child.*, **38**, 912.

W.H.O. (1950). Technical Report Series No. 27.

W.H.O. (1961). Technical Report Series No. 217.

YOUNG, I. M. (1962). *Clin. Science*, **22**, 325.

CHAPTER 2

CARE DURING PREGNANCY AND LABOUR, AND IMMEDIATELY AFTER BIRTH

THE obstetric care of a low-weight baby during pregnancy and delivery is just as important for its ultimate prognosis as the later paediatric care; and the close co-operation developing between obstetricians and paediatricians in perinatal care is most encouraging.

Management of Pregnancy

In addition to the usual routine prenatal care special attention must be paid to:

(1) Prevention (if possible) and treatment of all conditions which can result in a pre-term or growth-retarded infant (see causes of low birth weight, p. 244).

(2) Monitoring of the foetus in all conditions which may lead to intra-uterine death (pre-eclamptic toxaemia, hypertension, growth-retardation, antepartum haemorrhage, haemolytic disease, etc.) so that it is born alive, without after-effects of intra-uterine malnutrition or hypoxia, and as near term as the circumstances allow.

This entails booking all mothers likely to have a low-weight baby in a hospital with facilities for perinatal intensive care, i.e. with facilities for both obstetric and paediatric intensive care. In addition, any mother booked for her confinement at home (or in a hospital without special facilities) who is suspected of having a growth-retarded foetus, or who develops any condition which may result in a pre-term infant, should be transferred at once to a hospital with full facilities.

Estimation of gestational age. This is necessary if growth retardation is to be recognized. Information about the last menstrual period may not be available or it may be misleading (the increasing use of oral contraceptives can confuse withdrawal bleeding with true menstruation) and the mother may not have been examined early in pregnancy. In such cases other methods must be used to assess gestational age:

Radiology. The times of appearance of centres of ossification in the ankle and knee are most generally used, but unfortunately epiphyseal development is delayed in a growth-retarded foetus (Scott and Usher, 1964; Wigglesworth, 1966). In addition, radiology is not without risk.

Ultrasonics. Ultrasonic cephalometry is useful for estimating gestational age, especially between 20–30 weeks gestation (Campbell, 1969).

To establish growth retardation, ultrasonic cephalometry should be repeated at weekly intervals for 2–3 weeks.

Examination of liquor amnii. The concentrations of urea and creatinine increase as pregnancy progresses (Pitkin and Zwirek, 1967; Lind *et al.*, 1969). In addition, the cells in the liquor have been used to assess gestational age (Brosens and Gordon, 1966; Lind *et al.*, 1969). Unfortunately the cytological characteristics of the liquor amnii are not as closely linked to gestational age as was once hoped (Lind, 1970). This examination entails amniocentesis.

Methods of monitoring a foetus at risk. During recent years various techniques have been developed for monitoring the well-being of the foetus at risk during pregnancy.

Foetal heart monitors. Various kinds of apparatus are used to record the foetal heart, the uterine pressure changes, and the effect of the latter on the foetal heart. These include phonocardiography (Hammacher, 1962); the ultrasonic Doppler effect (Bishop, 1966; Brown and Robertson, 1968) and indirect foetal electrocardiography (Larks and Das Gupta, 1958; Mayes *et al.*, 1963; Friedman and Eckerling, 1969). The heart rate patterns are related to uterine activity by the use of tocography to record the uterine pressure (see Fig. 3).

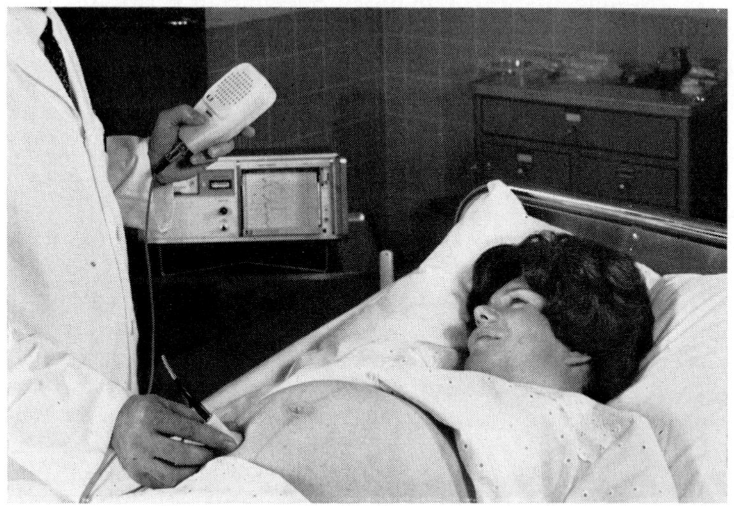

(Photograph by courtesy of Hewlett-Packard Ltd.)

FIG. 3. *Ultrasound Monitor and Cardiotocograph.* The ultrasound monitor uses the ultrasonic Doppler principle for easy auscultation of the foetal heart. The cardiotocograph (seen in background) provides a continuous display of foetal heart frequency and uterine activity when traducers are strapped onto the mother's abdomen over the foetal heart.

Oestriol assay. This is a valuable index of foetal growth and well-being, especially in relation to a growth-retarded foetus. It is also useful in the management of other high risk pregnancies, e.g. pre-eclamptic toxaemia, antepartum haemorrhage, etc. Absence of the normal rise in level between 32–34 weeks, or a falling level, indicate that the foetus is in danger (Coyle and Brown, 1963; Klopper, 1969).

Beicher *et al.* (1967) found oestriol levels useful when using conservative treatment for mothers with antepartum haemorrhage and they thought that the use of oestriol levels could prevent unduly early termination of pregnancy.

Amnioscopy has been used more frequently during the last few years to detect meconium staining of the liquor amnii, especially during the later weeks of pregnancy in cases of pre-eclamptic toxaemia, hypertension and foetal growth retardation (Henry, 1970). Henry thinks that the introduction of amnioscopy into antenatal departments would keep the rising incidence of surgical induction in check.

It is a simple and quick examination with few risks (Brown and Brennan, 1968), and can be repeated every alternate day if necessary. If there is a good volume of clear liquor the foetus is in no immediate danger.

Management of Labour in Specialized Hospitals

Ideally, all small pre-term infants and all growth-retarded babies should be delivered in a hospital with facilities for intensive obstetric care and with an intensive care neonatal nursery.

The chief hazards for a low-weight baby during delivery are:

(1) Hypoxia (especially growth-retarded babies).
(2) Intracranial birth injury.
(3) Infection.
(4) Danger from drugs given to mother during labour.

Prevention of hypoxia. To reduce the risk of hypoxia, drugs such as morphia and its derivatives, pethidine, scopolamine and barbiturates must be avoided as they cause neonatal respiratory depression (Snyder, 1949). Robert and Please (1958) and Rosen *et al.* (1969) have drawn attention to the depressant effect of pethidine on the respiratory centre.

The use of *regional analgesia and anaesthesia* (epidural block, pudendal block, local infiltration of the perineum, etc.), for the relief of pain during labour and delivery, is safer than inhalation analgesia and anaesthesia for a low-weight baby (Huntingford, 1963; Cavanagh and Talisman, 1969; Basford and Bonica, 1969).

If *inhalation analgesia or anaesthesia* have to be used, an adequate supply of oxygen must be insured. When an inhalation analgesia is necessary, gas and oxygen (50% nitrous oxide/50% oxygen) can be self

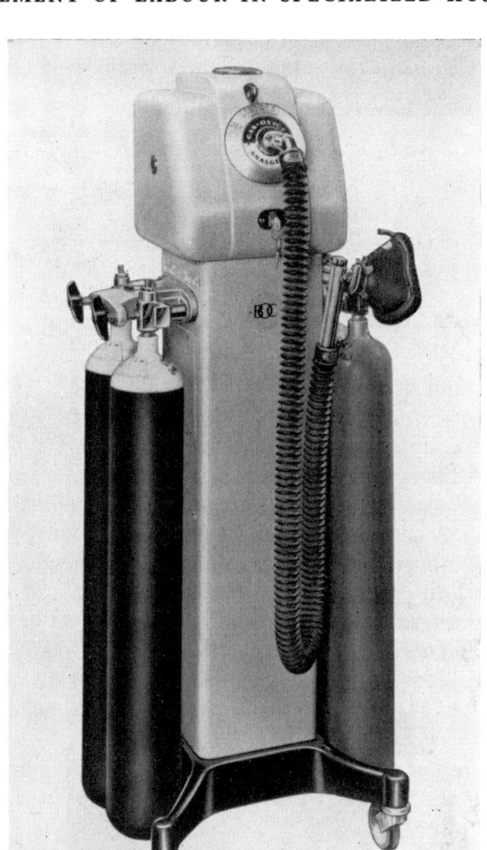

FIG. 4. Lucy Baldwin apparatus. (*British Oxygen Co.*)

administered by the patient, under the supervision of the midwife, by the use of either a Lucy Baldwin apparatus (see Fig. 4) or an Entonox apparatus. Methoxyflurane (Penthrane) and trichlorethyline (Trilene) should only be used with oxygen-enriched air when a low-weight baby is expected.

When inhalation anaesthesia becomes necessary, a very light concentration of such anaesthetics as cyclopropane, methoxyflurane or diethyl ether can be combined with muscular relaxants (Basford and Bonica, 1969).

The position of the mother during labour is important. The supine position leads to partial obstruction of the inferior vena cava and predisposes to compression of the aorta during uterine contractions. Signs of foetal distress can often be abolished, or decreased, by changing the mother's position from the supine to the lateral (W H O, 1965).

Signs of foetal hypoxia. These include:

(1) *Alterations in foetal heart rate.* The foetal heart is the most useful single guide to the well-being of the foetus during labour and should be monitored continuously with a foetus "at risk".

During the past decade, various techniques have been developed for this. The Hammacher cardiotocograph (Hammacher, 1962) combines a record of the foetal heart together with a record of the uterine contractions (see Fig. 3). It can be used with intact membranes; it involves a minimum of disturbance to the mother; and can be used by relatively unspecialized staff.

Foetal electrocardiography can be used indirectly from electrodes applied to the abdominal wall (Larks and Das Gupta, 1958; Mayes *et al.*, 1963; Friedman and Eckerling, 1969); or directly (after rupture of membranes) by attaching a clip electrode to the foetal scalp (Hon, 1967; Organ, 1968).

Using the Doppler effect, ultrasound has also been used to monitor the foetal heart (see Fig. 3) but there is some question as to its safety for continuous recordings. Bishop (1966) suggested a limit of 10 minutes for any examination. Recently Mackintosh and Davy (1970) found appreciable damage to the chromosomes in human blood cultures exposed to ultrasound from an ultrasound foetal heart detector for periods of one and two hours.

A combination of phonocardiography and direct electrocardiography is the most satisfactory, and probably the safest method at the present time (Pendleton, 1970).

(2) *The passage of meconium* is also a clinical sign of possible foetal anoxia. Before the rupture of membranes this can be diagnosed by amnioscopy.

(3) *Foetal acidosis.* If there are alterations in the foetal heart rate and/or meconium is passed, and delivery is not imminent, determination of the pH of the foetal blood has proved valuable in assessing the condition of the foetus. Saling (1962) first showed that foetal blood could be obtained from the foetal scalp and examined biochemically; and Huntingford (1964) was the first to describe the technique of foetal blood sampling in this country. The pH of the mother's blood must be examined at the same time because maternal acidosis affects the foetus and this type of foetal acidosis can be corrected by treatment of the mother (Jacobson and Rooth, 1969). The critical foetal pH level lies between 7·17 and 7·20 (Morris and Beard, 1965; Bretscher and Saling, 1967; Kubli, 1968; Paterson *et al.*, 1970). If the pH is 7·25 or over, the foetus is in no immediate danger, irrespective of changes in the foetal

heart rate or passage of meconium, but regular sampling should continue. When it falls below 7·20 preparations should be made for delivery of the foetus (Coltard *et al.*, 1969); and oxygen should be given to the mother because this can increase the foetal Po_2 (Newman *et al.*, 1967).

Foetal blood sampling is believed to reduce the perinatal mortality rate and also to reduce unnecessary Caesarean section by separating true foetal distress from clinical foetal distress (Saling, 1962; Beard, 1968). The avoidance of Caesarean section is particularly important when dealing with a pre-term infant because Caesarean section predisposes such an infant to idiopathic respiratory distress (see p. 129).

Prevention of intracranial birth injury. This is least likely to occur with a spontaneous vertex delivery aided by an adequate episiotomy. If the second stage is delayed, a carefully performed low forceps extraction reduces the risk to the child; but mid-cavity and high forceps, and forcible extraction of a breech should be avoided as they carry high foetal risks. Attempts to hasten delivery by the use of uterine stimulants are usually inadvisable.

Prevention of infection. To avoid this, the labour must be conducted with all the usual aseptic precautions. If gonorrhoea or thrush are present, the vagina must be treated early in labour. After the membranes have been ruptured for 24 hours, if the child has not been delivered, antibiotics may be given to the mother if infection is suspected (but long-acting sulphonamides must be avoided, also all antibiotics which compete with bilirubin for albumin binding and glucuronyl conjugation, as these may lead to jaundice in the newborn pre-term infant, see p. 187). Persons suffering from infection must be excluded from the labour room, and attendants must wear gowns and masks and wash their hands before handling the infant. The infant should be received into a sterile towel.

Prevention of danger from drugs. Drugs causing neonatal respiratory depression and drugs which depend on glucuronyl transferase have already been mentioned. Muscular relaxants given to the mother may lead to intestinal stasis and even obstruction in the pre-term infant; and barbiturates may cause coagulation defects and early neonatal bleeding.

The birth. As soon as the head has been delivered there is no need for haste. A controlled passage through the birth canal assists in draining fluid from the respiratory tract, which should be cleared as far as possible at this stage by suction, i.e. before the first breath is taken. If there is time, the closed eyelids can also be gently cleaned with moist sterile swabs, one for each eye.

During delivery of the body, all handling must be extremely gentle and reduced to a minimum. The infant should be received into a warm sterile towel in order to conserve heat and prevent contamination of the skin.

If not already done, the air passages must be cleared immediately, by oral and naso-pharyngeal suction. The cord can then be clamped and divided.

It is generally believed that a term baby's cord should not be clamped until it has ceased to pulsate, in order to allow blood to be transferred from the placenta to the baby and conserve the extra iron content. The temporary increase in total blood volume due to late tying of the cord is much greater in pre-term than in term infants, especially in those with the lowest gestational age because the proportion of blood in the placenta and umbilical vessels increases as the gestational age decreases. This increase in postnatal blood volume only lasts a few hours but during this time it might be harmful (Sisson and Whalen, 1960). James (1966) thought it reasonable to regard the distribution of blood between the foetus and the placenta during intrauterine life as being physiological for both foetus and newborn infant, rather than to regard blood in the placenta as the infant's birthright. Lind (1968) studied babies delivered by Caesarean section in which the cord was clamped *in utero*, and compared them with infants delivered vaginally with cord round the neck which was clamped before birth of the trunk. The blood volumes of the two groups were comparable and were considered to approximate to the foetal blood volume *in utero* at term. He found that infants who had their cords clamped early (within 10 seconds of birth) had greater blood volumes than this. Yao *et al.* (1969) found the following distribution of blood between the infant and the placenta: at birth 67% in the infant and 33% in the placenta; at 1 minute after birth these proportions were 80% and 20%; and at 3 minutes, or later, 87% and 13%. Because the placental transfusion is relatively larger in the pre-term infant, it would appear to be wise to clamp the cord early. The position may be different in regard to growth-retarded babies. More research is still required into this subject.

Care immediately after Birth

As soon as the cord has been divided, intensive paediatric care should commence. A medical member of the paediatric team should be present at the birth of all small low-weight babies. This person must of course wear a sterile gown and mask and wash the hands and forearms thoroughly with a suitable antiseptic soap (see p. 56) before receiving the infant.

The equipment required for the infant includes:

Heated incubator, or heated cot with warm sterile towels and blankets.

Equipment for laryngoscopy and suction.
Equipment for occluding and dividing the cord.
Means of identification for the infant; and also for the cot or incubator.
Equipment for the administration of oxygen (by face mask or endotracheal tube).
Glucose and sodium bicarbonate solutions for intravenous use, and equipment for their administration.
Drugs and equipment for their administration.
Equipment for giving intermittent positive pressure ventilation.

A resuscitation trolley which accommodates most of this equipment should be available (see Fig. 5); also a heated portable incubator should be available if the intensive care nursery is too far from the delivery

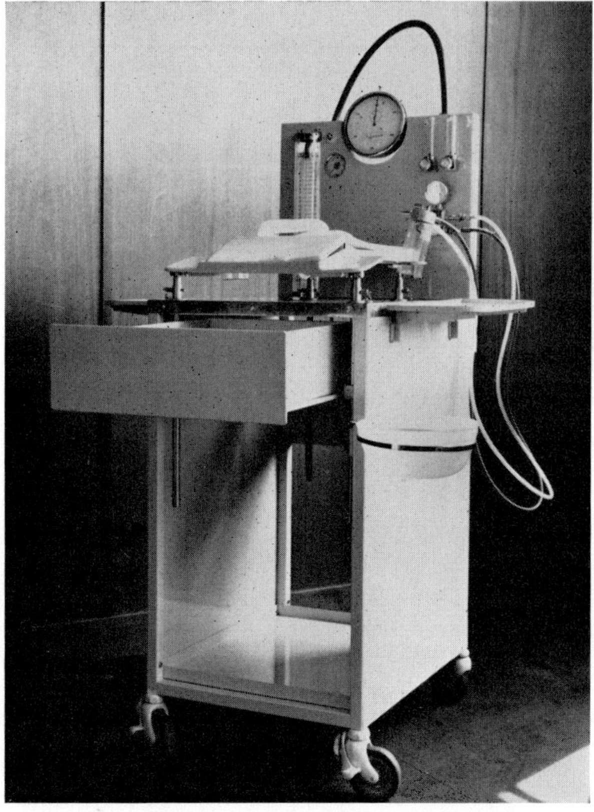

FIG. 5. Resuscitation trolley (*Oxygenaire Ltd.*)

room to permit the use of the ordinary incubator for transport of the infant.

The most important immediate care after birth is the prevention of loss of body heat. Kunnas (1968) has shown that the mortality rate among pre-term infants is significantly higher when their central temperature is allowed to fall to 34°C or below, during the first 24 hours of life. In order to avoid this, the infant should be placed at once in a heated incubator; or wrapped loosely in a sterile towel and blankets and placed in a heated cot.

The air passage must be cleared if and when necessary, and oxygen given by face mask if this is required. At the age of 1 minute the infant's condition is assessed by means of the Apgar Score (Apgar, 1955).

Apgar Score

Sign	0	1	2
Heart rate	Absent	Slow (below 100)	Over 100
Respiratory effort	Absent	Slow, irregular	Good, crying
Reflex irritability*	No response	Grimaces	Cough or sneeze
Muscle tone	Limp	Some flexion of extremities	Active motion
Colour	Blue, pale	Body pink, extremities blue	Completely pink

* Response to catheter in nostril tested after oropharynx has been cleared.

An alternative method of scoring has been suggested by Morrow and Myles (1969) which they call the ABC system: A for activity, B for breathing and C for circulation.

	0	1	2
A. Activity	No active movements	Some movement but sleepy and sluggish	Good active movement
B. Breathing	No spontaneous breathing	Unsatisfactory breathing, e.g. gasping, jerky, irregular	Unrestricted rhythmical sustained breathing
C. Circulation	No heart action	Heart rate less than 100. Facial cyanosis or pallor	Heart rate over 100. No facial cyanosis

They recommend that the result should be expressed as three individual numerals for A, B and C and not as a total score, e.g. a baby might be described as 0 1 1.

If the infant is breathing well and the Apgar score is seven or over, no special resuscitation is required; but if the score is six or less, further treatment is necessary because of the real risk of intraventricular haemorrhage from anoxia (see next section for treatment of asphyxia).

The Apgar score is repeated at the age of 5 minutes because the score at this time has been found to correlate well with the chances of survival and later neurological status (Drage and Berendes, 1966).

Meanwhile, vitamin K_1 (1·0 mg.) is given intramuscularly and the cord is occluded with a ligature or a latex rubber band (Vartan, 1964; Crowley, 1965). Whichever one is used must not be placed too close to the umbilicus in case catheterization of the umbilical vessels is required later. Plastic disposable clamps (Kariher and Smith, 1961) are not recommended by the author for small low-weight infants because they are uncomfortable when the infant is placed in the prone position.

The infant must be gently examined for signs of abnormality. This includes the introduction of catheters into the nose, stomach and rectum (to exclude atresias) and the examination of the cord (a single umbilical artery is often associated with congenital malformations, see p. 150).

Prophylactic drops should be instilled into the eyes if any vaginal infection is present or suspected.

As soon as respiration is well established, the infant should be moved to the special baby care unit; the earlier the commencement of specialized care the better is the prognosis for the baby.

The baby may be moved in its incubator, or cot, if the special care unit is near the delivery room; but a portable incubator carrier is preferred unless the distance is short. Facilities must be available for the administration of oxygen during the journey from the delivery room to the nursery.

Before leaving the delivery room, both the infant and its cot or incubator must be identified by whatever method is in use.

Birth Asphyxia

Low-weight babies, especially growth-retarded babies (light-for-dates babies), have a higher incidence of birth asphyxia than babies weighing more than 2,500 g. at birth. The main causes of low birth weight often predispose to intra-uterine hypoxia; and the babies themselves have relatively poor metabolic reserves and are badly equipped to face the stresses of labour.

Immediate recognition of any cause of asphyxia which requires special treatment is vitally important, e.g. congenital malformations (such as diaphragmatic hernia or choanal atresia); anaemic anoxia (due to haemolytic disease or, more rarely, foetal haemorrhage into the maternal circulation); drug anoxia (due to analgesics or anaesthetics given to the mother); intracranial birth trauma, etc.

During resuscitation the infant should not be allowed to lose body heat, nor should overheating occur. Both loss of heat and overheating increase metabolism and the need for oxygen (see p. 62). Heat loss at this time increases the later risk of acidosis (Gandy *et al.*, 1964); and of hypoglycaemia (Cornblath and Schwartz, 1966), especially in light-for-dates babies. The infant should be treated on a heated pad or under a source of radiant heat (Du and Oliver, 1969). The skin temperature should be monitored if possible and kept at 36·5°C.

Care must be taken to avoid infection and trauma during resuscitation, as low-weight infants are susceptible to both.

The main principles of resuscitation are:

(1) Ensuring an adequate airway.
(2) Initiation of respiration and administration of oxygen.
(3) Correction of any biochemical abnormalities.
(4) Supportive treatment.

Without a clear airway no success can be expected from other means of resuscitation, therefore the first step must be the clearing of the air passages by suction. In cases likely to develop idiopathic respiratory distress (small pre-term infants, babies delivered by Caesarean section, babies of mothers with diabetes, placenta praevia or meconium stained liquor) the stomach should also be aspirated to reduce the risk of regurgitation and inhalation of stomach contents. The best position for the baby during this procedure is flat on the back with a folded towel under the shoulders and the head fully extended. This allows drainage from the air passages and avoids pressure on the lung bases. The feet-up position limits expansion of the lung bases by pressure of the abdominal contents on the diaphragm, but after Caesarean section it may be necessary to place the infant in this position for a short time to obtain effective drainage of the air passages. If intracranial haemorrhage is suspected, the head-down position is contra-indicated. Twisting of the head should be avoided as this tends to decrease the lumen of the soft trachea. If the infant is atonic and the tongue tends to fall back and obstruct the air passage, a small airway should be inserted.

In some cases, e.g. if meconium has been aspirated, it is necessary to aspirate the larynx under direct vision. A sterilized infant laryngoscope should always be available; also personnel trained in its use.

If spontaneous respiratory efforts are being made, oxygen may be given by face mask but care must be taken not to depress the chin.

In the absence of respiratory effort, intermittent positive pressure ventilation is indicated. In mildly depressed infants this may be done with a mask and bag, e.g. with the Cardiff neonatal inflating bag (Mushin and Hillard, 1967) or with a Blease Samson neonatal resuscitator (see Figs. 6 and 7). If the infant is severely depressed (Apgar score two or less) intermittent positive pressure ventilation is best accomplished with endotracheal intubation, when a mask and bag or a mechanical ventilator can be used after tracheal suction. Care must be taken to avoid excessive pressure which might cause pneumothorax or pneumomediastinum.

If opiates or pethidine have been given to the mother during delivery, 0·1–0·2 mg. "Paediatric" Lethidrone (N-Allyl-normorphine) in 2 ml. sodium chloride, should be given into the umbilical vein. This drug must be used with care because if anoxia is due to any other cause it may be increased by Lethidrone (Eckenhoff *et al.*, 1956). Care must also be taken not to use an umbilical artery instead of the vein, in order to avoid possible vascular complications (Mills, 1949) and sciatic nerve palsy (San Agustin *et al.*, 1962). A mistake is particularly likely to occur if there is only one umbilical artery.

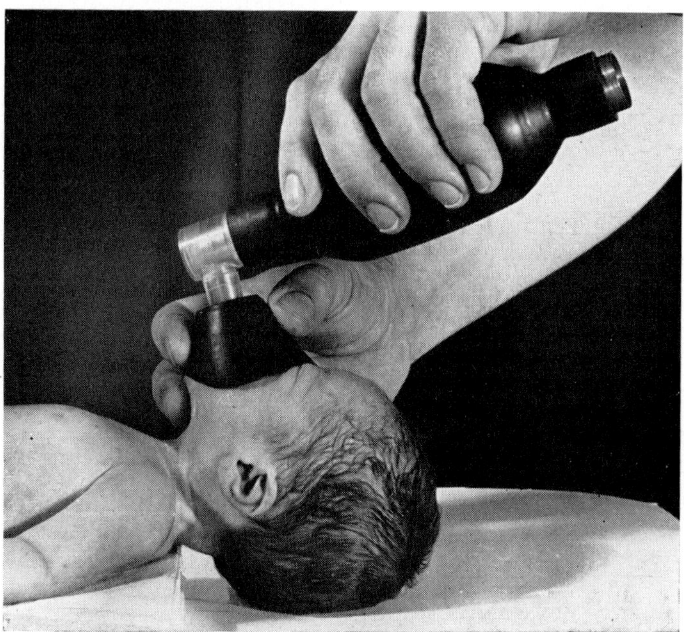

(Photograph by courtesy of Longworth Scientific Instrument Co. Ltd.)

FIG. 6. *The Cardiff Infant Inflating Bag.* This may be used with a mask or an endotracheal tube. An oxygen reservoir tube can be fitted to the inlet, allowing 100% oxygen to be given when required.

As soon as possible, the acid-base status of the infant should be estimated (by Astrup apparatus) also the blood glucose level (with Dextrostix). Both glucose and bicarbonate are exhausted during prolonged anoxia, and low-weight babies are particularly liable to acidosis due to their low carbohydrate reserves. Irreversible brain damage may result from anoxia when foetal reserves are insufficient and the administration of glucose and bicarbonate may reduce the severity of brain damage (W H O 1965). If the pH (scalp or umbilical vein) is less than 7·15 or if the infant is flaccid and pale or cyanosed after 5 minutes artificial ventilation, intravenous therapy with glucose and sodium bicarbonate should be commenced. Rapid intravenous injection of the usual 8·4% sodium bicarbonate is not without danger (Kravath *et al.*, 1969) and a panel on "Birth Asphyxia" (Behrman *et al.*, 1969) recommended the administration of 4 ml. 8·4% sodium bicarbonate (1 mEq/ml.) mixed with 2 ml. 5–10% glucose; of which 4 ml. is given rapidly and the remainder over 2–5 minutes. If there is no response, another 3–4 ml. of this mixture can be given. After this initial treatment the acid-base should be monitored and while awaiting the result 1–2 mg./kg. of 50% glucose may be given if there is no sustained response, then 10% glucose by intravenous drip (10 drops per minute).

Special care must be taken with light-for-dates babies as they tend to

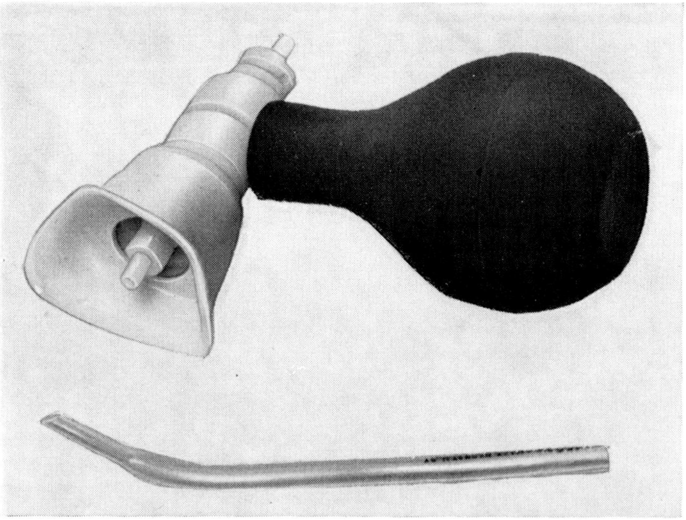

(*Photograph by courtesy of Blease Medical Equipment Ltd.*)

FIG. 7. *The Blease Samson Neonatal Resuscitator*. This may be used with a mask or an endotracheal tube (both shown). By connecting an oxygen supply to the oxygen inlet tube, up to 60% oxygen can be given.

become alkalaemic within a few hours of birth. Acidosis in these babies should only be treated if they are asphyxiated or if the blood pH has not risen above 7·25 by 2 hours of age, and all treatment must be carefully monitored for 6–12 hours after birth (Usher, 1970).

If the heart fails in spite of treatment, external massage of the heart must be performed. Compression of the middle portion of the sternum will massage the heart as it rests on the vertebral column (Thaler and Stobre, 1963). If combined with intermittent positive pressure ventilation, the pressure over the heart must coincide with expiration, or short-periods of massage can be alternated with periods of ventilation. As a last resort, 0·05–0·1 ml. of 1/1,000 adrenalin solution in 2 ml. of normal saline can be injected into the heart through the fourth intercostal space.

Stimulant drugs have little place in the treatment of asphyxia. Nikethamide (Coramine), cardiazol and lobeline are only effective in mild cases of apnoea when oxygen alone would stimulate respiration, i.e. when they are unnecessary. With marked hypoxia these drugs become ineffective and toxic; in addition lobeline is a cardiac depressant (W H O 1965).

Management of Birth of a Low-Weight Baby at Home or in a Small Hospital

The birth. Mothers selected as suitable for delivery at home (or in a small hospital or maternity home) who start labour after 36 weeks usually need not be transferred to a specialist hospital for delivery unless they have some complication, or the uterus is too small for the period of gestation.

If the mother is being delivered at home, her general practitioner obstetrician should be notified that she has commenced labour prematurely. Where there is a nurse responsible for the domiciliary care of low-weight babies in the district, she should also be notified so that she can be present at the birth and be responsible for the nursing care of the infant during the neonatal period. Meanwhile the room should be made as warm as possible (75–80°F or 24–26·5°C) and the cot should be warmed with well-covered hot water bottles and placed in a warm corner free from draughts.

In all small hospitals (or maternity homes) without facilities for special baby care, there should be at least one nurse with experience in the care of low-weight babies on the staff, and she should be notified of the expected birth in addition to notifying the doctor in charge of the case.

During labour the mother should be on her side, as this position is better for the baby (see p. 17). The liquor amnii must be watched for meconium staining and the foetal heart counted frequently. Sedatives and analgesics for the mother must be carefully chosen: morphia, pethidine, scopolamine and barbiturates must be avoided. An apparatus for giving gas and oxygen (Entonox) is approved by the Central Midwives Board for use by unsupervised midwives. This consists of an "on demand" inhalation unit which delivers premixed gas and oxygen at atmospheric pressure (50% nitrous oxide and 50% oxygen). The Lucy Baldwin apparatus (see p. 17) might also be available in a small hospital or maternity home.

As soon as the head is born, the air passages should be cleared with a sterile mucus catheter and the eyelids gently cleaned (a separate swab for each eye). The delivery of the body must be gently controlled. The infant should be received into a warm sterile towel to conserve heat and prevent infection. The cord should be clamped and divided at once and the infant handed to the doctor or special nurse (who must wear a sterile gown and mask and wash the hands and forearms before receiving the baby).

Care immediately after birth. The baby should be transferred to a clean warm sterile towel before it is loosely wrapped in a clean warm blanket and placed in the heated cot. Such a wrapped baby is usually placed on its right side at first, but after a little while it can be gently turned on to the left side in order to allow the lungs to expand equally. A wrapped baby must never be placed flat on its back because its head is not free to roll over to the side and this can lead to inhalation of any regurgitated fluid.

The Apgar score can be taken at the age of 1 minute; vitamin K_1 (1 mg.) should be given intramuscularly; and the cord can be ligatured, or occluded with a latex rubber band, and divided (not too near the umbilicus) and covered with a sterile dressing.

Birth asphyxia. If the infant is not breathing well, or if the Apgar score is low, the infant must be treated for asphyxia. Hospital treatment has already been described (see p. 23).

In domiciliary practice there must always be a prepared plan of action because asphyxia is an emergency. The midwife should have the following equipment for resuscitation:

- Mucus catheters for clearing the air passages.
- Equipment for administration of oxygen by face mask, or by bag and mask.
- Equipment for endotracheal intubation if this should prove necessary. (The Central Midwives Board has decided that a midwife trained in this procedure may carry out intubation in appropriate cases.)
- Sterile swabs, needles, syringes and certain drugs.
- A tongue clip.

A skilled general practitioner obstetrician should carry an oxygen set (Barrie, 1963) which includes an infant laryngoscope, a perspex water manometer, sterile disposable endotracheal tubes, and suction catheters.

The infant must not be allowed to lose body heat during resuscitation, so should be placed on well covered hot water bottles or on a well covered electric pad and the body should be kept covered as much as possible. The baby should be on its back on a level surface, with a folded towel under the shoulders and the head fully extended. If the tongue blocks the airway it may be held forward with a tongue clip (inserted into the sides of the tongue and not from above and below) or an endotracheal tube may be inserted.

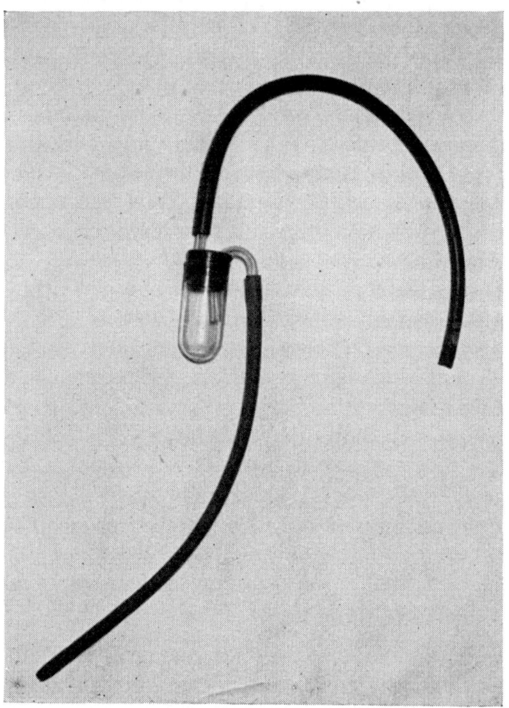

FIG. 8. Mucus catheter with large terminal opening, and trap for mucus.

The airway must be cleared and a simple mouth operated mucus catheter (rubber or disposable plastic, English size 12) can be very effective, especially if it has a terminal opening and a suitable trap for mucus (Fig. 8). Care should be taken not to pass the catheter past the pharynx into the oesophagus (unless the stomach is being aspirated) because this will not help in the clearing of the air passages. The catheter must be sterile and it should never be cleared by blowing down it because this contaminates the tube with organisms from the attendant's throat. As blockage easily occurs, several sterile mucus catheters should be available at every birth. If it is necessary to aspirate the larynx under direct vision a skilled general practitioner obstetrician should be able to use the laryngoscope in his oxygen set.

Oxygen can be given from a small oxygen cylinder (e.g. Sparklets Ltd.) by means of a soft rubber face mask placed over the nose and mouth and infrequent respirations can be increased by placing a hand under the infant's chest and arching the chest forward (see p. 142).

In the absence of respiratory efforts intermittent positive pressure ventilation can be performed by the mask and bag method using the Cardiff neonatal inflating bag (Mushin and Hillard, 1967) or the Blease Samson neonatal resuscitator (Figs. 6 and 7).

Where such equipment is not available mouth to mouth respiration should be tried. Several folds of gauze should be placed over the mouth to reduce the danger of infection, the infant's nose is held, and a hand is placed firmly over the infant's stomach to prevent air going into this organ instead of the lungs. The attendant then blows into the infant's mouth, with just sufficient force to expand the chest, at intervals of about 5–10 seconds.

If the heart fails, external massage should be performed (see p. 27) and as a last resort, 0·1 ml. adrenalin (1 in 1,000) in 2 ml. of saline may be injected into the heart, through the fourth intercostal space.

The need to treat birth asphyxia should be extremely rare in infants delivered at home or in a nursing home because all cases likely to result in an asphyxiated baby should have been booked for hospital delivery.

Decision on place of care. As soon as the infant is breathing well, the doctor must decide whether it can be nursed in the place of birth or whether it should be removed to a hospital with a special care unit. If the facilities in the home or hospital are inadequate the infant must be transferred; and even if the facilities are reasonably good, removal should be urged in the following circumstances:

(1) The birth weight is less than 2,040 g. (4 lb. 8 oz.).

(2) The colour is poor or cyanotic attacks are occurring, i.e. if there are any respiratory difficulties.

(3) The infant is incapable of sucking a bottle.

(4) The infant is suffering from an illness or birth injury, or is obviously underweight for its maturity.

Such infants require expert nursing and medical attention throughout the 24 hours of each day, supported by good equipment and good facilities for biochemical investigations, transfusions, etc.

When it is necessary to transfer the infant to hospital, arrangements must be made as soon as possible for its admission and transport.

Until removal can be arranged the respiration, colour, cord and general condition must be carefully watched. The air passages must be kept clear and oxygen given by face mask if necessary but with all the precautions set out on p. 134.

The temperature of the cot must be kept constant. In order to avoid bottle burns any hot water bottles used must be completely covered by placing them in bags or wrapping them in blankets. They should not be filled with boiling water and there should be several layers of blanket between the bottle and the infant. If an electric pad is used it should be placed *under* the infant, well covered with rubber or polythene sheeting and several layers of blanket. A thermometer should be placed between the blankets above the infant and checked at regular intervals. The thermometer should be kept at 95°F (35°C) if possible. The infant's temperature should also be watched, and this should not fall below 36°C (97°F).

In a home, where there may be difficulty in keeping a small infant warm until it is moved, it is better to use a "silver swaddler" (Baum and Scopes, 1968). This is a simple swaddling suit of polyester, laminated on the inside with a thin layer of aluminium, which prevents heat loss by evaporation, convection and radiation (see Fig. 9).

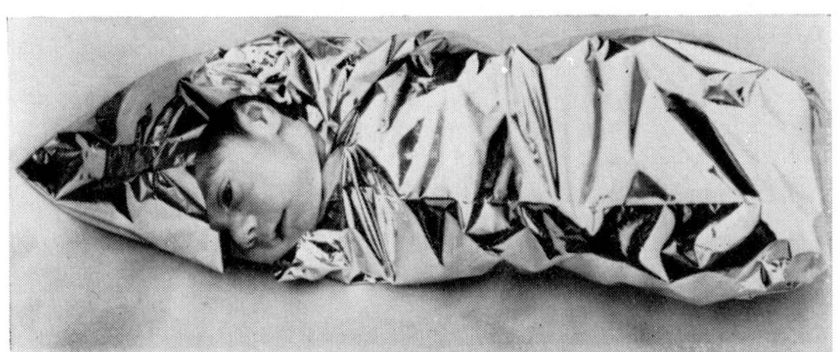

(Photograph by courtesy of Lewis Woolf Griptight Ltd.)

FIG. 9. *The Silver Swaddler.*

The infant should be disturbed as little as possible and no food should be given before removal.

REFERENCES

APGAR, V. (1955). *New York J. med.*, **55**, 2365.

BARRIE, H. (1963). *Lancet*, **1**, 650.

BASFORD, A. B. and BONICA, J. B. (1969). "Obstetric Analgesia and Anesthesia", p. 1273, ed. John J. Bonica. Blackwell Scientific Publications. Oxford.

BAUM, J. D. and SCOPES, J. W. (1968). *Lancet*, **1**, 672.

BEARD, R. W. (1968). *Proc. roy. Soc. Med.*, **61**, 488.

BEHRMAN, R. E., JAMES, L. S., KLAUS, M., NELSON, N. and OLIVER, T. (1969). *J. Pediat.*, **74**, 981.

BEICHER, N. A., BROWN, J. B., MACLEOD, S. C. and SMITH, M. A. (1967). *J. Obstet. Gynaec. Brit. Cwlth.*, **74**, 51.
BISHOP, E. H. (1966). *Amer. J. Obstet. Gynec.*, **96**, 863.
BRETCHER, J. and SALING, E. (1967). *Amer. J. Obstet. Gynec.*, **97**, 906.
BROSENS, I. and GORDON, H. (1966). *J. Obstet. Gynaec. Brit. Cwlth.*, **73**, 88.
BROWN, A. D. G. and ROBERTSON, J. G. (1968). *J. Obstet. Gynaec. Brit. Cwlth.*, **75**, 92.
BROWNE, A. D. H. and BRENNAN, R. K. (1968). *J. Obstet. Gynaec. Brit. Cwlth.*, **75**, 616.
CAMPBELL, S. (1969). *J. Obstet. Gynaec. Brit. Cwlth.*, **76**, 603.
CAVANAGH, D. and TALISMAN, M. R. (1969). "Prematurity and the Obstetrician". Appleton-Century-Crofts, New York.
COLTART, T. M., TRICKEY, N. R. A. and BEARD, R. W. (1969). *Brit. med. J.*, **1**, 342.
CORNBLATH, M. and SCHWARTZ, R. (1966). "Disorders of Carbohydrate Metabolism in Infancy", p. 35. W. B. Saunders Co. Philadelphia.
COYLE, M. G. and BROWN, J. B. (1963). *J. Obstet. Gynaec. Brit. Cwlth.*, **70**, 225.
CROWLEY, J. (1965). *Brit. med. J.*, **1**, 996.
DRAGE, J. S. and BERENDES, H. (1966). *Pediat. Clin. N. Amer.*, **13**, 635.
DU, J. N. H. and OLIVER, T. K. Jr. (1969). *J. Amer. med. Assoc.*, **207**, 1502.
ECKENHOFF, J. E., HOFFMAN, G. L. and FUNDERBURGH, L. W. (1956). *Amer. J. Obstet. Gynec.*, **71**, 1035.
FRIEDMAN, S. and ECKERLING, B. (1969). *Amer. J. Obstet. Gynec.*, **103**, 1160.
GANDY, G. M., ADAMSONS, K. Jr., CUNNINGHAM, N., SILVERMAN, W. A. and JAMES, L. S. (1964). *J. Clin. Invest.*, **43**, 751.
HAMMACHER, K. (1962). *Geburtsh. u. Frauenheilk.*, **22**, 1551.
HENRY, G. R. (1970). *Brit. J. hosp. Med.*, **3**, 516.
HON, E. H. (1967). *Obstet. and Gynec.*, **30**, 281.
HUNTINGFORD, P. J. (1963). *Brit. med. J.*, **1**, 1195.
HUNTINGFORD, P. J. (1964). *Lancet*, **1**, 95.
JACOBSON, L. and ROOTH, G. (1969). "Perinatal Medicine", p. 156. Academic Press, New York and London.
JAMES, L. S. (1966). *Pediat. Clin. N. Amer.*, **13**, 621.
KARIHER, D. Y. and SMITH, T. W. (1961). *Obstet. and Gynec.*, **17**, 648.
KLOPPER, A. (1969). "Foetus and Placenta", p. 471. Blackwell Scientific Publications, Oxford and Edinburgh.
KRAVATH, R. E., AHARAN, A. S. and FINBERG, L. (1969). *Pediat. Res.*, **3**, 354.
KUBLI, F. W. (1968). *Clin. Obstet. Gynec.*, **11**, 168.
KUNNAS, M. (1968). *Ann. Paediat. Fenn.*, **14**, 98.
LARKS, S. D. and DASGUPTA, K. (1958). *Amer. Heart J.*, **56**, 701.
LIND, J. (1968). *Ann. Paediat. Fenn.*, **14**, 1.
LIND, J. (1970). *Brit. J. hosp. Med.*, **3**, 501.
LIND, J., PARKIN, F. M., CHEYNE, G. A. (1969). *J. Obstet. Gynaec. Brit. Cwlth.*, **76**, 673.
MACKINTOSH, I. J. C. and DAVEY, D. A. (1970). *Brit. med. J.*, **4**, 92.
MAYES, B. T., BRADFIELD, A. and SMYTH, E. J. (1963). *Med. J. Aust.*, **2**, 905.
MILLS, W. G. (1949). *Brit. med. J.*, **2**, 464.
MORRIS, E. D. and BEARD, R. W. (1965). *J. Obstet. Gynaec. Brit. Cwlth.*, **72**, 489.
MORROW, W. F. K. and MYLES, T. J. M. (1969). *Brit. med. J.*, **2**, 820.
MUSHIN, W. W. and HILLARD, E. K. (1967). *Brit. med. J.*, **1**, 416.
NEWMAN, W., MCKINNON, L., PHILLIPS, L., PATERSON, P. and WOOD, C. (1967). *Amer. J. Obstet. Gynec.*, **99**, 61.
ORGAN, L. W. (1968). *Can. med. Ass. J.*, **98**, 199.

PATERSON, P., DUNSTAN, M., TRICKEY, N. R. A. and BEARD, R. W. (1970). *J. Obstet. Gynaec. Brit. Cwlth.*, 77, 390.
PENDLETON, H. J. (1970). *Brit. J. hosp. Med.*, **3**, 509.
PITKIN, R. M. and ZWIREK, S. J. (1967). *Amer. J. Obstet. Gynec.*, **98**, 1135.
ROBERTS, H. and PLEASE, N. W. (1958). *J. Obstet. Gynaec. Brit. Emp.*, **65**, 33.
ROSEN, M., MUSHIN, W. W., JONES, P. V. and JONES, E. V. (1969). *Brit. med. J.*, **3**, 263.
SALING, E. (1962). *Arch. Gynäk.*, **197**, 108.
SAN AGUSTIN, M. S., NITOWSKY, H. M. and BORDEN, J. N. (1962). *J. Pediat.*, **60**, 408.
SCOTT, K. E. and USHER, R. (1964). *New Engl. J. Med.*, **270**, 822.
SISSON, T. R. C. and WHALEN, L. E. (1960). *J. Pediat.*, **56**, 43.
SNYDER, F. F. (1949). "Obstetric Analgesia and Anaesthesia". Saunders, Philadelphia and London.
THALER, M. M. and STOBRE, H. C. (1963). *New Engl. J. Med.*, **269**, 606.
USHER, R. H. (1970). *Ped. Clin. N. Amer.*, **17**, 169.
VARTAN, C. K. (1964). *Brit. med. J.*, **2**, 944.
W H O (1965). Technical Report Series 300.
WIGGLESWORTH, J. S. (1966). *Brit. med. Bull.*, **22**, 13.
YAO, A. C., MOINIAN, M. and LIND, T. (1969). *Lancet*, **2**, 871.

Chapter 3

NEONATAL CARE IN HOSPITAL

Special Neonatal Care Units and Intensive Care Nurseries

Low-weight babies have an increased susceptibility to infection, they have difficulty in maintaining an adequate body temperature, and they require gentle handling and special methods of feeding. In addition they are prone to certain complications (jaundice, respiratory distress, hypoglycaemia, etc.) which require constant expert observation and treatment, expensive equipment and a 24-hour laboratory service. For these reasons, the best results are obtained if babies weighing less than $4\frac{1}{2}$ lb. (2,040 g.) at birth are treated in a specially equipped self-contained unit with its own staff of nurses (trained in the care of low-weight babies), under the direction of a consultant paediatrician, and supported by laboratory and radiological facilities.

These units should be large enough to allow for economic use of staff and equipment, for research and for training of nursing and medical personnel, i.e. 20–30 cots.

The Report of the Sub-Committee on "Prevention of Prematurity and the Care of Premature Infants" (Ministry of Health, 1961. H.M. Stationery Office, London) recommended the provision of special baby care units in large and medium sized maternity hospitals and departments catering for abnormal obstetrics and having sufficient prenatal beds and emergency beds for unbooked cases in labour. This Committee stressed the importance of concentrating specialized baby care into one or two of the larger maternity departments in each area, rather than having a small unit in every maternity department. These specialist centres should accept mothers in premature labour, also low-weight babies and non-infected sick babies after birth in their own homes or in smaller maternity units. This means the acceptance of the principle of transfer from one maternity department to another in the interests of the baby.

Small maternity departments, and maternity nursing homes, should transfer all babies weighing less than $4\frac{1}{2}$ lb. (2,040 g.) to a specialist centre. However, small maternity departments must make provision for the care of low-weight babies in the labour room, because they will not always have time to transfer the mothers who go into labour before 36 weeks gestation. The accommodation required for low-weight babies in large, medium sized, and small maternity departments is discussed later in this chapter.

Intensive care nurseries. The need for intensive care for certain adult patients has been recognized for some time but it has only recently been realized that if the incidence of handicaps is to be reduced a minority of the newborn (including the smallest pre-term and other low-weight babies) may require much more intensive care than can usually be given in the majority of the existing special care units.

New techniques have been developed for the intensive care of the newborn, including continuous monitoring of the vital signs; monitoring of the blood gases and pH; intermittent positive pressure ventilation for respiratory failure, etc. These techniques are very specialized and time consuming and they demand an even larger staff of highly skilled nurses and doctors, and even more specialized services (such as a laboratory capable of dealing with micro- and ultramicro-samples and a portable radiological service on a 24 hour basis), than can be provided in many of the special care units. Indeed it would be uneconomic for all existing special care units (which vary in size and facilities) to provide such an expensive service which may only be required by a small minority of the babies they are treating. The most economic method is to include intensive care nurseries in selected special care units which can provide intensive care for the area.

When all the recommendations of the sub-committee on "Domiciliary midwifery and Maternity Bed Needs" (Department of Health and Social Security, 1970. H.M. Stationery Office, London) have been implemented, all small obstetric units will have been replaced by larger combined consultant and general practitioner units in general hospitals; and the district general hospital will be the focus of all maternity services in its area. When this has been achieved the obvious place for the intensive care unit is in the district general hospital. Until then, the hospitals chosen should be those which also provide intensive *obstetric* care, i.e. those which:

(1) Book mothers with a high risk of having a baby which will need intensive care.

(2) Provide beds for mothers requiring intensive care during pregnancy in order to protect the baby.

(3) Provide emergency beds for unbooked mothers in labour with babies requiring intensive care during and after birth.

The principle of transfer of mothers from one maternity department to another must be accepted if the best treatment is to be obtained for the baby.

Stahlman (1969) reported a marked fall in mortality when intensive care facilities were introduced into the Jefferson Davis Hospital in

1960; the mortality of pre-term babies being reduced more than that of term babies.

Usher (1970) investigated the results of intensive care among babies weighing 1,001–2,500 g. when started from birth, and when started after transfer from one hospital to another. The babies born in the hospital with an intensive care nursery had a first week mortality of 5·47%; babies born in the hospitals which transferred those requiring intensive care (but the transferred babies were included in the results of the hospital in which they were born) had a death rate of 8·45%, while the babies born in hospitals with no intensive care nursery and no arrangements for transfer had a mortality of 8·93%, i.e. practically the same as the hospitals which transferred cases. The incidence of low birth weight was the same in all three groups of hospitals. Usher stated that these figures indicate that, for the low-weight baby, intensive care is most effective if it begins at birth in the maternity hospital, rather than after transfer to another hospital; and that low-weight babies need care the earliest and tolerate transport least well.

Low-weight babies should only be transferred from a good special care unit to an intensive care unit in another hospital if they require techniques and equipment not available in their own unit; and the risk of transfer must always be balanced against the extra facilities provided in the intensive care nurseries. It is also desirable that the mother and baby should not be separated unnecessarily.

Because intensive care is required from birth, every effort must be made to deliver "high-risk" babies in a hospital with an intensive care nursery. For this reason every large maternity hospital or department which books large numbers of mothers with babies "at risk" should have an intensive care nursery in their special care unit.

Special care units with intensive care nurseries should be used for training medical and nursing personnel, and for research.

Special care units without intensive care nurseries should also be able to train personnel if part of the training is taken in the intensive care nursery of the area. These units should also be able to train nurses for domiciliary care of low-weight babies delivered and nursed at home or after their discharge from hospital.

Developing countries will have to consider the economics of intensive care very carefully. Large sums of money could be spent on the intensive care of a very small percentage of the total number of low-weight babies of which only a relatively small proportion will survive and some of the survivors may be handicapped. The majority of low-weight babies will survive and have a good chance of developing normally without intensive care, provided there is adequate skilled nursing care. All other facilities for the care of low-weight babies should be provided before embarking on an intensive care programme (see p. 276).

Transport

Since July, 1948, under the National Health Service Act, each local health authority has been responsible for the provision of an ambulance service in its area and this service includes suitable arrangements for the transport of low-weight infants. During transit chilling and infection must be avoided, and facilities must be available for keeping the respiratory passages clear and for giving oxygen, humidity and, if necessary, intermittent positive pressure ventilation.

At the present time two types of low-weight babies will have to be transported, i.e.

(1) Healthy babies weighing less than 2,040 g. (4½ lb.), born at home or in a small maternity unit, being taken to a special care unit.

(2) Very small (or sick) pre-term or light-for-dates babies being transferred to an intensive care unit.

If transferring an infant to an intensive care nursery, the ambulance should collect a nurse and doctor from this nursery, together with their emergency equipment, before collecting the infant. Such an infant may require specialized treatment before and during transfer, e.g. treatment for hypoglycaemia, intubation and administration of oxygen, and perhaps even intermittent positive pressure ventilation (Storrs and Taylor, 1970). Fig. 10 shows a portable ventilator.

If transferring a baby to a special care unit a nurse experienced in the care of low-weight babies can accompany the baby in the ambulance (see Frontispiece). This could be achieved by training some ambulance midwives; or by arranging for the ambulance to pick up a domiciliary baby care midwife, or a nurse from the special care unit, before calling for the baby. Such a midwife or nurse must be able to intubate the baby if necessary (The Central Midwives Board have decided that if a midwife has been trained in this procedure she may carry out intubation in appropriate cases). She should also be able to use a resuscitator, such as the Blease Samson neonatal resuscitator or the Cardiff neonatal inflating bag (Mushin and Hillard, 1967), either of which can be used with a mask, or with an endotracheal tube if this is necessary (see Figs. 6 and 7).

The ambulance should be heated, and portable incubators or carriers which can be plugged into the ambulance battery (or a separate battery) are now generally available (Fig. 11). In these carriers the temperature, humidity and oxygen concentration can all be controlled. Such a carrier should now be considered indispensable for transportation of low-weight infants for long distances and, if possible, it should also be used for short distances.

If the infant is being collected after birth at home, it should already be in a warm cot, wrapped loosely in a sterile towel and clean blankets; or in a silver swaddler (Fig. 9).

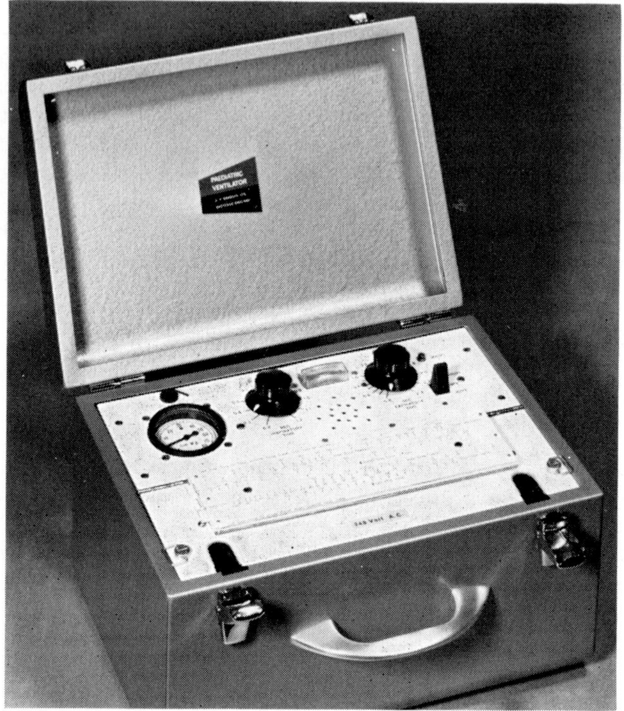

(*Photograph by courtesy of H. G. East and Co. Ltd.*)

FIG. 10. *The Sheffield Infant Ventilator.* A compact portable ventilator which can be operated from the main electric supply or from batteries. The storage compartment holds the humidifier and other accessories.

In the City of Birmingham all midwives carry special case history sheets which they use when transferring infants to a special care unit. In other areas the ambulance nurse or doctor must complete a case history sheet provided by the unit concerned before removing the baby. The details required include:

(1) Name, address and telephone number.
(2) Nationality, age and health of parents.
(3) History of present pregnancy and birth.
(4) History of previous pregnancies and births.
(5) Health of other children.
(6) Mother's blood group and result of Wasserman and Rhesus tests.
(7) Birth weight of infant and expected date of delivery.
(8) Possible cause of low weight.

(9) Drugs given to infant, with dosage.
(10) If oxygen given, length of time and amount given.
(11) Passage of urine and meconium.
(12) Feeding, if any.
(13) Home conditions.
(14) Presence of infection of any kind in the home.
(15) Religion and if infant has been baptized.
(16) Husband's occupation.
(17) Name, address and telephone number of midwife and doctor.
(18) Signed permission for any operation which might become necessary.

The address and telephone number of the hospital should be given to the parents who are told that arrangements will be made to admit the mother to the hospital when the baby is ready to feed from the breast. Instructions are given to the mother in regard to the collection of her milk; and she is told of the importance of maintaining her supply. In the City of Birmingham, nurses from the human milk bank pay daily visits to these mothers. They lend the necessary equipment, advise the mothers and collect the milk.

If the infant is being collected from a hospital, in addition to completing the case history sheet from the special care unit, the hospital case notes (and X-ray films if any) should be borrowed if possible.

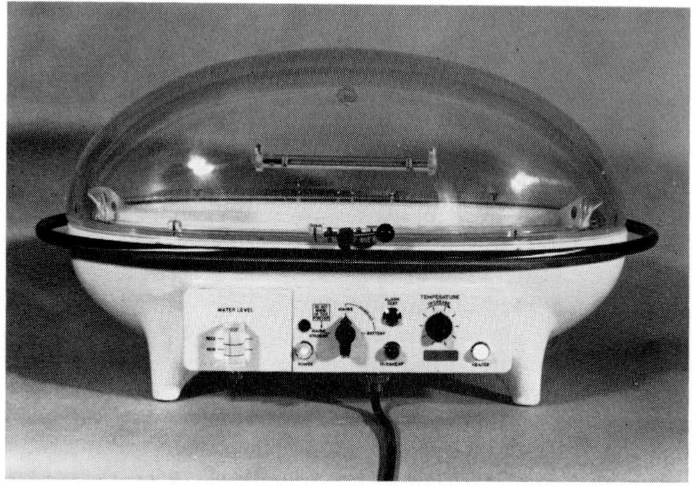

(Photograph by courtesy of Vickers Ltd. Medical Engineering)

FIG. 11. *Portable Incubator.* A portable incubator with controlled oxygen administration (oxygen cylinder is carried in space under infant), temperature and humidity, which can be used on batteries or the main electric supply.

Before handling the infant, the doctor and/or nurse must wash their hands. They must make sure that the infant is fit to travel, i.e. that the air passages are clear and that the infant is a good colour and breathing well. Any necessary treatment is given before the infant is transferred to the incubator.

If the baby is being collected from its home, the portable incubator is kept plugged into the ambulance battery until the baby is ready to be transferred; in other cases it is plugged into the electric supply of the nursery of the hospital or nursing home.

If the baby is in a good condition (e.g. a healthy small baby being transferred early to a special care unit) and the journey is short, it can be wrapped loosely in a sterile towel and a small light sterile blanket in the incubator; but if the journey is long and the baby is cold, or if it is likely to need treatment on the journey which will necessitate opening the incubator, it is better to use a silver swaddler (Baum and Scopes, 1968).

If available, the placenta should also be taken to the special care unit.

During transit the condition of the child must be carefully watched and an electric torch is useful for this. The air passages must be cleared by suction when necessary, and oxygen given if required. If respiration fails, intermittent positive pressure ventilation must be undertaken and suitable equipment must be carried in case any of these procedures become necessary. An electrocardiographically actuated heart rate meter has been found useful when transporting very sick infants to an intensive care nursery (Storrs and Taylor, 1970).

The prevention of infection is important, so separate portable incubators and ambulances should be kept for transporting infected infants. All incubators must be carefully sterilized after each use.

In countries where such elaborate methods of transport are not justifiable, good results can be obtained with simple improvisations. When the first English unit caring for low-weight infants was started at Sorrento Maternity Hospital in the City of Birmingham in 1931, large wicker baskets were originally used as carriers, several being kept ready for use at the ambulance station. These baskets were fitted with a strong washable lining. In the lining were three pockets for hot-water bottles, one each side and one at the foot. The hot-water bottles were filled and placed in the basket before the ambulance set out to fetch the infant. Lightweight sterilizable blankets were provided as coverings. A basket once used was not put into service again until it had been scrubbed, relined and provided with clean blankets. This simple carrier was cheap and proved useful for the transportation of babies from within the city boundary. Because of the relatively short distances involved, the method of heating was adequate, and the risk of retrolental fibroplasia from the administration of pure oxygen to cyanosed babies was not great but unfortunately the open basket offered no protection from droplet infection by attendants and provided no extra humidity.

Admission to Special Care (or Intensive Care) Unit

It is important to arrange for admission of the infant before it is moved to ensure than an incubator or cot is available in the unit and to enable preparations to be made for the infant's reception.

On arrival at the unit, the portable incubator is handed over to the unit nurses who take it into the admission room (in the absence of an

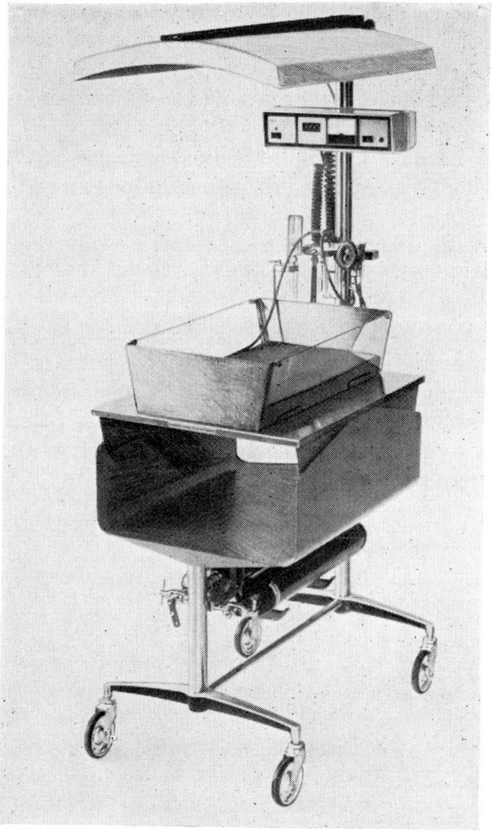

(Photograph by courtesy of Becton, Dickinson UK Ltd.)

FIG. 12. *Complete Neonatal Care Unit.* This unit is mobile and includes an over-table radiant heater, an adjustable (also removable) bassinet with four fold-down sides, facilities for the administration of oxygen, and roomy storage space. It can be used in the delivery room, admission room of the special baby care unit, or in the treatment room.

admission room, an empty observation room may be used instead) and the resident doctor is notified of the arrival.

If the infant's condition is good, it can be weighed and transferred to an incubator or cot at a suitable temperature (see p. 61). The identity of the infant should be checked and both infant and incubator (or cot) labelled. The respiration, heart rate and temperature are recorded. The cord is inspected for bleeding and, if necessary, is re-ligatured. The passage of urine and meconium is noted.

If the condition is poor, the resident doctor must see the infant immediately in case emergency treatment is required. All equipment necessary for resuscitation and emergency treatment must be available in the admission room, and it is useful to have over-table heating (Fig. 12).

The resident doctor should examine every infant as soon as possible after admission for signs of abnormality or disease; and the gestational age should be assessed (by length, body-weight, proportions, etc.). This examination should be made in the incubator or cot, with the minimum of handling.

Certain infants should be screened for hypoglycaemia (with Dextrostix), i.e. asphyxiated babies, light-for-dates babies, babies of diabetic mothers, and very small babies.

A decision must be made as to the type of nursery to which the infant should be admitted. Infants known to have been in contact with a source of infection, or infants admitted from their homes later than the first few hours after birth, should be regarded as potentially infected and admitted to a suspect or isolation nursery where they can remain until proved free from infection.

The Nurseries

Type of nursery. The following types of nursery should be available for the care of low-weight babies:

(1) Hot nurseries for incubators (85–88°F or 29·5–31°C, not humidified), the warmer temperature being required for the smallest infants.

(2) Warm nurseries (75–80°F or 24–25°C, with a relative humidity of 60–65%) in which the larger infants can be nursed in heated cots.

(3) Cool nurseries (65°F or 18·5°C, not humidified) in which infants can be acclimatized to natural conditions before being sent home.

In countries where incubators are not available, the smallest infants can be nursed naked in a hot humidified room (see p. 64), or clothed in heated cots in a slightly cooler room.

Size of nursery. The smaller the number of babies in any one nursery, and the greater the air space per cot, the less is the risk of infection. If possible, a minimum floor space of 50 square feet ($4\frac{1}{2}$ square metres) should be provided for each cot; and 30 square feet ($2\frac{3}{4}$ square metres) for each incubator. Up to 12 incubators may be allowed in any one nursery, but no cots should be allowed in such a large incubator nursery because any baby in a cot would be exposed to air emerging from too many incubators. (The infants in the incubators are breathing clean air, i.e. outside air, or nursery air cleaned by a bacterial filter.)

The maximum number of cots in any cot nursery should be four to six. This limitation reduces the risk of cross infection.

Unless cots can be well spaced (at least 5 ft. or $1\frac{1}{2}$ m. between centres, see Fig. 13) they should be separated by partitions or screens, but each cot must stand 6 in. (15 cm.) from any side wall or partition and at least 2 ft. (60 cm.) must be left on one side of a cot for nursing care. The upper portion of the partition or screen should be made of glass, or other transparent material, to allow for easy inspection of the babies and good lighting in all parts of the nursery. Some authorities believe that each of the infants should be in a completely separate cell (partitions reaching the ceiling and floor and each cell ventilated and heated separately). This is not a good plan for the smallest infants, among whom the risk of death from unnoticed regurgitation and inhalation is far greater than the risk from infection: these infants can be more safely isolated by the use of incubators in a room which is never left unattended. In any case, even a cell does not prevent cross infection by dust (brought in on feet and blown up by currents of air), droplet or contact, unless special precautions are taken against each. In the author's opinion the risk of infection in open nurseries is very small if the cots are well spaced (see Fig. 13), the number of cots in each nursery is limited, dust is controlled, and barrier nursing is conscientiously carried out.

Heating and ventilation. The temperature in each nursery must be as constant as possible. This is achieved ideally by installing an air-conditioning plant, but such a plant is expensive and can easily go out of order. In case of failure of the plant, means of obtaining natural ventilation and heating must be available. Fortunately, simpler methods can give equally good results. Central heating by hot water or steam radiators, augmented if necessary by well ventilated gas fires or electric radiators, can be used for heating purposes.

To avoid loss of heat from the baby by radiation via the incubator to cold walls, ceilings and windows, all external walls should be insulated (cavity walls) and all windows double-glazed. The nursery temperature and humidity must be checked and recorded at regular intervals; and if a more sophisticated method is not available, each room should be

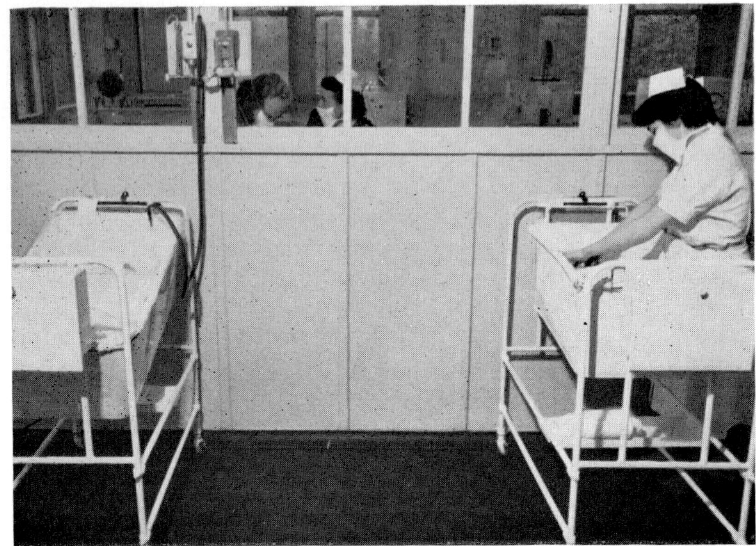

(*Photo by Camera Talks*)

Fig. 13. Part of a nursery in Sorrento Special Care Unit. The cot spacing is well shown (5 ft. or 1½ m. between cots, and 50 sq. ft. or 4½ sq. m. floor space for each cot).

provided with a hygrometer by which both temperature and humidity can be checked (Fig. 14).

Ventilation must be adequate (10–12 changes per hour) but freedom from draughts is essential. Ideally, fresh air should enter high up and be extracted at floor level carrying dust downwards, and this should be arranged if an air-conditioning plant is installed. In the absence of air-conditioning, window ventilators (inlet from outside air) and extraction fans are cheap and effective. If there is any possibility of draughts, the cots must be screened.

Humidity. The relative humidity should not fall below 50% if drying of the mucous membrane of the respiratory passages is to be avoided; and it only needs to be over 60% when the nose is by-passed, e.g. with endotracheal intubation. A relative humidity over 50% decreases the thermoneutral environmental temperature required by 0·5°C (Hey and Katz, 1970); but within the thermoneutral range infants are not affected by alterations in the relative humidity (Hey and Maurice, 1968), nor does the relative humidity affect the mortality rate if the environmental temperature is correct (Dawes, 1968). Finally, bacterial growth is minimal when the relative humidity is 50–65% (Brück, 1968).

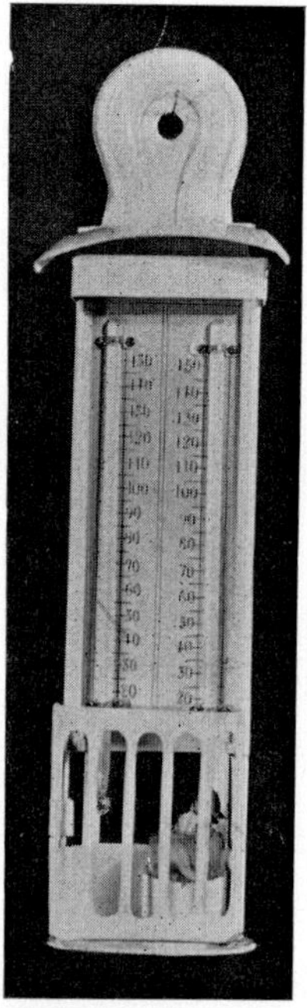

FIG. 14. Wet and dry bulb hygrometer.

If an air-conditioning plant is installed, the humidity of the nurseries is controlled with the heating and ventilation, but the correct humidity can also be obtained by simpler methods: for instance a humidifier or even a pan of water can be heated on a well-guarded gas or electric ring and the results checked by means of a wet and dry bulb hygrometer (Fig. 14). To ensure a humidity of 60% the wet bulb thermometer should register 65°F (18·5°C) in a nursery kept at 75°F (24°C), and 62°F (17°C) in a nursery kept at 70°F (21°C). Below these figures the air will be too dry. The hygrometer must be observed frequently to ensure a constant temperature and humidity throughout the 24 hours. The correct humidity is easily maintained during the summer months, but during the cold weather a larger amount of steam is required, and in a large nursery more than one humidifier or pan may be needed.

Incubators and Cots

Incubators. Various makes of incubators are now available (see Figs. 15 and 16). They are all expensive, therefore it is fortunate that they are not indispensable for the successful rearing of low-weight babies. There is, however, no doubt that incubators save much valuable nursing time. They can supply the correct heat, humidity, and concentration of oxygen to suit any individual baby; they allow easier

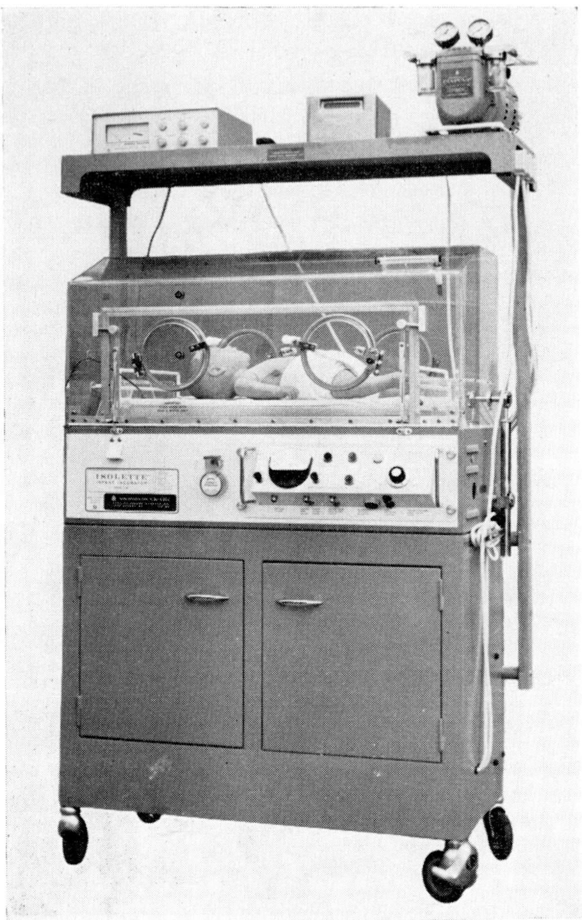

(*Photograph by courtesy of Air-Shields* (*UK*) *Ltd.*)

FIG. 15. *Isolette Infant Incubator*. Servo-control of the infant's temperature is available. This illustration shows a space-saving shelf attached above the incubator for any necessary apparatus.

observation of the baby from a distance and eliminate the need for dressing the baby. In addition, if correctly used, they can reduce the incidence of air-borne infection.

It is now realized that incubators allow naked infants to lose heat by radiation, and special precautions must be taken to avoid this (see temperature control, p. 61). In addition they are difficult to clean, the water containers are potential sources of bacterial growth, and some procedures are difficult in a closed incubator.

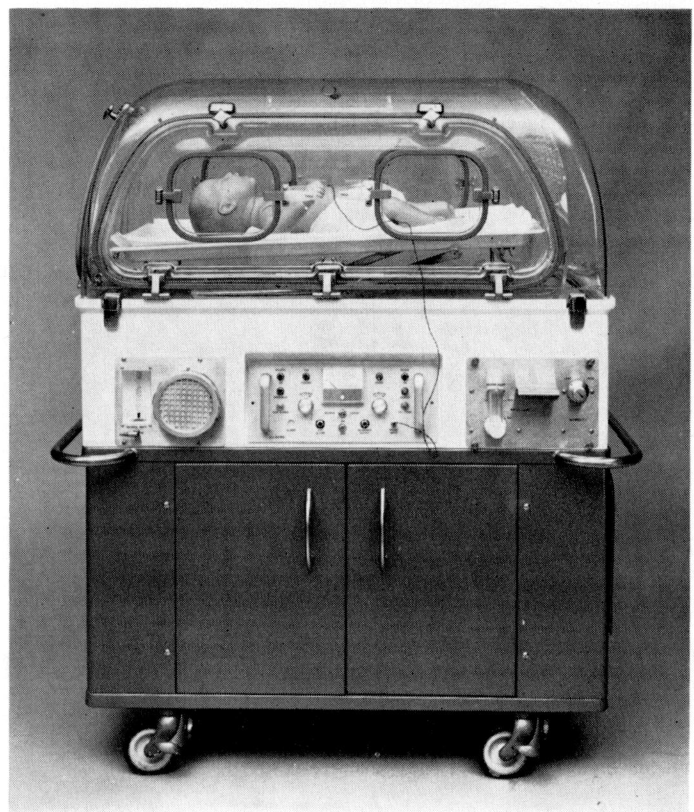

(Photograph by courtesy of Vickers Ltd. Medical Engineering)

FIG. 16. *Incubator with servo-control of infant's temperature.*

An incubator can never be regarded as a substitute for a good nurse; it requires careful handling and it is as well to remember that any incubator is only as good as the nurse who is managing it.

Incubators should certainly be provided in special care units and in intensive care nurseries, i.e. the units which handle the majority of the smallest infants born in each area.

Some incubators are more efficient than others. The minimum requirements for an incubator are:

(1) Adequate ventilation with air free from bacteria and at a stable temperature.

(2) Facilities for the administration of a controlled percentage of oxygen.

(3) A unit which can produce various degrees of humidity.
(4) Easy access to the infant for all nursing procedures.

In order to secure a satisfactory minimum standard of safety from electrical risks, overheating and fire risks and to ensure accessibility for cleaning purposes and a proper control of oxygen concentration, all British incubators have to comply with the specifications of the British Standards Institution for "Electrically heated incubators for babies" (B.S. 3061: 1965).

A good incubator is ventilated with clean air (from outside the building, see Fig. 17; or from nursery air through an adequate bacterial

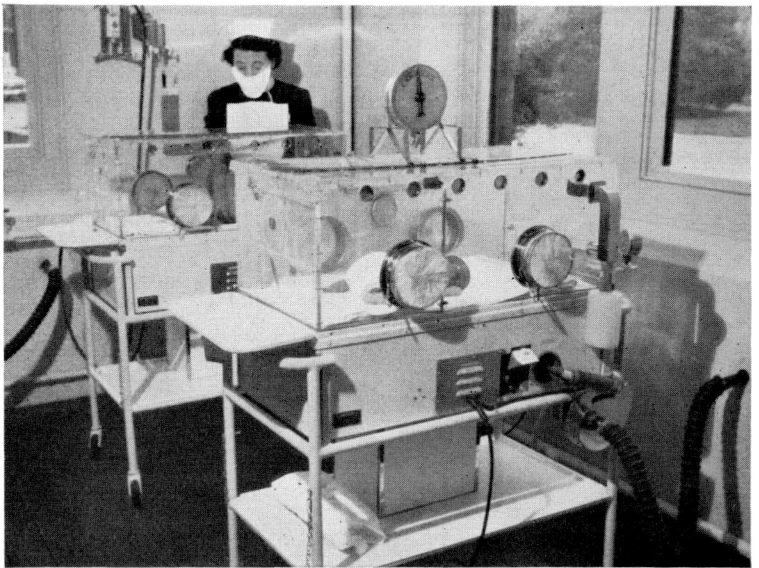

(*Photo by Camera Talks*)

FIG. 17. Incubators with air supply from outside the building.

filter) by means of an electrically driven fan, so that the pressure inside the incubator is slightly greater than that in the room. Such an incubator provides reasonably good but not complete protection from air-borne infections and there will be little fluctuation in the temperature or concentration of oxygen in the incubator if the baby is cared for in the correct way, i.e. through the port-holes. Even weighing must be done inside the incubator (see p. 65). If required, a relatively high humidity should be obtainable without difficulty and there should be facilities for the occasional use of a nebulizer (with compressed air, *not* unfiltered nursery air).

Incubators should be kept in a relatively hot room (85–88°F or 29·5–31°C) to avoid condensation inside the cover (which obscures the view of the baby) as well as to avoid loss of heat by radiation.

If nursery air is being used, the filter in the air-inlet must be changed at regular intervals. Care must be taken with the use of the port-holes and sleeves to prevent them from becoming a source of infection. In the Sorrento unit the portholes on one side of the incubator are used for "clean" procedures (feeding, extracting mucus from the pharynx, or giving sterile injections) and the other side for "dirty" procedures (changing, cleaning, and taking rectal temperatures). If sleeves are used, they must be changed and sterilized frequently if they are not disposable. Disposable thin plastic gloves can also be used on the ports (Segal, 1966).

Open heated cots. It is possible for even the smallest infants to be reared successfully in open cots in a hot nursery, if incubators are not available. Cots are cheap and can be heated easily, they allow easy handling of the infants, and oxygen can be given by face mask or a Gairdner head box (see p. 134 for safe administration of oxygen); but ideally cots should only be used for the larger babies not requiring oxygen.

Cots should be made of metal, or plastic material, which can be disinfected easily. They should be sufficiently deep to be draughtproof, and of a height and size to enable easy handling of the infant. Means must be available for tilting the baby either head-up or head-down, and sufficient locker space must be available. Fig. 18 shows the cot in use in the Sorrento unit. It is made of white enamelled steel, and the hanging bassinet measures 32 in. (81 cm.) in length, 18 in. (46 cm.) in width and 12 in. (30·5 cm.) in depth. It is easily adjustable to three levels at either end by means of three pairs of hooks. It is fitted with a strong washable lining, in which there are three pockets for hot-water bottles, one each side and one at the foot. When additional heat is required an electric blanket is used. A Dunlopillo mattress is used, enclosed in an impervious cover to prevent contamination. All blankets are sterilizable and a blanket, once used, is not issued to another infant until it has been washed. Pillows are forbidden. The cot is disinfected and the lining changed at least once a week throughout a baby's stay in hospital. In order to avoid undue handling or cooling of the babies, the child is transferred, with its mattress and blankets, into a clean, warm cot, the original cot being removed from the nursery for cleaning and disinfection before being put into service again.

Each cot is provided with a locker, in the form of a metal box attached to the foot of the cot. This is used for the storage of the individual equipment belonging to each baby.

The cot is also provided with a shelf, on which is kept the gown to be worn by the nurse when she attends to this particular baby.

In order to keep the heat of the cot as uniform as possible, a routine method of changing the hot-water bottles should be adopted. To maintain a high cot temperature for a small baby the following method can be used: each hour one of the side bottles (alternately) is transferred to the pocket at the foot of the cot, the one previously at the foot being removed, refilled, and placed in the empty side-pocket. As the baby gets bigger and maintains a higher body temperature the bottles can be filled less frequently. Each bottle should be covered completely by being placed in a washable flannel bag; by the use of these bags, and the placing of the bottles in the pockets of the cot-lining, all danger of bottle burns is avoided. Great care should be taken to ensure that the bottles from the various babies do not come in contact with each other during the re-filling, and on no account should the flannel bags be removed from the cots in case they also become a source of cross-infection. Carelessness as regards these points leads to breaks in the technique of barrier nursing.

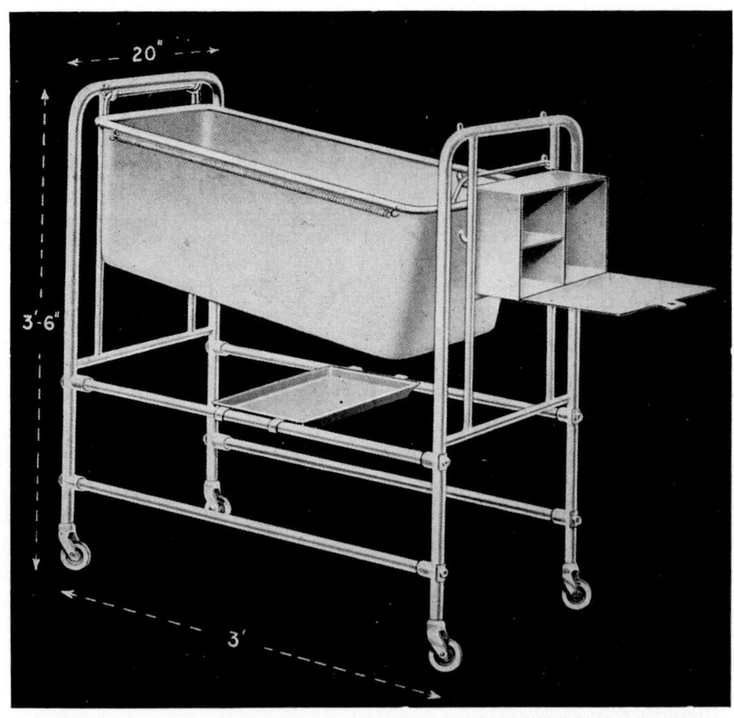

(Photograph by courtesy of John & Joseph Taunton Ltd.)

FIG. 18. "Sorrento" Cot.

An electric blanket or pad is most useful for heating up a cot quickly before the arrival of a new admission. If the pad is used under the baby as an extra means of heating the cot, special precautions must be taken to avoid the three possible dangers of cross-infection, electric shock and overheating. As regards infection, it should be remembered that it is

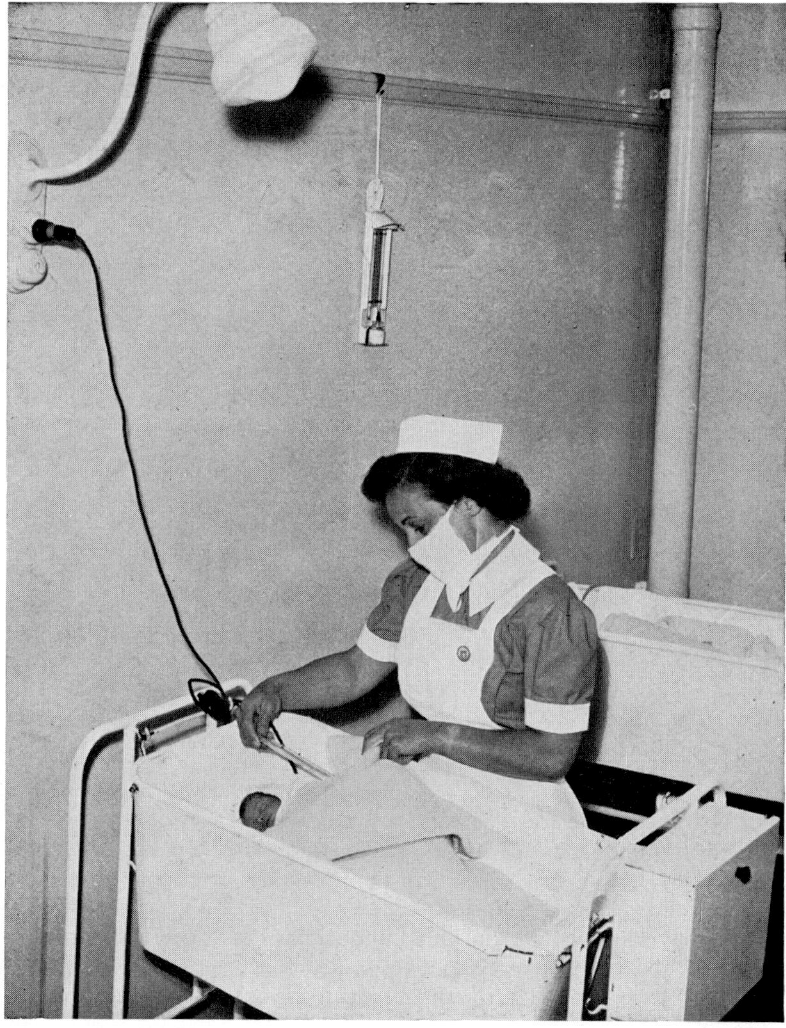

(*Photo by Camera Talks*)

FIG. 19. Electric pad in use. Photograph shows the control switch, the red light over the cot and the cot thermometer.

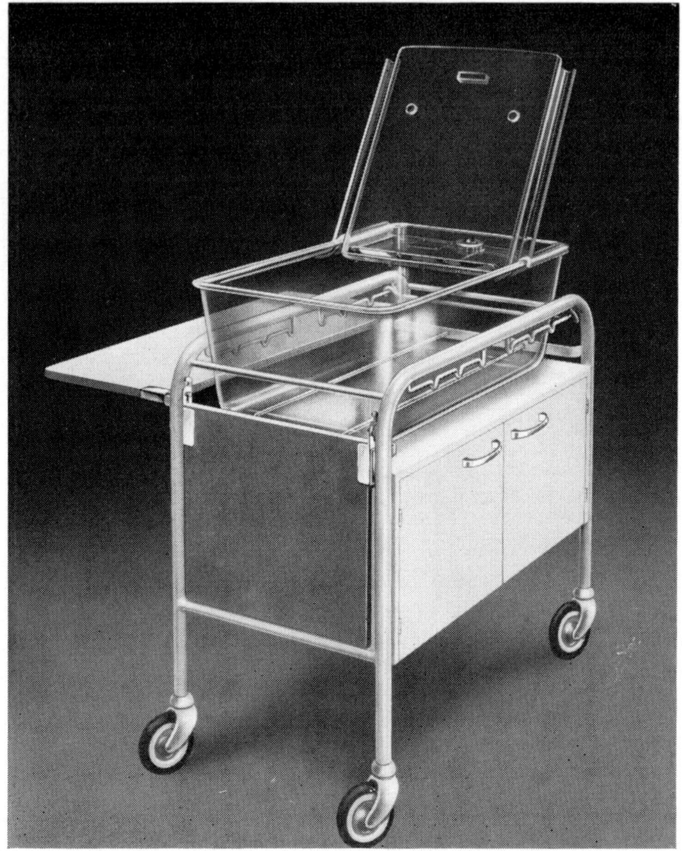

(*Photograph by courtesy of Hoskins and Sewell Ltd.*)

FIG. 20. *Another type of Cot.* The bassinet can be converted into an oxygen tent by means of the drop-on lid.

impossible to sterilize such a pad, therefore, in addition to the use of a washable cover, it should be completely covered with strong rubber or polythene sheeting so that contamination is impossible. This sheeting will also serve to prevent the possibility of electric shock. To prevent overheating, the electric pad should be well covered with several layers of blanket and an additional layer of rubber or polythene sheeting and the temperature of the pad should be automatically controlled. All infants who are being treated in heated cots (whether heated by hot bottles or electric blankets) should be provided with a cot thermometer (wall type), which is placed between the blankets on top of the infant, and when the temperature on this thermometer rises above the required level the heating of the cot is reduced. As an additional precaution, the electric blanket can be used on a two-way switch, a red electric light bulb being fixed on the second socket. A red light will then show over the cot when the blanket is in use, and this reminds the nurse of the need to inspect the cot thermometer at frequent intervals (see Fig. 19). On no account should the temperature of the coolest part of the cot (on top of the infant) rise above 37°C (98·4°F) or heat stroke will develop.

As a general rule, the smallest infants require a cot temperature of 32–35°C (90–95°F); as they become larger and stronger, and their level of stabilization of the body temperature higher, the temperature of the cot is gradually reduced (see Temperature Control, p. 61).

Another type of cot is shown in Fig. 20. The crib is made from clear perspex and can be raised at either end. A locker and shelves are provided. The bassinet is slightly smaller than that of the Sorrento cot, being 27 in. (68·5 cm.) long, 15 in. (38·0 cm.) wide and 10 in. (25·5 cm.) deep. It has the advantage of allowing good observation of an infant not requiring a heated cot, but loses this advantage if a lining, with pockets for hot water bottles, has to be inserted. It can be converted into an oxygen tent by means of a drop-on hinged perspex lid which is fitted with an oxygen mixer valve allowing any required concentration (between 25% and 90%) to flow into the crib.

Prevention of Infection

(1) **General precautions.** As few people as possible should enter a special care unit; usually only healthy people concerned with the care of the infants, i.e. nurses, doctors, laboratory technicians, X-ray personnel, domestic cleaners and, of course, mothers. Special short-sleeved uniforms or gowns must be worn while working in the unit, and the correct use of masks in certain nurseries is of value if the technique is good (see p. 59).

No one with a cold, sore throat, skin infection, diarrhoea or other form of infection should be allowed in the unit. No nurse should commence duty in a special baby care unit unless she is healthy and free from infection. New nurses who have been working in sick children's wards, isolation wards or children's nurseries (day or residential) should have nose, throat and rectal swabs taken before commencing duty in the unit. Visiting doctors, medical students and nurses may occasionally be admitted to the nurseries if they are free from infection and wear both gown and mask, but usually they stay outside the nurseries and observe the infants through the viewing panels.

As parents cannot be admitted to certain nurseries, a viewing window or glass panel should be provided, either in the door or wall of these nurseries, to enable them to see their infants (see Fig. 21). This is not

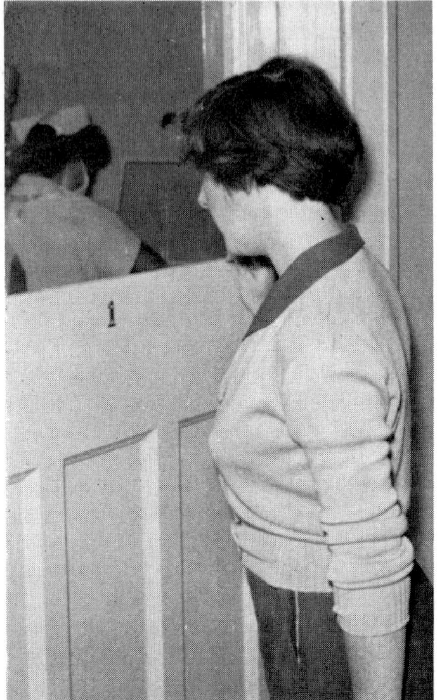

(*Photo by Camera Talks*)

FIG. 21. A mother viewing her baby.

necessary, of course, if the upper part of all interior walls is made of glass.

Infants should not be admitted to the main nurseries unless newly born and free from exposure to infection. Any infant who has been exposed to a known infection, or who has not been admitted to the unit immediately after birth, should be kept in a "suspect" nursery until proved free from infection.

The cleaning of the nurseries is a most important factor in the prevention of infection. The walls and ceilings must be washed at least four times a year and also after any infection. Furniture and equipment must be wiped daily with a damp cloth (soap and water or disinfectant) and thoroughly cleaned once a week. If curtains or screen covers are used, they must be washed frequently. Ayliffe *et al.* (1966) showed that it was impossible to sterilize floors by washing or disinfecting because of continuous re-contamination, so efforts must be made to prevent infected dust rising. These include the application of spindle oil to wooden floors and linoleum, and the mopping of impervious floors with

Triton oil emulsion (Krugman and Ward, 1951) after washing or disinfecting. Vacuum cleaners (which will filter the air before it leaves the bag, or are connected to outlets outside the nursery) should be used instead of sweeping. Dusters must be used damp (with hexachlorophane solution) and be sterilized after use. Cotton cellular blankets produce as much dust as woollen ones but they can be boiled or autoclaved more easily (Rountree *et al.*, 1962; Rubbo, 1963).

Clean linen should be kept in cupboards *outside* the nurseries (if possible in autoclaved packets) until required for use, and care must be taken in its handling. Neither clean nor dirty linen should be allowed to come in contact with the nurse's uniform, and no dirty linen should be put on the floor or into the hand basin. All dirty linen should be put into bins lined with disposable plastic bags and with lids operated by foot pedals. Packets containing sterile dressings, swabs, instruments, etc., should be protected from contamination. All unused packets should be re-sterilized at specified intervals and at any time if contamination may have occurred.

Because of the recent increase in infections due to the *Pseudomonas* group (normal inhabitants of water and soil) particular care must be taken to eliminate them from water reservoirs. All sinks must slope sufficiently to empty completely. All taps should be removable for sterilization, and traps under sinks and hand basins should be disposable or removable for sterilization.

Finally, adequate isolation facilities must be provided, and any baby showing the slightest signs of a possible infection should be isolated at once by the nursing staff if medical advice cannot be immediately obtained.

(2) **Barrier nursing.** Careful barrier nursing is required when a nurse is dealing with more than one infant. If cross-infection is to be avoided it is essential to ensure that each baby shall come in contact only with the nurse's washed hands and forearms, and its own individual "cot gown" (never with the nurse's unprotected uniform).

As far as possible, equipment should be disposable or kept separate for each individual baby. All other equipment and linen (i.e. not disposable and not kept for the use of the one baby only) must be adequately cleaned or sterilized before use, e.g. stethoscopes, tape measures, clothing, napkins, bed-linen, blankets, bathing bowls and towels, etc.; or protected, e.g. paper on weighing scales. Nebulizers should only be used with sterile distilled water and be carefully disinfected after use. All equipment used for suction and resuscitation should be capable of being dismantled and autoclaved.

Incubators and cots must be suitably sterilized at least once a week as well as between babies. To combat *Pseudomonas, Aerobacter Klebsiella*, etc., especially among babies treated in incubators, Kresky (1964) suggested that all nursery equipment should be cleaned with 1% Povidone iodine. Barrie (1965) only eliminated bacteria from incubators by washing with soap, water and 1% cetrimide, then steeping the sleeves and sleeve rims in Milton 1:80 (125 parts per million of hypochlorite) for 1 hour also leaving Milton 1:80 in the lower deck tanks for 1 hour. In some incubators, the reservoir and water taps can be detached and autoclaved. Incubators may also be fumigated with formaldehyde vapour before cleaning; and some hospitals operate their incubators dry (without a baby) for 24 hours in order to interrupt cycles of bacterial growth. Filters on the air-inlet must be changed and the oxygen tubing autoclaved.

All nursing care should be given at the cot side: communal changing tables must be avoided. Babies should be bathed in boiled or autoclaved bowls and not in communal fixed baths. Special precautions for the prevention of cross-infection during the various nursing procedures will be discussed in the section on nursing care.

(3) **Hand washing.** This cannot be too greatly stressed as a means of preventing the spread of infection because indirect contact is the usual method of transmission; pathogens from an infected infant or from the nose of a carrier being transferred to the hands and so to another infant. "Hand" washing entails washing the *hands and fore-arms* under running water.

Lowbury *et al.* (1964), divide bacterial flora into:

(1) Resident flora which is virtually unaffected by washing or scrubbing with soap and water.

(2) Transient flora which can easily be removed with soap and water.

They showed that certain antiseptics such as a liquid soap containing 3% hexachlorophane or a detergent cream containing 3% hexachlorophane (PhisoHex) or Povidone iodine scrub (Betadine) can considerably reduce the resident flora. The hexachlorophane acts slowly on the skin after the hands have been dried while povidone iodine scrub disinfects at the time of application. They found that the use of 1% chlorhexidine cream (Hibitane) to dry hands produced no reduction of skin flora. The most suitable routine for a special baby care unit would seem to be the use of a liquid soap containing 3% hexachlorophane for all routine hand washing. Povidone iodine scrub could be reserved for the first hand washing when coming on duty, before any operative procedure, and after caring for an infected baby.

Nurses must use their common sense as to when to wash, but the following list may act as a guide:

On entering the unit.
Before preparing feeds or putting teats on bottles.

Before giving a feed or supervising a breast-feed.
Before handling clean linen or equipment.
Before and after any handling of an infant.
After handling soiled linen and equipment, or the telephone.
After using a handkerchief, or putting the hand into a pocket which contains or has contained a handkerchief.
After any adjustment to the mask.

Much washing of the hands can be saved by avoiding unnecessary handling of infants, cots and equipment. Each infant should be dealt with from above downwards, because once a nurse has touched the napkin area, the upper portion of the baby must not be touched until the nurse has washed her hands. Doctors, laboratory technicians, etc., must be equally careful in regard to washing, especially on entering the unit, and before and after touching either an infant or the inside of its cot or incubator. Running water should be available in every nursery and, if possible, paper towels (or towels for use once only before being rewashed) for drying the hands after washing (see Fig. 22 (*a*) and (*b*)). If elbow taps, or knee or foot pedals are not provided, the taps must be turned off with the towel before this is discarded, to prevent re-contamination of the hands from the tap.

(4) **Use of gowns.** *Nursing staff.* Before changing, cleaning, or dressing a baby, and before lifting it out of its cot, the nurse must put on the short sleeved "cot gown" belonging to the baby with which she is dealing. These individual "cot gowns" can be kept on a rail or shelf on each cot, or on a hook near the cot. They should be folded or hung with the outer side inwards, so as to keep this outer side, which comes in contact with the infant, free from contamination (the outer side should be clearly marked in some way). After removing the "cot gown", the nurse must wash her hands carefully before going on to the next baby. If nurses are working in the special care unit only, they wear these "cot gowns" directly over their special uniform, i.e. uniform worn only while on duty in the unit. If nurses work in other wards in addition to the special baby care unit (maternity wards, or the term baby nurseries —a practice not to be encouraged), then a special gown must be put on over the uniform (or the uniform changed), before entering the special baby care unit. This gown must be used in addition to the "cot gowns".

A "cot gown" need not be worn while handling an infant inside an incubator but if the baby is taken out of the incubator, or if the side of the incubator is opened and the baby pulled out on its mattress, a gown must be worn.

Medical staff, technicians, etc. On entering the unit, medical and other staff must put on clean white coats or gowns (with short sleeves to prevent cross infection when handling the babies);

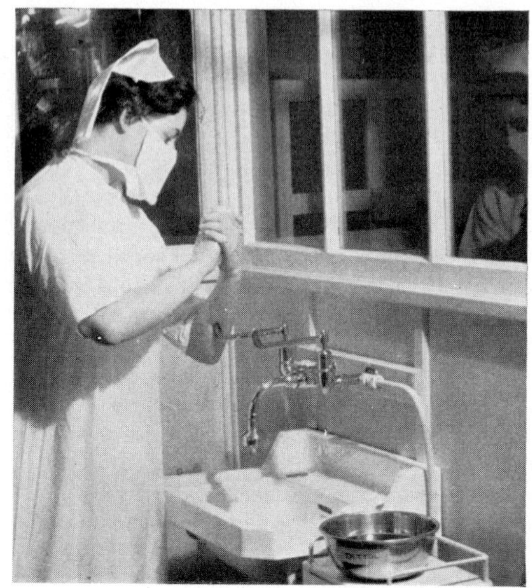

FIG. 22 (*a*). "Hand" washing. Elbow taps are used.

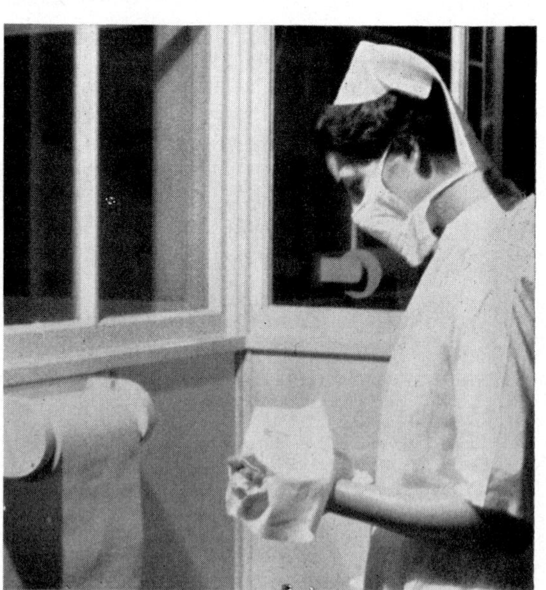

FIG. 22 (*b*). "Hand" washing. Hands are dried on paper towels.

(*Photos by Camera Talks*)

and use an infant's "cot gown" if the infant or any of the cot blankets, etc., will come in contact with more than the washed hands and forearms.

All staff must use special gowns for the "suspect" or isolation nurseries, and full details as to the use of the isolation gowns will be considered later.

(5) **Use of masks.** The author still believes that the correct use of masks in certain situations can be a means of preventing infection. Of course if they are used carelessly they may even cause infection.

It is likely that the use of masks has little effect on the incidence of staphylococcal infections (Forfar and Maccabe, 1958) because the hands provide the main source of transmission of staphylococci (Wolinsky *et al.*, 1960). The wearing of masks when dealing with small infants in open cots should reduce the risk of infection from an attendant's nasopharyngeal organisms which can cause infections in low-weight babies. Obviously it is unnecessary to wear a mask in an incubator room unless an infant is taken out of the incubator.

A clean mask should be put on before entering a nursery with open cots. Disposable masks are usually provided but they must be proved to be impervious to bacteria. The Promask (Smith and Nephew-Southalls Limited) has passed rigorous tests and may be regarded as safe (Rogers, 1959). If these are not available, masks may be made with two layers of a sterilizable close-meshed absorbent material, with an opening so that a piece of cellophane or thick paper can be placed between the two layers to render the mask impervious (Medical Research Council, 1948).

Both nose and mouth must be completely covered by the mask, and it is most important that any adjustment of position should be made *by means of the elastic or tapes only* if contamination of the fingers is to be avoided. If the mask is touched by mistake, at any time, the hands must be washed immediately. On leaving the nurseries, the mask is removed (by manipulation of the elastic or tapes only) and dropped into disinfectant. All non-disposable masks must be well sterilized before they are re-issued for use, and masks must be available in a sufficient quantity to allow a fresh one every time one is required.

(6) **Ventilation and cot spacing.** Ventilation should be adequate (10–12 changes per hour) and overcrowding of nurseries avoided (see p. 43).

(7) **Feeding and infection.** Breast fed infants are less likely to become infected than bottle fed babies so, when the baby is strong enough, the mother (if she has kept up her milk supply) should be admitted for breast feeding. Before receiving her infant, a mother must wash her hands with a suitable antiseptic, e.g. soap containing 3% hexachlorophane. For the smaller babies, unable to feed at the breast, scrupulous care must be taken in the preparation and administration of formulae and, if possible, human milk should be used (see p. 104).

The use of human milk eliminated *E. Coli* 0.111 from a premature nursery after failure to control an epidemic of diarrhoea by antibiotics or closure of the nursery (Svirsky-Gross, 1958).

Nursing Care

Clinical observations. The procedure followed on admission to the special baby care unit is described on p. 41. The nurse will continue to observe the following:

Respiration—rate, type, regularity.
Colour—pallor, cyanosis, jaundice.
Rectal temperature (and skin temperature if requested).
Heart rate (apex beat).
Activity and cry.
Umbilical cord—haemorrhage, signs of infection.
Feeding behaviour—amount taken, regurgitation.
Passage of urine—character of urine.
Passage of stools—character of stool.
Any abnormal signs, e.g. oedema, haemorrhage, etc.

She should observe and control the temperature and humidity inside the incubator (or temperature in the cot) so as to ensure a rectal temperature of 36–37°C (97–98·6°F) in the baby, and maintain the prescribed temperature and humidity in the nursery.

The nurse will record her observations at regular intervals and notify the doctor of any abnormalities or new developments.

General handling. The shorter the gestational age the less is the infant's vitality and the more carefully must it be handled. When regurgitation occurs in infants who are nursed naked in incubators, the regurgitated fluid runs out of the mouth because the head always rolls over on to one or other side. There is, however, a great danger of inhalation of regurgitated fluid when infants are clothed and their heads are thus prevented from rolling over to one side. A clothed infant in a cot must therefore always be placed on its side, and never flat on its back. In order to allow equal expansion of both lungs, it is a good rule to place the infant on its right side during and after a feed, and to turn it carefully over on to the left side midway between feeding times. With this exception, small feeble infants should be handled as little as possible because of the danger of precipitating a cyanotic attack. In incubators, the smallest infants tend to be on the side (foetal position) at first, but soon roll over on to their backs. If they are not moving freely, it is a good thing to turn them over into the prone position from time to time. The stomach empties more rapidly in this position and, according to Bruns *et al.* (1961), neither the ventilation nor the respiratory rate are affected in healthy low-weight babies, but may be improved in babies with periodic respiration (Kravitz *et al.*, 1958; Bruns *et al.*, 1961). Infants also bring up wind better in the prone position because the oesophagus enters the stomach posteriorly (Hughes-Davies, 1967). After any alteration in position, the baby must be watched carefully to make sure that no harm has been done by the handling.

For babies in incubators, all nursing care should be carried out inside the incubator. Babies in cots should not be removed from the cot for changing, feeding, cleaning or dressing until they are strong enough to allow of handling without regurgitation or change of colour, and careful handling is required when taking the infant out of the cot for weighing. Any necessary handling, such as weighing, should take place *before* and *not after* a feed if regurgitation is to be avoided.

When infants are nursed in cots, the position of the cot should be altered rather than the position of the baby in the cot: for example, during a feed, the head of the cot should be raised; and if the baby has a cyanotic attack due to inhalation, the head of the cot should be lowered to drain the inhaled material from the air passages. Incubators should be provided with a mechanism for tilting the platform on which the mattress is placed.

Maintenance of respiration. Respiratory distress is the commonest complication of low birth weight. Careful observation of the respiratory rate (hourly for the first 6 hours, then 2-hourly until the rate settles at about 40/minute) can lead to early diagnosis and treatment of respiratory distress. The respirations must be counted while the child is quiet and counted for a complete minute because of the tendency to irregular respiration. A rising respiration rate or the development of rib recession or grunting must be reported at once to the doctor.

The nurse must use suction when necessary to keep the air passages clear and she must administer oxygen if cyanosis develops in spite of a clear air way (see p. 134 for safe administration of oxygen). The doctor must be notified if cyanosis develops and also if there is an undue secretion of mucus.

Temperature control. In the pre-term infant all normal responses to heat (vasodilatation and sweating) and cold (vasoconstriction and increased heat production) are reduced, the responses decreasing as the gestational age decreases. Pre-term infants also have little brown fat (see p. 3). Light-for-dates babies have normal responses if born after 37 weeks gestation. All low-weight infants have large surface areas relative to their small body mass, little subcutaneous fat, and poor glycogen reserves so they rapidly lose body heat unless proper precautions are taken.

Ideally, low weight infants should be nursed in a thermoneutral environment, i.e. an environmental temperature in which a normal body temperature (rectal 36–37°C or 97–98·6°F; and skin 0·5°C or 1·0°F lower) is maintained with minimal metabolic effort (Adamsons, 1966; Scopes and Ahmed, 1966; Dawes, 1968).

In ordinary, or increased, oxygen levels the basal metabolism (and oxygen requirements) rise as the temperature of the environment, and body, falls (McCance, 1959; Pribylova and Znamenacek, 1964; Silverman, 1964; Adams *et al.*, 1964; Brück, 1968; Dawes, 1968; Hey and Katz, 1970). If much heat is lost, "cold injury" can occur (Mann and Elliott, 1957; see p. 219); and Calmari *et al.* (1959) found a sharp rise in morbidity and mortality when the body temperature was allowed to fall below 34°C (92·2°F).

Many investigators have reported better survival rates when the rectal temperature is kept above 36°C, or 97°F (Silverman *et al.*, 1958; Buetow and Klein, 1964; Day *et al.*, 1964). Glass *et al.* (1968) showed that the rate of increase in body weight was significantly faster if infants were nursed in a thermoneutral environment. In the author's experience, the incidences of idiopathic respiratory distress (Crosse, 1957, 1959a and 1959b) and jaundice (Crosse *et al.*, 1955; Crosse, 1959b) were increased in low-weight babies if the rectal temperature was low on admission to the special care unit.

It is now realized that the control of the body temperature of a low-weight baby is much more critical than was formerly believed. Brück (1961) and Brück *et al.* (1962) found the thermoneutral environment for pre-term babies was 32–34°C (89·6–93·2°F) but they did not distinguish between large and small infants. Mestyán *et al.* (1964) found the thermoneutral environment for babies weighing 1,500–2,000 g. was at least 34·5°C (94°F); and for those under 1,500 g. it was 36°C (96·8°F).

Scopes and Ahmed (1966) reported that the thermoneutral environment varied with the size, postnatal age and clinical condition of the infant; being highest for the smallest, youngest and sick infants. They also stated that babies who were light-for-dates needed a temperature appropriate for their weight rather than for their gestational age. These investigators also divided the low-weight babies into two groups but at a higher weight level, i.e. above and below 2,000 g.; and they gave thermoneutral ranges, not temperatures. From the results of these two investigations it would appear that the thermoneutral environmental temperature lies between 31–35°C (88–95°F), the higher temperature being necessary for the smallest and youngest infants.

Within the thermoneutral range, changes in the relative humidity do not affect heat loss (Hey and Maurice, 1968); while at a lower temperature, a high relative humidity can reduce heat loss (Silverman and Blanc, 1957).

When an infant is nursed naked in an incubator, it loses heat by radiation to the hood of the incubator; and the hood radiates heat to the ceiling, walls and windows of the room (especially the windows in cold weather). If the room is cold, the operative temperature in the incubator is less than the air temperature recorded by the incubator thermometer. The operative temperature in the incubator falls 1°C below the incubator air thermometer for every 7°C by which the incubator thermometer exceeds the room temperature (Hey and Mount, 1967). If the windows are double-glazed and the room temperature is high, this loss is reduced. Heat loss by radiation can also be reduced by using a double walled incubator (Bardell *et al.*, 1968); by placing a perspex radiation reflecting shield over the infant in the incubator in such a way that it does not interfere with the nursing (Levison *et al.*, 1966; Hey and Mount, 1967); or by swaddling the infant in a transparent material (Dawes, 1968). Another method of maintaining the body temperature is the use of low energy infra-red radiation (Agate and Silverman, 1963; Buetow and Klein, 1964; Day *et al.*, 1964).

Servo-controlled incubators have now been developed and these provide a more sensitive temperature regulation, the regulating system being controlled by a thermister probe taped on to the infant's anterior abdominal wall. The skin temperature is more reliable than the rectal temperature because the latter will only rise and fall when the infant's own thermostatic mechanism is failing, while the skin temperature gives a reading on which the incubator temperature may be adjusted before the infant is subjected to an unnecessary stress (Scopes, 1970). However, Segal (1966) has drawn attention to the possibility of a servo-control concealing a rise in temperature due to infection; and also to the undue delay in reheating an incubator which has been open for some time.

After the need for continuous observation is over, light clothing can be used to minimize the effect of fluctuations in the incubator temperature (Hey and O'Connell, 1970).

Overheating also increases the metabolic rate and oxygen requirements (Adamsons *et al.*, 1965). Direct sunlight should never be allowed to fall on an incubator, as this may cause over-heating.

If clothed low-weight babies are nursed in unheated cots, the temperature of the nursery should be over 25°C (77°F) for infants weighing less than 2,000 g. and up to 30°C (86°F) for really small infants (Hey and O'Connell, 1970) but the temperature inside the clothing is the important one. Scopes and Ahmed (1966) found the temperature of ambient air inside the clothing was frequently as high as 35°C (95°F) when the nursery temperature was 26°C (78·8°F).

Variations in the room temperature have to be fairly large before a clothed infant in a cot is affected (i.e. between 19°C and 31°C) while 1°C change in the incubator temperature can be important to a naked baby (Hey and O'Connell, 1970).

Jonxis (1967) has described an alternative to incubator care which allows good observation, good facilities for investigations and medical procedures, and is easier for nursing procedures. Babies are nursed naked in a room kept at 32°C (90°F) with a relative humidity of 60%. Loss of heat by radiation is avoided by means of electric heating in the ceiling, as well as central heating, and by the use of a small perspex "bell" over the infant if a higher environmental temperature is necessary. Oxygen is given by means of a small tent when required. This would seem to be an excellent method of treatment in the tropics because the infants could be covered with bells during the cooler hours of the night.

Unless it is necessary to monitor the skin temperature the temperature is usually taken in the rectum, and when there is a reasonable degree of stabilization it need only be taken twice daily. If however, the temperature is unstable it must be taken more frequently. If, at any time, a baby feels too hot or too cold to the hand, it is wise to take the temperature. Also, if a baby is found to have either a very high or very low temperature, it should be taken frequently during the appropriate treatment, in order to check the result of the treatment. The thermometer must be well inserted to obtain an accurate reading, the whole of the bulb being carefully inserted half an inch inside the anus. The thermometer should be inspected before each insertion to ensure that the bulb is intact.

Temperatures taken in the axilla or groin are approximately 0·5°C (1°F) lower than the rectal temperature. There are no contra-indications to taking rectal temperatures, indeed there are some advantages:

(1) The regular mechanical stimulation of the rectum prevents constipation (it cannot cause diarrhoea).

(2) The disturbance to the infant is less than the axillary method in a clothed infant because the temperature is taken when the napkin is changed.

Each infant should have its own thermometer and this can be kept in disinfectant in the infant's locker. A low-reading thermometer is necessary, to give readings down to 24°C (75°F).

Weighing. In order to avoid unnecessary handling of small infants, weighing should not be frequent, twice a week being sufficient in the case of healthy infants. The procedure should be carried out in such a way as to avoid undue handling, exposure and cross infection. The pan of the scales must be washable and should be washed at least once a day with hexachlorophane soap and water; and boiled or autoclaved if used for an infected baby. Before placing the baby on the scales the pan should be covered with a sheet of clean paper so as to avoid contamination of the scales, a fresh sheet of paper being used for each infant. If weights have to be handled, this should be done with disposable paper. The scales are most conveniently kept on a trolley so that they can be taken to the cot side. Each infant is weighed in one of its own blankets, the blanket being weighed after removal of the baby and this weight deducted.

In an incubator, the baby is placed in its individual sling and weighed by hanging the sling on the hook which passes through a hole in the top of the incubator to be attached to a special spring balance (see Fig. 23). An allowance must be made for the weight of the sling. The sling is kept in the infant's locker.

Changing and dressing. Clothing should be simple and easily adjustable, so that an infant can be undressed and re-dressed with as

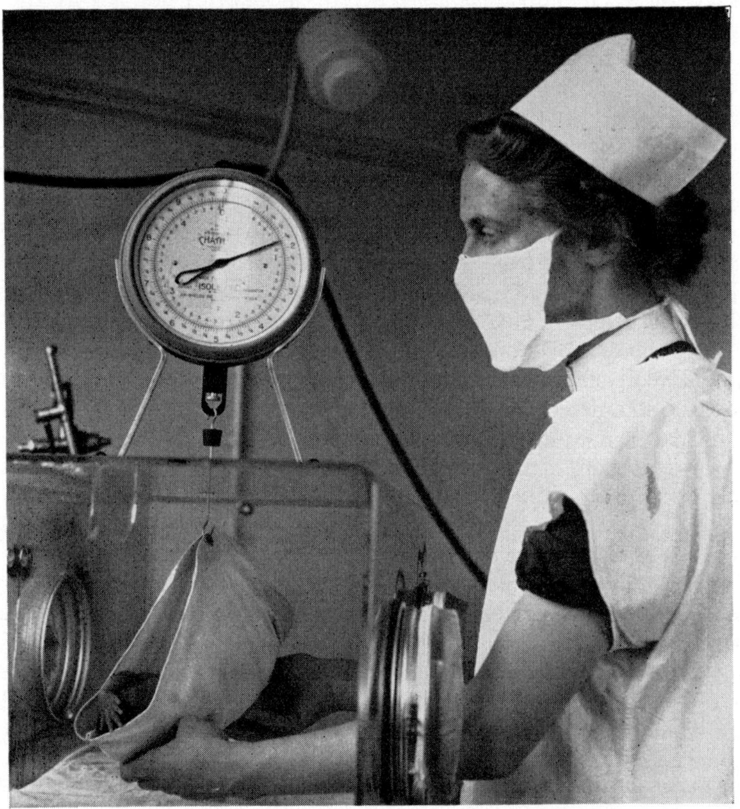

(*H.M.S.O.*)

FIG. 23. Weighing in an incubator. Each baby is weighed in its own individual washable sling. After weighing, the hole in the top of the incubator is closed with the rubber cork and the hook is drawn up.

little disturbance as possible. Suitable clothing is described in a later chapter.

Infants nursed in incubators require only a small napkin. Naked nursing has many advantages, e.g. less need to disturb the infant; absence of any restriction to breathing and other movements; and ease of observation of respiration, spontaneous movements and such signs as abdominal distension, oedema, jaundice and cyanosis.

Small feeble infants nursed in cots should be changed and dressed in their cots with the minimum of handling and exposure; the older and stronger infants can be lifted out on to the nurse's knee. This cot side treatment is less likely to spread infection than the use of communal changing tables. The nurse must put on the "cot gown" designated for each individual baby before she carries out any of these procedures.

All soiled napkins and clothing should be placed at once in covered receptacles and not placed on the floor or elsewhere; on no account must they be put into the hand-basin. A separate receptacle must be provided for soiled napkins.

The smaller infants should be changed *before* a feed (when they are less likely to regurgitate). Changing of napkins and cot linen is known to increase the bacterial count of the air, so all soiled napkins and linen must be removed from the nursery before feeding is commenced. Sufficient napkins and linen must be provided to allow for frequent changing. If possible napkins should be disposable.

Bed-linen and clothing should not be stored in the nursery, but in autoclaved packets in a special linen room. Sufficient must be provided to meet all emergencies. Clean linen dropped on the floor, by mistake, must not be used until it has been re-sterilized. Soiled linen must never be carried against a nurse's uniform as this will lead to contamination of the uniform. Sorting of soiled linen and sluicing of napkins should never be done by the nursing staff. The use of disposable napkins and sheets eliminates most of this work.

After handling a soiled napkin the nurse must not touch the baby's face, bib, or any part of the top of the bed until she has washed her hands.

Care of skin. It is important to avoid mechanical irritation of the skin, both in the pre-term and light-for-dates baby, because their skins are easily infected. Loss of heat and undue disturbance must also be avoided.

On the first day, after the baby has recovered from the ordeal of birth and if it is in a good condition, the blood and debris may be gently wiped away from the body with a warm solution of 3% hexachlorophane in a liquid detergent base (PhisoHex), or 1 in 500 cetrimide, on sterile swabs; the face is washed with sterile swabs wrung out in warm sterile water, then dried with sterile swabs; and a dusting powder containing 0·33% hexachlorophane in a pre-sterilized base (Sterzac) is applied liberally to the whole body. On succeeding days the skin folds (axillae, groins, neck and backs of ears) are similarly treated once daily, and the napkin area at each "change". Because of the risk of loss of heat by exposure, or regurgitation and inhalation following the handling, and of mechanical irritation of the skin, cleaning is reduced to this minimum. If the infant is too feeble to allow of even this amount of cleaning, it is left undisturbed. As the baby grows stronger it can be cleaned more thoroughly.

When a healthy infant reaches the weight of about 4½ lb. or 2,040 g., it should be possible to give a water bath every third day, in addition to the cleaning already described. The use of hexachlorophane soap (Cidal) or the addition of hexachlorophane (1 in 50,000) to the bath water, and a dusting powder containing hexachlorophane all help to reduce the incidence of skin infection. At first the baby should be bathed on the nurse's knee, being completely covered with a warm towel with the exception of the part being washed. Later, the infant can be put into the bath in the ordinary way. The temperature of the water for a "knee-bath" should be 40·5–43·5°C (105–110°F), but if the baby is to be put into the bath the temperature should not be above 40·5°C (105°F). For water baths individual bowls should be used because they can be sterilized before use. It is doubtful if a fixed bath can ever be satisfactorily sterilized and therefore boiled or autoclaved bowls provide a simple alternative. Ideally, a clean towel should be used for each bath. Failing this, each infant must have its own bath towel, this being kept in the infant's locker to avoid contamination with dust and the possibility of getting mixed with other infants' towels.

When bathing or cleaning, the nurse must wear the "cot gown" kept for the individual infant and she must remember to commence with the cleaning of the face and work downwards, dealing with the thighs and buttocks last of all.

Care of the eyes. The closed eyelids should be cleaned daily with sterile swabs wrung out in warm boiled water which has been poured into a disposable gallipot or small sterilized bowl. Separate swabs are used for each eye.

Care of the mouth. The mouth should be inspected at each feeding time (not just once daily at the bathing time), as it is most essential to recognize thrush in its earliest stages and to secure prompt treatment. A healthy mouth should never be cleaned, as the mucous membrane is very easily injured and infected.

Care of the nose. As the nasal mucous membrane is also easily injured and infected, the nostrils should be left untouched. The outer nares only may be cleaned, if necessary, with a swab wrung out in warm boiled water; on no account should twisted wool be inserted up the nostril. Obstructed nasal passages can be cleared by using bland nose drops to make the baby sneeze.

Care of the cord. Unless the umbilical cord is properly protected (by a sterile dressing, or by daily painting with bactericidal dyes or 1% chlorhexidine in spirit, or by using a powder containing hexachlorophane) it rapidly becomes a reservoir for staphylococci (see p. 168) and often also for haemolytic streptococci (Boissard and Eton, 1956; Kwantes and James, 1956; Fairchild *et al.*, 1958) and for *E. Coli*, *Pseudomonas*, *Klebsiella-Aerobacter* and *Proteus* (Light *et al.*, 1968). A useful method of cord care is to spray the umbilical stump, and an area of the abdominal wall for 1 in. round the base of the stump, with Octaflex Aerosol (Ward, Blenkinsop & Co. Ltd.) which forms a film containing 1% octaphen. Hexachlorophane powder (Sterzac) is then applied and this powder is re-applied each time the napkin is changed. In developing countries, where infection is likely, the treated stump can be covered with a sterile dry dressing and a *loose* binder to keep this in place. Care must be taken to protect the umbilical stump from contamination during cleaning or bathing. If a polyp is left when the cord separates, this may be treated with methylated spirits and, if necessary, with a silver nitrate or copper sulphate stick.

Methods of Isolation

If several infants are being cared for in the same nursery, adequate facilities must be available for isolation. The Sister-in-charge should have authority to move a sick baby out of a nursery on her own responsibility if medical advice cannot be obtained at once. If spread of infection is to be avoided, it is extremely important to isolate a sick baby at the earliest possible moment, and all nurses working in the unit should be instructed to report the slightest sign of abnormality.

Conditions requiring isolation include infection of the respiratory and gastro-intestinal tracts, and of the skin, mouth or eyes, as well as generalized infections. It is normally possible to isolate most of the infections in the isolation nurseries attached to the special care unit, so that the babies can still be looked after by nurses trained in the care of low-weight babies; but proved cases of diarrhoea due to *E. Coli* must be completely removed from the unit, and the affected nursery closed to all new admissions until all contacts have been discharged. Facilities should be available for separating the various forms of illness so as to prevent cross-infection. It is therefore useful to have several small isolation nurseries. If only one room is available the cots or incubators must be well spaced. Isolation nurseries should be planned with a separate utility room and they should be isolated from the other nurseries.

Each infant in the isolation nurseries should be provided with

When it reaches the weight of 2,000 g. (4 lb. 6 oz.) the baby can usually be transferred to a cool nursery. It is then lifted out of the cot for all nursing procedures such as changing, bathing and dressing, and it is carried to its mother for feeding as soon as this becomes possible. For some time care will be required to prevent undue cooling when the baby is removed from the cot, and all nursing procedures should be carried out in a warm room, screened from draughts, and with as little exposure as possible.

As infection is the greatest cause of death after the first 4 weeks of life, there should be no relaxation in the aseptic technique, and every care should be taken to avoid exposure of the child to infection of any sort.

Infants are not normally discharged until they reach a weight of 5–5½ lb. (2,270–2,500 g.) and are making good progress. However, some healthy babies may be discharged at 4–4½ lb. (1,800–2,040 g.) for breast feeding if the home is good and the domiciliary special care baby service can take over the case.

Before discharge, the eyes should have been examined to exclude retrolental fibroplasia and other abnormalities of the eye, a screening test for phenylketonuria should have been performed and the haemoglobin level estimated. On the day of discharge the infant should have a full medical examination. The weight, body length and head circumference should be recorded.

Home inspection. This is usually done by the health visitor (public health nurse) of the area, and an infant should not be sent home until a good report has been received, both as regards the preparations made for the reception of the child and the health of the other members of the family. If the home conditions are unsuitable for any reason, arrangements will have to be made to transfer the baby to another institution until it is strong enough to cope with the difficult home conditions. The risks of infection in an institution should, however, be carefully weighed against the risks of the home conditions, and every effort should be made to improve the home so that the infant can return there as soon as possible. The baby can be breast fed more easily at home; it will receive more individual attention and, most important of all, the mother's interest in the baby will be kept up.

Education of the mother. The education of the mother in the care of her infant is of extreme importance, and in every hospital that deals with low-weight infants adequate arrangements should be made for this essential part of the work. Whenever possible, the mother should be admitted for several days before the baby is discharged so that she can take over complete charge of her infant under supervision: small rooms (each for one mother and her baby) should be provided for this purpose. For mothers unable or unwilling to be admitted, a room is set aside as a demonstration room, and here the mothers are taught how to feed their infants and manage them generally (Fig. 25), including the avoidance of infection and the reporting of early signs of infection, or other abnormalities, to their doctor. The teaching consists of practical demonstrations and personal discussion, as well as printed instructions.

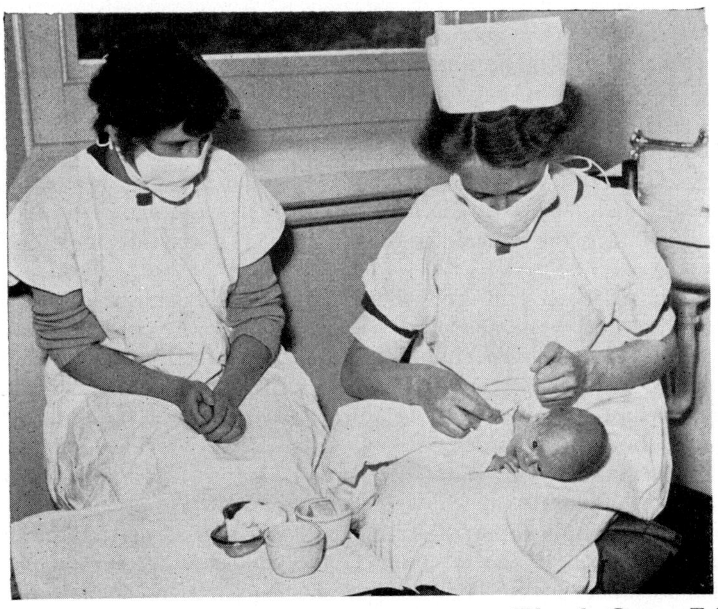

(*Photo by Camera Talks*)

FIG. 25. Education of mother. A mother is shown how to bath her infant. Before she takes him home she will bath him herself under supervision.

Arrangements for follow-up care. The mother is advised to take the baby at regular intervals to her own doctor or to the Maternity and Child Welfare Centre. At these visits the baby is weighed and examined and the mother advised. Special attention is given to the maintenance of breast feeding and the prevention of rickets and anaemia. Advice is also given as regards vaccination against smallpox and immunization against diphtheria, measles, whooping cough, poliomyelitis and tetanus.

Babies who weighed less than 1,500 g. at birth and those who had complications during birth or the neonatal period (birth trauma or asphyxia, neonatal anoxia from any cause, hyperbilirubinaemia, hypoglycaemia, etc.) should be given an appointment to return to the hospital follow-up clinic where they can receive a general medical examination and an assessment of mental and physical development. This is in order to ensure early diagnosis and treatment of any abnormality.

Arrangements must be made for the ophthalmic examination, at the age of 3 months, of all babies weighing less than 2,000 g. at birth and who required oxygen during the first 2 weeks of life.

A full medical report is sent to the family doctor and to the Medical Officer of Health; the latter for the use of the health visitor (public health nurse) so that she can visit the home, advise the mother, and make sure that the baby is taken regularly to the doctor, the Welfare Clinic or the hospital clinic.

Personnel

Nursing staff. The appointment of a good nursing staff is the first step towards obtaining good results in a special baby care unit.

The nursing is very specialized and the quality of the nursing staff is as important as the quantity. Great attention to detail is necessary and results depend largely on the reliability, enthusiasm and diligence of the nursing staff. In addition to the careful management of incubators, such details as the regular filling of hot-water bottles, the regulation of the nursery temperature and humidity, the watching of the cot thermometers, and the regular turning of clothed infants from side to side, play a very important part in maintaining a high survival rate. Conscientious barrier nursing, correct wearing of gowns and masks (when necessary), a careful aseptic technique, and the reporting of colds or other infectious conditions reduce the incidence of infection; while careful control of oxygen concentrations eliminates the risk of blindness due to retrolental fibroplasia (see p. 206).

Nurses dealing with low-weight babies must be prepared to take responsibility and deal with emergencies, such as cyanotic attacks. They must be prepared to modify feeding instructions if the baby's condition warrants this and the doctor is not immediately available. They must be able to recognize early signs of illness in the baby and have authority to isolate such babies until medical advice can be obtained. They must also know the indications for catheter feeding, and the administration of oxygen; they must be experts in the regulation of the infant's body temperature and in suitable methods of resuscitation. They must recognize (and report) early or deepening jaundice, tremors which may indicate hypoglycaemia and all the various deviations from normal which may occur.

Nurses working in intensive care nurseries must understand and be able to use monitoring equipment; they must know how to care for a baby with an indwelling umbilical catheter, and for a baby with endotracheal intubation (suction, assessment of position of tube, irrigation of tube and even replacement of tube if necessary). They must be able to manage a mechanical respirator and other complicated apparatus.

A healthy permanent staff reduces the risk of infection among the babies: nurses should never be borrowed from departments which deal with potentially infected patients.

Considering all these things, it is obvious that a constantly changing staff is a great disadvantage. A certain amount of change is unavoidable if the unit is being used for training in special baby care nursing. The only way to get over this difficulty is to ensure a sufficient number of permanent trained staff (trained in special baby care nursing) to supervise those in training. Ideally the ratio of specially trained nurses to nurses in training should be one to one in a special care unit, and higher in an intensive care nursery.

The number of nursing staff to be provided is also of great importance, for however reliable the nurses may be they cannot give the necessary attention to detail if they are too few in number. The correct proportion of staff to babies depends on the type of baby admitted and the number of hours per week worked by the nursing staff. As nurses in England will soon only work 40 hours per week, approximately 4½ nurses will be required to keep 1 nurse on duty throughout the week (these figures should allow for annual leave but will not allow for sick leave, or for study periods for those in training).

In a *special care unit*, each baby requires at least 5 hours of nursing time daily (Dunham, 1955), therefore the ratio of nurses to cots should be one to one, i.e. 30 nurses for a special care unit with 30 cots.

In an *intensive care nursery* the nursing time required for each baby will be greatly increased, and the ratio of nurses to cots must be much higher, i.e. 2 or 3 nurses per cot.

A nursing officer (Salmon No. 7) should be in charge of the unit and she must be supported by a sufficient number of specially trained staff, i.e. half the total nursing staff in a special care unit, and a much higher proportion in an intensive care nursery. Specially trained staff may include State Certified Midwives, Registered Sick Children's Nurses, State Registered Nurses, State Enrolled Nurses and trained Nursery Nurses (NNEB), who have taken a course in special baby care nursing.

Nursing auxiliaries, who have received an in-service training, can be employed in such duties as the feeding and changing of the older and larger babies, and the cleaning of equipment. This releases the specially trained staff for the nursing of the smaller and younger infants, and for the supervision of nurses in training.

Medical staff. All members of the medical staff must set a good

example in aseptic technique and should pay special attention to such points as the sterilization of the chest-piece of the stethoscope between cases (unless the chest piece is disposable, or an individual stethoscope is provided for each baby), the sterilization of the tape measure (if not disposable) which is used to measure the body length, the washing of hands and forearms on entering a nursery and after touching a baby, and the correct use of gowns and masks. It is important to recognize early signs of illness in the infant and to encourage early isolation in infective cases. A full knowledge of the nursing difficulties is essential in order to be able to guide the nursing staff. Above all, the paediatrician in charge should be really interested in the work and able to convey his or her enthusiasm to the medical and nursing staff.

The consultant paediatrician in charge of the special baby care unit should visit the unit at regular intervals, conducting nursery rounds and discussing current problems, and be available at other times for consultation. This paediatrician should be responsible for the plan of care (which should be available in writing, for the use of both medical and nursing staff), for the preparation of annual statistics, and for the follow-up of "at risk" infants discharged from the unit. At least one other consultant paediatrician should be available to cover the periods when the paediatrician-in-charge is off duty. The consultants should be supported by at least two registrars or senior house officers, one of whom must be on call, day and night (resident in the hospital during their periods on duty). These doctors must visit the unit daily, examine each infant on admission and before discharge, and answer emergency calls to babies in the labour ward and maternity wards as well as in the special care unit.

Ideally, the paediatrician in charge of a unit with an intensive care nursery should be a specialist in the care of the newborn (a neonatologist). He, or she, should be responsible for the training of medical personnel in special care for the newborn (including intensive care), and for the organization of research projects.

In units with an intensive care nursery, consultant anaesthetists should be available to advise on respiratory difficulties; and there must be a full supporting pathological, biochemical and radiological medical service.

There should be full co-operation between the various members of the medical staff, and it is useful to have regular staff conferences at which paediatricians, obstetricians, anaesthetists (when applicable) and nurses discuss the cause of each death with the pathologist.

Care of Low-weight Babies in various Types of Maternity Accommodation

Small maternity hospitals or departments (including private nursing homes). These are expected to disappear in the future (see p. 35). No mother expecting a very small baby should be delivered in a small maternity department. An observation nursery with some draught proof cots should be available for babies weighing 2,040–2,500 g. (4½–5½ lb.) and one heated cot should be provided for the use of an unexpected smaller baby until transfer can be arranged. A heated cot is better than an incubator, which could be dangerous in the hands of unskilled personnel. Whenever possible, at least one nurse with experience in the care of low-weight babies should be on the staff. Booked cases going into labour before 36 completed weeks of gestation and mothers with growth retarded babies should be transferred to a specialist centre for delivery whenever this is possible.

Medium sized maternity hospitals or departments. (These will all be part of general hospitals in the future; see p. 35.) At present, these include hospitals or departments catering for abnormal obstetrics and producing more than 100 low-weight babies per year; but not having accommodation for unbooked prenatal cases, unbooked mothers in premature labour or low-weight babies born at home or in smaller hospitals. These should be able to deal with the majority of their own low-weight babies if suitable accommodation, sufficient specially trained nursing and resident medical staff and consultant paediatricians are available. At least one room should be set aside for low-weight babies. The maximum number of cots (or cots and incubators) in one room should be six and if more are required, two rooms must be provided. A floor space of 50 sq. ft. (4½ sq. m.) must be allowed for each cot or incubator. Babies requiring intensive care must be transferred.

Large maternity hospitals and departments. (These will all be in district general hospitals or university centres in the future, see p. 35.) These hospitals should provide special care units (with intensive care nurseries) to accommodate:

(1) The babies weighing less than 2,040 g. (4½ lb.) born in their own hospital.

(2) Babies weighing less than 2,040 g. born in smaller hospitals without a special unit.

(3) Babies weighing less than 2,040 g. born in their own homes.

(4) Non-infected sick newborn infants over 2,040 g. born in their own hospital or elsewhere (e.g. babies suffering from birth injury, asphyxia, haemolytic disease or jaundice and infants of diabetic mothers, etc.).

These hospitals must provide intensive perinatal care, i.e. intensive obstetric care in addition to intensive neonatal care.

Accommodation required in a Special Baby Care Unit

The unit should be self contained, provide accommodation for 20–30 infants, and be situated near the labour rooms. If possible, all external walls should be cavity walls and all outside windows should be double-glazed. All doors should open in both directions (push-doors) and close automatically. The upper portion of all the internal walls of the nurseries should be made of glass, or other transparent material, to allow easy inspection of the babies and good lighting in all parts of the unit.

The following accommodation is required whether the unit provides an intensive care nursery or not. If intensive care is included, extra incubator nurseries are required.

(1) **Entrance lobby.** Doctors and technicians should be able to change their coats in the lobby. Facilities should be available for all staff to wash before entering any nursery.

(2) **Accommodation for babies.**

(a) *Admission nursery.* (29·5–31°C or 85–88°F, with a relative humidity of 60–65%.) All babies should be examined in the admission room before a decision is made as to which nursery they will be admitted. Facilities should be available for all first aid treatment (oxygen, suction, etc.) and for monitoring vital signs. Over-table heating should be provided (see Fig. 12 for a neonatal care unit).

(b) *Incubator nurseries.* (29·5–31°C or 85–88°F, not humidified.) The maximum number of incubators in one nursery is 12 (if correctly used with outside air or bacterial filters); and 30 sq. ft. (2¾ sq. m.) should be allowed for each incubator.

(c) *Warm humidified nurseries.* (24–26°C or 75–80°F with a relative humidity of 60–65%) for infants nursed in open cots. The number of cots in one nursery should be limited to 6 and 50 sq. ft. (4½ sq. m.) allowed for each cot.

(d) *Cool nurseries.* (15·5–18·5°C or 60–65°F not humidified.) For acclimatizing low-weight babies to natural conditions before discharge; and for treating non-infected sick mature babies.

Note. It is useful if all the warm and cool nurseries can be interchangeable, i.e. any one usable either as a warm or a cool nursery according to the need at any time.

(e) *Suspect and isolation nurseries.* These should be planned in conjunction with a utility room and be separated from the rest of the unit. These nurseries should be capable of being heated and humidified as required; and 50 sq. ft. (4½ sq. m.) must be allowed for each cot or incubator; one isolation cot is usually required for every five cots or incubators in the unit, and the maximum number of cots in each isolation nursery should be two.

(f) *Treatment and transfusion nursery.* This should be capable of being heated to any required temperature; and facilities must be available for all forms of treatment.

In all these nurseries, the following facilities are required:

Full visibility of babies.
Adequate ventilation and heating.
Temperature and humidity control.
Hand-washing facilities, with elbow or foot controlled taps.
Piped oxygen and compressed air (Fig. 26).
Electric points for incubators, suction, extra heating, respirators, humidifiers, monitoring equipment, etc.
Cupboards for the day's supply of linen (opening into the corridor and into the nursery).
Emergency communication system.

In the incubator nurseries there might also be a system to monitor the infants' temperatures, connected to a control panel outside the nursery.

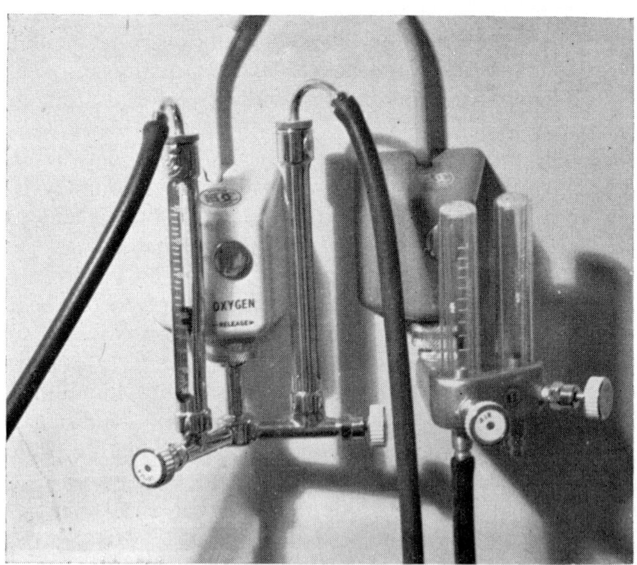

(*Photo by Camera Talks*)

FIG. 26. The piped supply of oxygen and air (each capable of supplying two incubators). The special oxygen flowmeter can indicate as small a flow as one tenth of a litre per minute.

(3) **Accommodation for mothers.**

(a) *Single rooms for mothers.* These should be at least 120 sq. ft. (11 sq. m.) to allow the infant to be with its mother when it is fit for a cool nursery. In units where low-weight babies are only admitted if they are less than 5 lb. (2,270 g.) at birth, the mother is usually admitted for a few days before the infant is discharged, and one room is required for every 10 cots used for infants admitted under 5 lb. If, however, the baby is over 5 lb. on admission, the mother should be admitted with her baby; and an appropriate number of rooms provided.

Each room for a mother and baby requires:

Adequate ventilation and lighting.
Temperature control.
Handwashing facilities.
Electric points.

(b) *Day room for mothers.*
(c) *Sanitary facilities for mothers.*
(d) *Demonstration room.* Mothers living at home can breast feed their infants in this room and have demonstrations on the care of their infants before taking them home.
This room can also be used for teaching nurses, and should be separated from the main nurseries.

(4) **Ancillary rooms.**

(a) *Clean utility room.* If supplies are available from a central sterilizing department, this room is used for storage of sterile supplies and setting trolleys for cotside care, etc. A basin with elbow taps, a work top and storage facilities are required.
(b) *Dirty utility room.* For storage of material awaiting disposal, and for rinsing of bowls, instruments, etc., before return to the central sterilizing department. A sink is required, and provision for disposal bins, laundry bags, etc.
(c) *Linen room or cupboards.*
(d) *Storage room for equipment.*
(e) *Ward kitchen or pantry.* For preparation of beverages and light meals only.
(f) *Milk kitchen or milk pantry.* If there is a central milk kitchen (see p. 120) only a small milk pantry will be required for storage and warming of prepared feeds.
(g) *Laboratory.* For estimating blood gases, etc.

(5) **Staff accommodation.**

(a) *Changing room for nurses.* This must open off the lobby near the entrance to the unit. Facilities for hand washing must be available.

(b) *Duty room for nursing staff.* This should be in a position from which all the main nurseries can be seen.

(c) *Doctor's office.* This room can also be used for tutorials for medical staff and students.

(d) *Cleaner's room.*

(e) *Sanitary facilities for staff.*

(6) **Accommodation for follow-up clinic.** This clinic need not be held in the same buildings as the special care unit. If it is held in the hospital out-patient department, arrangements must be made to separate the follow-up babies from other out-patients.

Intensive Care Nursery

The only additional accommodation required is one, or more, extra incubator nurseries. The important extra requirements are: an increased expert nursing and medical staff; additional equipment, e.g. monitors for vital signs, mechanical ventilators, etc.; and increased laboratory and radiological services.

REFERENCES

ADAMS, F. H., FUJIWARA, T., SPEARS, R. and HODGMAN, J. (1964). *Pediatrics*, **33**, 75.

ADAMSONS, K. Jr. (1966). *Pediat. Clin. N. Amer.*, **13**, 599.

ADAMSONS, K. Jr., GANDY, G. M. and JAMES, L. S. (1965). *J. Pediat.*, **66**, 495.

AGATE, F. J. and SILVERMAN, W. A. (1963). *Pediatrics*, **31**, 725.

AYLIFFE, G. A. J., COLLINS, B. J. and LOWBURY, E. J. L. (1966). *Brit. med. J.*, **3**, 442.

BARDELL, E., FREEMAN, J. and HEY, E. N. (1968). *Arch. Dis. Childh.*, **43**, 172.

BARRIE, D. (1965). *Arch. Dis. Childh.*, **40**, 555.

BAUM, J. D. and SCOPES, J. W. (1968). *Lancet*, **1**, 672.

BOISSARD, J. M. and ETON, B. (1956). *Brit. med. J.*, **2**, 574.

BRÜCK, K. (1961). *Biol. Neonat. (Basel).*, **3**, 65.

BRÜCK, K. (1968). *Pediatrics*, **41**, 1027.

BRÜCK, K., PARMALEE, A. H. and BRÜCK, M. (1962). *Biol. Neonat.*, **4**, 32.

BRUNS, W. T., LOREN, K. O. and SIEBENS, A. A. (1961). *Pediatrics*, **28**, 388.

BUETOW, K. C. and KLEIN, S. W. (1964). *Pediatrics*, **34**, 163.

CALAMARI, A., PIERACCINI, P. and BORGOGNI-BECHERELLI, E. (1959). *Riv. Clin. Pediat. Firenze*, **63**, 59.

CROSSE, V. M. (1957). *Ann. Paediatr. Fenn.*, **3**, 153.

CROSSE, V. M. (1959a). *Pediatria Internazionale*, **9**, 115.

CROSSE, V. M. (1959b). Report of IX International Congress of Paediatrics, Montreal.

CROSSE, V. M., MEYER, T. C. and GERRARD, J. W. (1955). *Arch. Dis. Childh.*, **30**, 501.

DAWES, G. S. (1968). "Foetal and Neonatal Physiology". Year Book Publications, Chicago.

DAY, R. L., CALIGUIRE, L., KAMENSKI, C. and EHRLICH, F. (1964). *Pediatrics*, **34**, 171.

DUNHAM, E. C. (1955). "Premature Infants", 2nd ed. Hoeber-Harper, New York.

FAIRCHILD, J. P., GRABER, C. D., VOGEL, E. H. Jr. and INGERSOLL, R. L. (1958). *J. Pediat.*, **53**, 538.

FORFAR, J. O. and MACCABE, A. F. (1958). *Brit. med. J.*, **1**, 76.

GLASS, L., SILVERMAN, W. A. and SINCLAIR, J. C. (1968). *Pediatrics*, **41**, 1033.

HEY, E. N. and KATZ, G. (1970). *Arch. Dis. Childh.*, **45**, 328.

HEY, E. N. and MAURICE, N. P. (1968). *Arch. Dis. Childh.*, **43**, 166.

HEY, E. N. and MOUNT, L. E. (1967). *Arch. Dis. Childh.*, **42**, 75.

HEY, E. N. and O'CONNELL, B. (1970). *Arch. Dis. Childh.*, **45**, 335.

HUGHES-DAVIES, T. H. (1967). *Brit. med. J.*, **4**, 172.

JONXIS, J. H. P. (1967). *Acta. Paediat. Scand. Suppl.* 172.

KRAVITZ, H., ELEGANT, L., BLOCK, B., BABAKITIS, M. and LUNDEEN, E. (1958). *Pediatrics*, **22**, 432.

KRESKY, B. (1964). *Amer. J. Dis. Child*, **107**, 363.

KRUGMAN, S. and WARD, R. (1951). *J. Amer. med. Assoc.*, **145**, 755.

KWANTES, W. and JAMES, J. R. E. (1956). *Brit. med. J.*, **2**, 576.

LEVISON, H., LINSAO, L. and SWYER, P. R. (1966). *Lancet*, **2**, 1346.

LIGHT, I. J., SUTHERLAND, J. M., COCHRAN, M. L. and SUTORIUS, J. (1968). *New. Engl. J. Med.*, **278**, 1243.

LOWBURY, E. J. L., LILLY, H. A. and BULL, J. P. (1964). *Brit. med. J.*, **2**, 531.

MANN, T. P. and ELLIOTT, R. I. K. (1957). *Lancet*, **1**, 229.

MCCANCE, R. A. (1959). 31st Ross Conference on Pediatric Research.

MEDICAL RESEARCH COUNCIL. (1941). War Memorandum No. 6, London.

MEDICAL RESEARCH COUNCIL. Special Reports Series No. 262 (1948). "Studies in Air Hygiene", p. 224.

MESTYÁN, J., FEKETE, M., BATA, G. and JÁRAI, I. (1964). *Biol. Neonat. (Basel)*, **7**, 11.

MUSHIN, W. W. and HILLARD, E. K. (1967). *Brit. med. J.*, **1**, 416.

PRIBYLOVA, H. and ZNAMENACEK, K. (1964). *Biol. Neonat. (Basel)*, **6**, 324.

ROGERS, K. B. (1959). Personal communication.

ROUNTREE, P. M., LOEWENTHAL, J., TEDDER, E. and GYE, R. (1962). *Med. J. Aust.*, **2**, 376.

RUBBO, S. D. (1963). "Infections in Hospitals", p. 231. Blackwell Scientific Publications, Oxford.

SCOPES, J. W. (1970). *Brit. J. hosp. Med.*, **3**, 579.

SCOPES, J. W. and AHMED, I. (1966). *Arch. Dis. Childh.*, **41**, 407.

SEGAL, S. (1966). *Pediat. Clin. N. Amer.*, **13**, 1149.

SILVERMAN, W. A. (1964). *Pediatrics*, **33**, 276.

SILVERMAN, W. A. and BLANC, W. A. (1957). *Pediatrics*, **20**, 477.

SILVERMAN, W. A., FERTIG, J. W. and BERGER, A. P. (1958). *Pediatrics*, **22**, 876.

STAHLMAN, M. T. (1969). "Problems of Neonatal Intensive Care Units". Report of 59th Ross Conference on Pediatric Research.

STORRS, C. N. and TAYLOR, M. R. H. (1970). *Brit. med. J.*, **3**, 328.

SVIRSKY-GROSS, S. (1958). *Ann. Paediat. Basel*, **190**, 109.

USHER, R. H. (1970). *Pediat. Clin. N. Amer.*, **17**, 199.

WOLINSKY, E., LIPSITZ, P. J., MORTIMER, E. A. and RAMMELKAMP, C. H. (1960). *Lancet*, **2**, 620.

CHAPTER 4

DOMICILIARY NEONATAL CARE

Need and Advantages

THE expert group on prematurity (W H O, 1950) recommended that any care programme for babies weighing 2,500 g. and less should be related to the pattern of maternity care in the country or area concerned, depending on the proportion of births occurring in hospitals and at home.

During 1968, 54,180 babies weighing 2,500 g. and less were born alive in England and Wales (Annual Report of Department of Health and Social Security for 1968). Of these, 7·4% were born, and nursed, in their own homes so it is still necessary to provide a domiciliary care service for the larger low-weight infants born at home. The excellent results that can be obtained with a good home care service for carefully selected low-weight babies were well demonstrated in Newcastle-on-Tyne by Miller as early as 1948.

The advantages of home care are obvious, i.e. the normal mother-baby relationship, the easy education of the family in the care of their own baby, and the higher incidence of breast feeding which becomes possible. In addition, unless a continuous day and night service is required, home care is much cheaper to provide than hospital care.

Results

The results of home care depend largely on the skill of the nurse. Specialized home care has been provided in Birmingham since 1933. At first midwives were given a short extra training in the care of the low-weight baby, but in 1950 the Newcastle plan was adopted in Birmingham and eight specially trained midwives are now employed full-time in the home care of low-weight babies. These special nurses take over the care of the mother and baby as soon as possible after birth and work in close contact with the family doctor. They also take over the care of low-weight babies after discharge from special care units until they feel that the mother can deal with the situation. During 1969, 1,063 low-weight infants were cared for by the eight special midwives; 70 after home delivery and 993 after discharge from hospital (Report on the Health of Birmingham in 1969).

It is difficult to obtain comparable mortality rates for home and hospital deliveries. Low-weight babies born at home tend to have a lower mortality rate than those of comparable birth weights born in hospital (wherever they are cared for) because abnormalities of pregnancy and labour, and congenital malformations of the infant increase the mortality rate and low-weight babies associated with such complications are more likely to be born in hospitals. In the British Perinatal Mortality Survey (Butler and Bonham, 1963) it was found that the mortality rate for low-weight babies born to women booked and delivered in hospital did not differ significantly from the Survey average for such babies, in spite of the high-risk selection for hospital delivery.

To obtain the best results with low-weight babies, mothers with complications of pregnancy and labour should not be delivered at home, neither should mothers going into labour before 36 completed weeks gestation. If a baby weighing less than 2,040 g. (4 lb. 8 oz.) is born at home, it should be transferred at once to a special baby care unit. Any baby weighing between 2,040 and 2,500 g. need only be transferred if suffering from some complication such as cyanotic attacks, respiratory distress, feeding difficulties, cerebral irritation, early jaundice, haemolytic disease, inability to maintain body temperature, etc.; or if facilities for home care are inadequate.

During 1968, 24·4% of the low-weight babies born at home in England and Wales had to be transferred to special care units, showing that the selection for home delivery was not as good as it should have been.

Facilities Required

Facilities necessary for home care are:

(1) A suitable room.
(2) Suitable equipment.
(3) An intelligent mother or attendant.
(4) Attendance by a specially trained nurse or midwife.
(5) Medical supervision by the family doctor.
(6) The services of a home help if required.

Domiciliary care must be supported by:

(1) Facilities for admission to a special care unit for:
 (a) Sick infants.
 (b) Infants with a birth weight below 2,040 g. (4 lb. 8 oz.).
 (c) Infants with poor home conditions.
(2) Transport for moving infants to hospital if this is required.
(3) Facilities for advice from a consultant paediatrician.
(4) A supply of human milk from a human milk bank, or other source, if necessary.

The principles of home care for low-weight babies are the same as hospital care in regard to nursing care, for feeding, prevention of infection and early recognition and treatment of complications. It is generally assumed that the risk of infection is less in domiciliary care, but this is not true. The baby cared for at home is less exposed to cross-infection but more exposed to the risk of respiratory infections, probably acquired from relations and visitors (Crosse and Mackintosh, 1953), and this danger must be realized and guarded against. Williams (1961) found that staphylococcal infections were just as numerous among babies born at home as among babies born in hospital.

The Room

A separate room should be provided for the baby whenever possible, but if only one room is available for both mother and child the mother cannot be permitted to receive visitors until she is able to get up and meet them in another room. An even room temperature must be maintained (night as well as day): clothed infants over 2,040 g. require a room temperature of 24°C (75°F) at first, even when in a heated cot. The room can be heated by any type of fire, but it is difficult to maintain an even temperature with a coal fire. In cold weather, it is advisable to increase the relative humidity of the heated air by placing a kettle or pan of water on the fire or on a gas or electric ring if the baby is under 5 lb. (2,270 g.) as a higher relative humidity reduces heat loss when the infant is not in a thermoneutral environment, and in cold weather the air can get very dry when heated.

Constant draughtless ventilation is most easily ensured by fitting a board under the lower frame of a sash window. This allows the upper and lower frames to overlap and creates an upward current of air.

A screen should be placed round the cot to protect it from draughts when the door is opened, and the cot should not be in a direct line between the door and window.

All unnecessary furniture should have been removed and dusty carpets taken up. Dry dusting and sweeping should not be allowed. Damp dusters should be used, floors washed, and carpets vacuum-cleaned, or sprinkled with damp sawdust or tea leaves before being swept.

Equipment

In the British Isles, the local health authority is responsible for the domiciliary care of low-weight babies (Ministry of Health Circular 20/44), and this authority should supply any necessary equipment which is not provided by the family. Such equipment includes:

(1) Folding draught-proof cot with pockets for hot-water bottles, mattress, blankets and rubber or polythene sheeting (Fig. 27).
(2) Hot water bottles and covers.
(3) Cot screen.
(4) Suitable clothing for the infant.

(5) Basket or table for infant's personal equipment.
(6) Portable bath or bathing bowl.
(7) Emergency tray with disposable mucus catheters and suitable stimulants.
(8) Low reading rectal thermometer.
(9) Two thermometers (one for cot and one for wall).
(10) Receptacles for soiled napkins and for other soiled linen.
(11) Equipment for the preparation and administration of feeds.
(12) Gowns for attendants.
(13) Facilities for hand washing (paper towels if possible).
(14) Suitable temperature, weight and feeding charts.
(15) Other items, such as vitamin preparations, and dried milks (if human milk is not available).

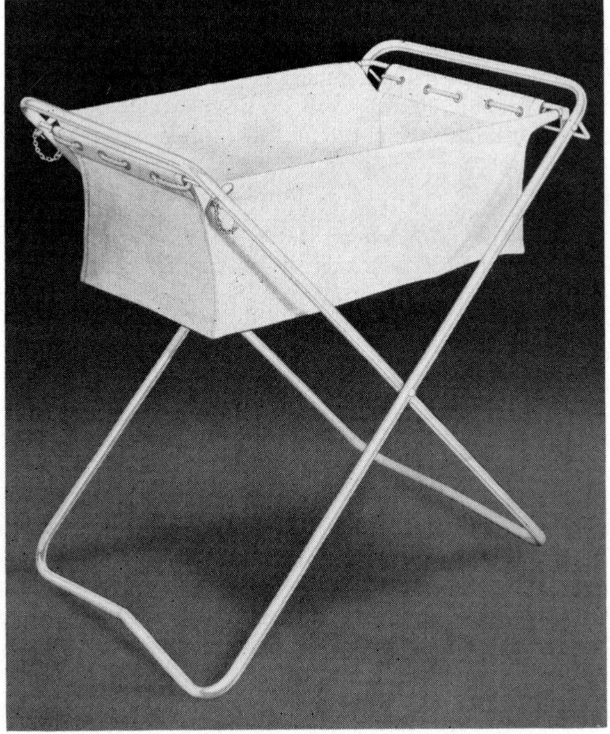

(Photograph by courtesy of Hoskins and Sewell Ltd.)

FIG. 27. *Folding Cot.* The canvas sling can be provided with a pocket on each side for hot water bottles. A towel rail is fitted to one end.

The visiting nurse carries resuscitation equipment and weighing scales.

The cot. If a suitable cot is not available, one can be improvised by using a washing basket, wooden box, portable bath, or even a drawer from a chest of drawers. This should be provided with a washable lining, which must be changed when soiled. The lining should have pockets for hot-water bottles, one on either side and one at the foot of the cot. Such a cot can be tipped up at either end as required by placing books or other similar objects under the end to be raised. The cot should have a firm mattress, so that the infant cannot smother itself if it rolls over on to its face. A pillow should *never* be used. A large rubber or polythene sheet should be provided to keep the mattress dry; all blankets must be light in weight and washable. Hot-water bottles should be sufficient to heat the cot. The bottles should be placed in bags which completely cover the stopper: bottles should not be filled with boiling water and at least two layers of blanket should be between the bottle and the baby. An electric pad should never be used in the home (see p. 51 for dangers). A thermometer must be provided for all heated cots, the ordinary wall type making a good cot thermometer.

Clothing. Suitable clothing will be discussed in the next chapter. Mothers must be warned not to use tight binders, as these can lead to death (Emery, 1967).

Attendants

If every midwife who delivers a low-weight baby is to look after that baby, *all* midwives will have to be trained in the care of such babies. In practice this is extravagant but may have to be done in rural areas. The most practical method in urban areas is to have a team of specially interested and specially trained domiciliary midwives working in association with their colleagues, to take over the care of low-weight infants born at home (this includes care of the mother). These midwives should continue to visit until the infant reaches a weight of 6 lb. (2,720 g.).

The chief function of these domiciliary nurses is to educate the family and help them to care for their own infant. Because the nurse cannot be in constant attendance, the mother and other members of the family must be taught how to look after the baby between the visits of the nurse. The nurse should undertake such procedures as temperature-taking, weighing, cleaning or bathing, and dressing; but definite instructions must be given to the family on the following subjects:

(1) How to keep the baby warm:

Heating and ventilation of the room.
Heating of the cot (routine filling and use of hot water bottles).

Screening of the cot.
Clothing.
The importance of avoiding exposure during changing and feeding.

(2) How to protect the baby from infection:

Cleaning of room without raising dust.
Exclusion of visitors.
Use of gown (and mask if the attendant has a cold or sore throat).
Hand washing.
Protection from flies.

(3) General handling of the baby.

Minimum of handling, especially after feeds.
Position of child in cot.

(4) Feeding:

Breast feeding.
Preparation and administration of feeds, vitamins, etc.
Care of bottles and teats.

(5) Necessity for continuous observation and immediate notification of any signs of illness or abnormality, e.g.

Early or severe jaundice.
Cyanosis.
Bleeding.
Vomiting.
Loose stools.
Skin rashes.
Thrush.
Nasal discharge.
Distressed respiration.
Twitching.

(6) How to deal with certain emergencies, e.g.

Inhalation of vomitus.
Haemorrhages.
Convulsions.
Overheating.
Abdominal distension.

(7) Record keeping:

Amount of feed taken.
Regurgitation.
Passage of urine and stools.

Good results may be expected from home care of the larger infants (over 2,040 g. at birth) who are free from congenital malformation and birth injury, who do not require oxygen or special methods of feeding (i.e. they can suck and swallow) and who do not develop jaundice or other complications; provided that the home conditions are reasonable, a proper feeding and nursing technique is used, and the infant is protected from infection. It is known that the mortality rate between the ages of 1 and 6 months is reduced by breast feeding (see p. 260) and the higher incidence of breast feeding likely to be obtained among the larger babies kept at home may add an advantage to home care for this group of babies.

The problem is quite different for the smaller babies who are liable to cyanotic attacks, feeding difficulties, hypothermia and other complications of low birth weight such as the development of respiratory distress, hypoglycaemia or jaundice (with the possibility of kernicterus). In these cases, continuous care by specially trained and experienced nurses is required day and night, and the infants will have a better chance of survival in a well equipped special baby care unit under expert paediatric supervision, and where good laboratory services are readily available.

The existence of a good home care service allows earlier discharge of low-weight babies from specialized hospital units and so reduces the number of cots required in such units.

In a complete programme for low-weight babies, both hospital care and home care must be provided, with full co-operation between these two services. (See p. 277.)

REFERENCES

Annual Report of Department of Health and Social Security for 1968. H.M. Stationery Office, London.

Butler, N. R. and Bonham, D. G. (1963). "Perinatal Mortality". E. & S. Livingstone Ltd., Edinburgh and London.

Crosse, V. M. and Mackintosh, J. M. (1953). *Brit. med. J.*, **1**, 1374.

Emery, J. L. (1967). *Proc. roy. Soc. Med.*, **60**, 1003.

Miller, F. J. W. (1948). *Lancet*, **2**, 703.

Ministry of Health Circular 20. (1944). "Care of Premature Infants". H.M. Stationery Office, London.

Report on the Health of Birmingham in 1969 by the Medical Officer of Health.

Williams, R. E. O. (1961). *Lancet*, **2**, 173.

World Health Organization (1950). Technical Report Series No. 27. Expert Group on prematurity.

Chapter 5

CLOTHING

The advantages of nursing the smaller infants naked in incubators have been discussed (p. 45). In this country, the majority of the larger low-weight babies are nursed in open heated cots and require clothing. Clothing must fulfil certain requirements. It must:

(1) Cover the baby completely, with the exception of the face.

(2) Be simple in design, so that it can be changed easily with a minimum of exposure and handling of the infant.

(3) Be made of a material which conducts heat badly, so that the body heat is conserved.

(4) Be washable.

(5) Be loose in order to allow free movement of the chest and limbs.

(6) Be smooth, soft and non-irritating.

Cotton is inferior to wool in preventing heat loss and for this reason should not be used for permanent clothing. In emergencies, a woollen blanket lined with a towel is better than gamgee. Ordinary cotton wool should never be used because it sticks to the body and its later removal entails much exposure of the child; in addition, the cotton wool may get into the child's mouth and even into the air passages. Flannel is the ideal material for clothing for low-weight babies, the variety called "union" flannel containing just enough cotton to prevent the shrinkage which occurs with pure flannel.

In the Sorrento Unit three types of clothing are in use (Fig. 28).

First type. This is only occasionally used for the smallest infants (if they are not being nursed in incubators) and consists of:

(a) A flannel vest, open but overlapping in front, with tape fastenings over the shoulders to allow for easy changing.

(b) A flannel cape, open down the front, with plenty of overlap and provided with a hood to prevent loss of heat from the head (which is large in proportion to the body), the front of the hood being adjustable.

(c) A soft napkin.

Second type. This is used when the infants are more active. It consists of:

(a) A vest as before.

(b) A cape with a hood as before, but with the addition of sleeves to enable the child to move its arms more easily.

(c) A soft napkin.

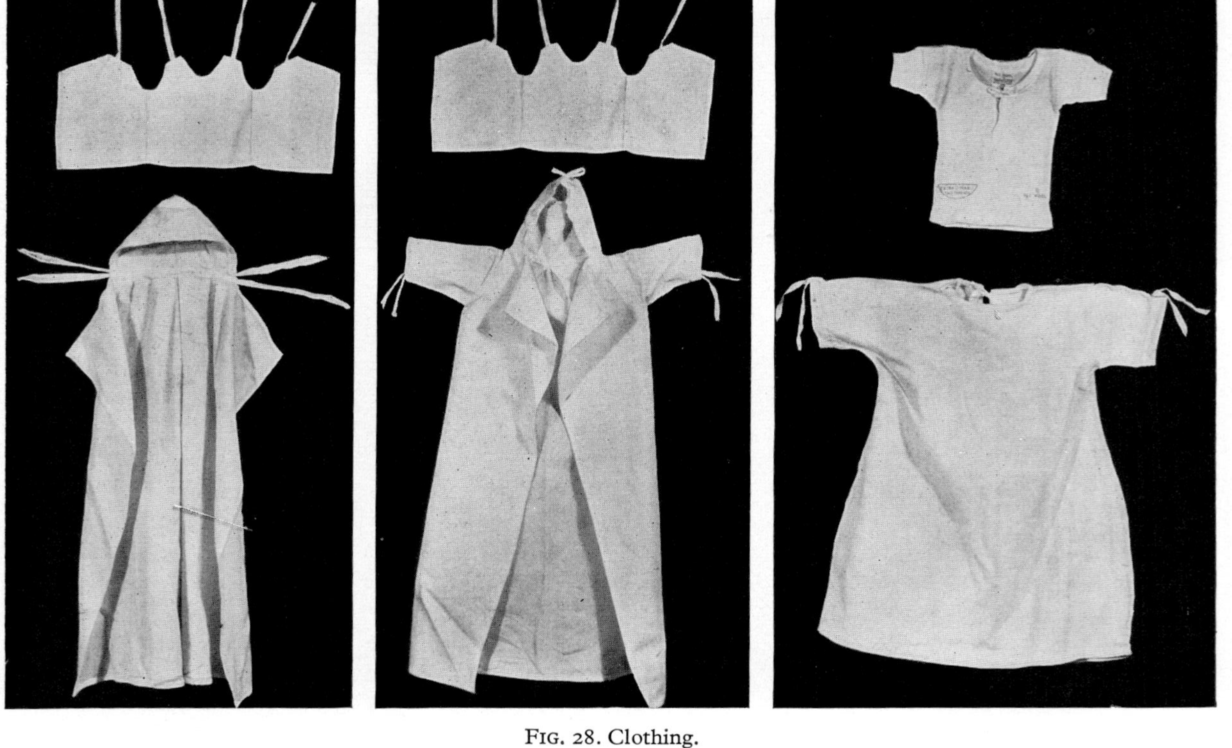

FIG. 28. Clothing.

Left. Vest and gown of first type. *Centre*. Vest and gown of second type. *Right*. Vest and gown of third type.

Third type. This is used for the larger infants after their body temperature has become stabilized and it is no longer necessary to prevent loss of heat from the head. It consists of:

(a) A vest.
(b) A flannel gown with sleeves.
(c) A soft napkin.

If only one type of clothing is desired, the second type is recommended, because the sleeves need not be used for the smaller babies and the hood is easily turned back for the larger babies.

Napkins. For reasons of cleanliness a napkin may be worn even if the infant is otherwise naked. Disposable napkins should be used if possible.

Bibs. Bibs (if used) must *never* be made of an impervious material (e.g. plastic) which might suffocate the baby if it got over the face. Bibs should be tied loosely round the body, as well as the neck, to keep them in place.

Gloves. The hands need only be covered if the infant develops paronychia or other infections of the fingers. If gloves are home made, they should be worn with the seams outside to prevent strangulation of the fingers with loose threads.

Silver swaddler. This is a simple plastic hooded sheet lined with a thin layer of aluminium, which prevents loss of heat by radiation, conduction and convection (see Fig. 9). It is expensive and hyperpyrexia is a theoretical hazard if one is worn for a long period so it should not be used as routine clothing. However, it has proved extremely useful for low-weight babies awaiting, and during, transport (Storrs and Taylor, 1970).

Marking of clothing. If marking ink is employed, all clothing (especially napkins) must be washed before use, otherwise methaemoglobinaemia may occur from absorption of aniline (Howarth, 1951).

REFERENCES

Howarth, B. E. (1951). *Lancet*, **1**, 934.
Storrs, C. N. and Taylor, M. R. H. (1970). *Brit. med. J.*, **3**, 328.

Chapter 6

FEEDING

Feeding Difficulties

CERTAIN difficulties may be met with, in connection with the feeding of pre-term infants. Due to the weak buccal, tongue and palate muscles, and the incomplete development of the nervous system, the power of suction is weak and, in the smallest infants, is virtually absent in regard to ability to feed. Moreover, if the sucking reflex is inadequate the swallowing reflex is also inadequate. Special methods of feeding are therefore required to overcome these difficulties.

The mechanism for closure of the cardia is poorly developed and regurgitation of food may occur; the regurgitated food, owing to the absence of the cough reflex, may be inhaled. Large feeds should therefore be avoided and the infant handled as little as possible after feeds.

The lower the gestational age, the weaker is the power of digestion, especially with regard to the fat of cow's milk, and unless a suitable formula is given digestive upsets will result. Abdominal distension may also occur and give rise to attacks of cyanosis.

Both pre-term and term low-weight babies have small carbohydrate reserves (Shelley, 1964). In addition they both have less available body fat than infants weighing more than 2,500 g.

A good knowledge of infant feeding, including the correct use of catheter feeding (gavage) is essential for anyone who undertakes the care of low-weight babies. A healthy term infant may thrive in spite of unsuitable feeding, but a weakly or pre-term infant is unlikely to do so.

General Principles of Feeding

The following general principles must be considered for each individual baby:

- Kind of food to be given.
- Amount of food required daily.
- Method of giving feeds.
- Frequency and size of feeds.

Kind of food. Human milk is the natural food for the human baby and every effort should be made to obtain it. For babies weighing less than 4½ lb. (2,040 g.) cow's milk should only be resorted to when human milk is unobtainable. The advantages and disadvantages of human milk are further discussed in the section on human milk feeding (p. 104).

Amount required daily. Sufficient food must be given to maintain good nutrition. Underfeeding, which may result in undue loss of weight, dehydration, hypoglycaemia, hyperbilirubinaemia and hypothermia, must be avoided; but overfeeding must also be avoided, with its associated dangers of abdominal distension, vomiting (with possible aspiration, apnoea and cyanosis) and diarrhoea, leading to loss of weight and dehydration, etc.

There has been considerable controversy as to the early requirements of low-weight infants. In the early 1950's it became the custom to delay the first feed until the 2nd or 3rd day (or even 4th day in sick or very small infants) in order to reduce the death rate from aspiration. In the early 1960's late feeding came under suspicion, due to the relationship which was found between late feeding and mental impairment (Freedman, 1961; Drillien, 1964) and between the degree of neonatal weight loss and spastic diplegia (Churchill, 1963). Various trials of early and late feeding have since shown that, in comparison with late feeding, early feeding results in high levels of blood glucose and lower levels of unconjugated bilirubin, less initial loss of weight and a more rapidly regained birth weight (Hubbell *et al.*, 1961; Smallpeice and Davies, 1964; Keitel *et al.*, 1965; Beard *et al.*, 1966; Wennberg *et al.*, 1966; Cornblath *et al.*, 1966; Wu *et al.*, 1967; Rabor *et al.*, 1968) and a greater early increase in head circumference (Davies and Davis, 1970). Because hypoglycaemia and hyperbilirubinaemia may both cause damage to the brain, the advantage of early feeding seems very great. The only disadvantage is the possibility of regurgitation and inhalation in the pre-term infant (Wharton and Bower, 1965; Barrie, 1968) and this danger can be reduced by giving small frequent feeds or even an intra-gastric drip if necessary. However, the danger of regurgitation and aspiration must not be underestimated as it can cause death. This danger is minimal in low-weight babies born after 37 weeks gestation.

In spite of a number of studies, the optimum food intake for low-weight babies remains unsettled (W H O, 1968). In the author's experience, pre-term infants need about 130 calories/kg./day (60 calories/lb./day) if they are to gain satisfactorily, but these values need not be reached until the second week of life.

It is generally agreed that the malnourished group of the light-for-dates babies require more calories than pre-term infants with the same birth weight. Such a baby will get the extra calories required if the calories are calculated on its "expected" birth weight, i.e. the mean birth weight for its gestational age.

Pre-term infants usually lose about 10% of their birth weight and do not regain this weight until the second week of life. The majority of light-for-dates babies (the malnourished group) lose less weight and regain it more rapidly if they are fed for their "expected" weight. But the light-for-dates dwarfs gain less well than a pre-term infant whose birth weight is consistent with its maturity (Black, 1961): in fact, most of the hypoplastic group of babies who are light-for-dates do not gain well.

In order to assess the progress of any particular baby, it is convenient to plot the birth weight, and subsequent weights, at the appropriate gestational age on an average *in utero* weight curve, i.e. a curve showing the average weight of the foetus at different gestational ages. Weights which could be used for this purpose have been quoted by Anderson (1946), Huggett (1946), Lubchenco *et al.* (1963), Hendricks (1964), Kitchen (1968), Usher and McLean (1969) but it is probably better to construct one's own curve because birth weights vary from country to country and even area to area. Fig. 29 shows the curve used by the author. The progress of (a) a normal pre-term baby and (b) a light-for-dates term baby have been plotted against this curve to show what loss and gain might be expected in these two types of baby.

This method of charting the birth weight against the gestational age is useful in many ways. If the infant is unduly large for dates, it may be oedematous, have a diabetic mother, or suffer from some malformation (e.g. hydrocephalus), or the dates may be incorrect or the maturity wrongly calculated. If the infant is small for dates, it may be malnourished or suffer from some malformation (e.g. anencephaly), or again the dates may be incorrect or the gestational age wrongly calculated. If subsequent progress is slow, underfeeding or disease should be suspected; if it is too rapid, oedema may be the cause (e.g. from excessive electrolytes in the feed). The chart also indicates the expected weight (average weight for the gestational age) of a light-for-dates baby which can be used for calculating food requirements.

Methods of giving feeds. Generally speaking, if an infant can suck, it is put to the breast (if strong enough) or given a bottle. If it cannot suck well, it will not be able to swallow well either and catheter feeds must be given.

In actual practice, the method of giving feeds may be varied from feed to feed according to the condition of the individual baby at the time of each feed.

During feeds, the head end of the cot or incubator mattress should be raised. This is done for three reasons:

(1) To reduce the possibility of regurgitation.
(2) To avoid middle ear infection.
(3) To prevent swallowed air passing out of the stomach into the intestines.

The necessity for warming feeds has been questioned by Holt *et al.* (1962), who found no disadvantages from feeding low-weight babies

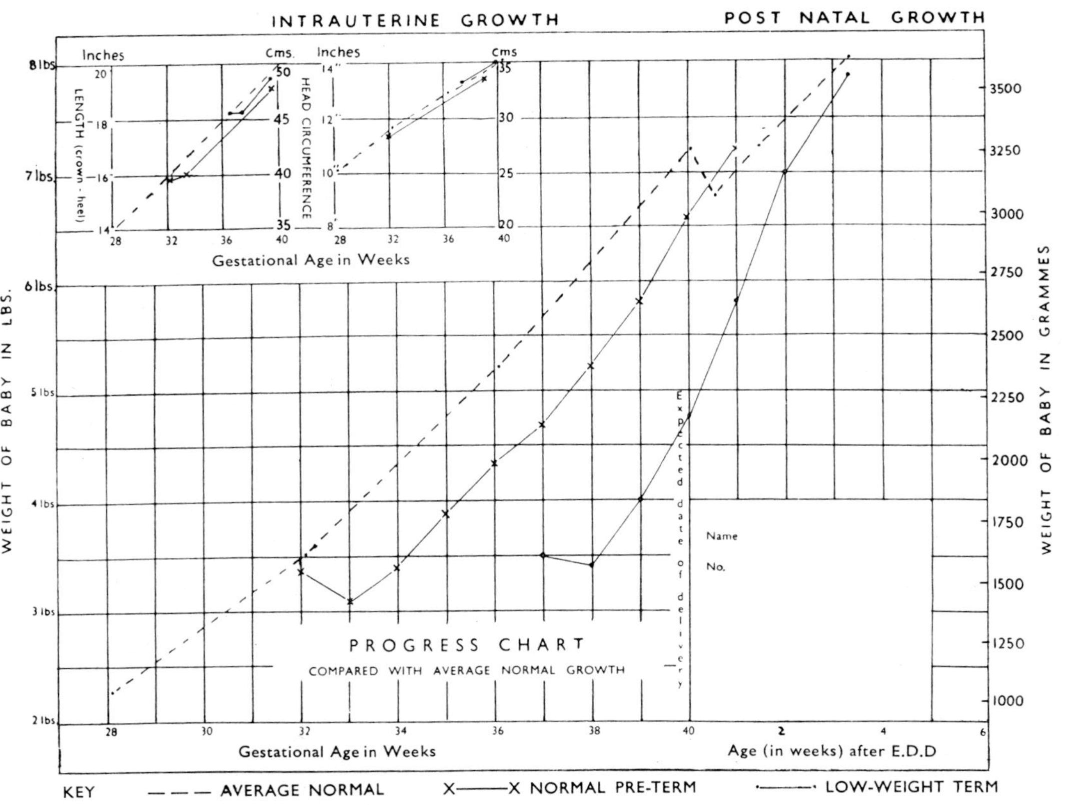

FIG. 29
The progress of a normal pre-term baby and a term low-weight baby have been plotted against the average weight, length, and head circumference at different gestational ages

with milk from a refrigerator at 4°C. They reported a fall in body temperature of 0·1°C (0·2°F) only. However, recognizing the importance of avoiding any increase in metabolism, it would seem advisable to warm feeds before administration when facilities are readily available.

Breast feeding. This will be dealt with later in this chapter.

Bottle feeding. The ordinary upright feeding bottle may be used if the baby sucks well. To prevent excessive air swallowing the teat should not be too hard and the hole in the teat should be large enough to allow a rapid flow of drops (not a stream) when the bottle is inverted.

The boat-shaped bottle is useful for infants with poor powers of suction, because the valve can be either removed or replaced by a teat with a large hole in it. If this is done the formation of a vacuum is avoided and less suction is required, but care is necessary to prevent the flow being too free which may lead to choking and inhalation. However, these bottles are awkward to store and transport, if feeds are prepared in a central milk-kitchen. Some experienced nurses find a Belcroy feeder useful in such cases. If this feeder is used, *no pressure should be made on the bulb*, because this may force milk into the infant's mouth before it is ready to swallow and lead to inhalation. Because of this very real danger, the author does *not* recommend the use of this feeder.

Before commencing a bottle feed, the head end of the cot or incubator mattress should be raised and the baby turned on to its right side. In this position regurgitation is less likely, and if it should occur the regurgitated fluid can run out of the corner of the mouth; the stomach can empty more easily into the duodenum; and there is less pressure on the heart by the dilated stomach.

When the mouth is opened in the usual way by pressure on the lower jaw or on the cheeks, the tongue tends to stick to the roof of the mouth, and the nurse must make sure that the teat is placed *above* the tongue.

When attempting to stimulate suction the nurse must avoid the temptation of *twisting* the bottle in the mouth, as this may injure the mucous membrane and so predispose to thrush. Permissible methods to stimulate suction are: to press the teat down on to the tongue (without twisting the bottle) or to apply gentle upward pressure under the chin. The bottle should always be held and not "propped" as the latter may lead to regurgitation and inhalation. It is also important to hold the bottle in such a position that the teat is kept full if excessive air-swallowing is to be avoided (Fig. 30).

At the end of a feed the infant should be supported in the sitting position until the "wind" comes up. It should then be placed on its right side, and before leaving it the nurse must open and inspect the mouth to satisfy herself that the whole of the feed has been swallowed. The head end of the cot, or incubator mattress, should remain tilted

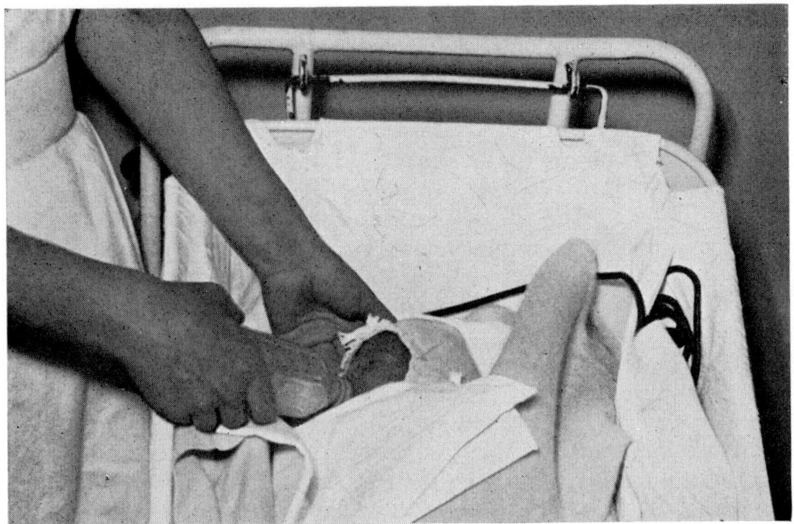

(*Photo by Camera Talks*)

FIG. 30. Bottle feeding. The bottle is held by the nurse, not "propped". The tilt of the bottle (to keep the teat full and reduce air-swallowing) is shown. The head end of the cot is raised and the infant lies on its right side. A disposable tissue is placed under the chin in case regurgitation occurs.

up for half an hour after feeds; and the baby should remain on its right side until half way through the interval between feeds, when it is turned on to its left side.

As the infant becomes larger and stronger, and able to stand more handling, it may be lifted out of the cot and fed on the nurse's knee.

Catheter feeding. This has three main uses:

(1) It is a means of feeding small infants who can neither suck nor swallow, or who become cyanosed when fed by means of a bottle.

(2) It is a useful method of feeding sick infants, e.g. cases of intracranial birth injury or respiratory distress, since it demands the least effort on the part of the child and so conserves strength.

(3) It can be used as a means of giving additional food to infants who are unable to take sufficient for their needs by bottle. In some cases an occasional catheter feed may suffice, while in others a catheter feed may replace a bottle feed every 4, 6 or 12 hours, according to the needs of the child.

Finally, it must be emphasized that *catheter feeding has definite dangers, and should never be used as a means of saving time or trouble.* Catheters should only be introduced by trained attendants.

Interrupted catheter feeding. This older method of catheter feeding is generally only used for the larger infants, but can also be used for the smaller active babies who cannot tolerate an indwelling catheter.

Both oesophageal and stomach feeds can be given by this method, but the former are preferable because they can be repeated at regular intervals without any risk of causing vomiting or gastric irritation. If stomach feeding is practised, there is an additional risk of distension, due to the air in the apparatus becoming trapped in the stomach.

A polyvinyl catheter is commonly used, but any catheter of the correct size (English size 4, American size 8, and French sizes 10–12) and approximately 14 in. long, can be employed.

It is important to know how far to pass the catheter, so as to ensure that the tip reaches the correct position in the lower end of the oesophagus, i.e. about ½ in. (1·25 cm.) above the cardiac sphincter, and the method described by Hess and Lundeen in 1949 is recommended. The infant is measured in a straight line, from the bridge of the nose to the tip of the ensiform cartilage, and this measurement is marked off on the catheter (from the tip) before sterilization. When the catheter is passed as far as this mark, the tip reaches the lower end of the oesophagus, and when it is passed a further 1–1½ in. (2·5–4 cm.) the tip is well within the stomach. Each infant must have its individual catheter, not only to avoid cross-infection but also to ensure the correct measurement. The catheters can be marked with different coloured cottons or silks and, in order to make sure that each infant is fed with its own measured catheter, a piece of cotton or silk of the same colour as that used to mark the catheter may be tied to the end of the incubator or cot. This practical detail is of great value when a number of infants are on catheter feeds. Instead of a wide funnel, a small pipette (fountain-pen filler without the rubber bulb) is attached to the upper end of the catheter. The small size of this glass tube allows easy observation of the rate of flow of the feed, the importance of which will be referred to later. The glass barrel of a small syringe is sometimes recommended, but the pipette is a more economical proposition.

Before giving a catheter feed, the head end of the cot, or incubator mattress, should be raised at least 30 degrees and the infant placed on its right side. The empty sterilized catheter is introduced through the mouth, and *not through the nose*, since the nasal passages are too narrow for this size of catheter and the mucous membrane might easily become injured and infected. The catheter is passed down the oesophagus until the cotton mark is on a level with the infant's gums; the tip will then be about ½ in. (1·25 cm.) from the stomach. There is no danger of the catheter entering the larynx, but in rare cases of oesophageal atresia the passage of the catheter is arrested. The catheter is tightly compressed and the feed poured into the pipette until the apparatus is full. The catheter is then released and the feed allowed to flow slowly, the pipette being refilled each time before it becomes empty so as to avoid the introduction of air. When the whole of the feed has been given, the catheter is tightly pinched and gently extracted (see Fig. 31).

One of the dangers of catheter feeding, and it is a very real one, is the risk of overflow into the air passages. This can, however, be avoided if the head is raised and the feed given sufficiently slowly. It is important to remember that the feed is being put into the lower end of the oesophagus and has to run into the stomach by gravity. If time is not allowed for this, the feed will overflow into the larynx because of the poorly developed cough reflex. This accident may either cause immediate suffocation or lead to inhalation pneumonia or atelectasis from an obstructed bronchus. If inhalation occurs, the baby must be tilted head-down, the catheter pinched and withdrawn, and the oropharynx cleared by suction.

Another danger in this method of feeding is the careless extraction of the catheter at the end of the feed. Unless it is firmly compressed, any residual milk will flow out as it is being removed and may run

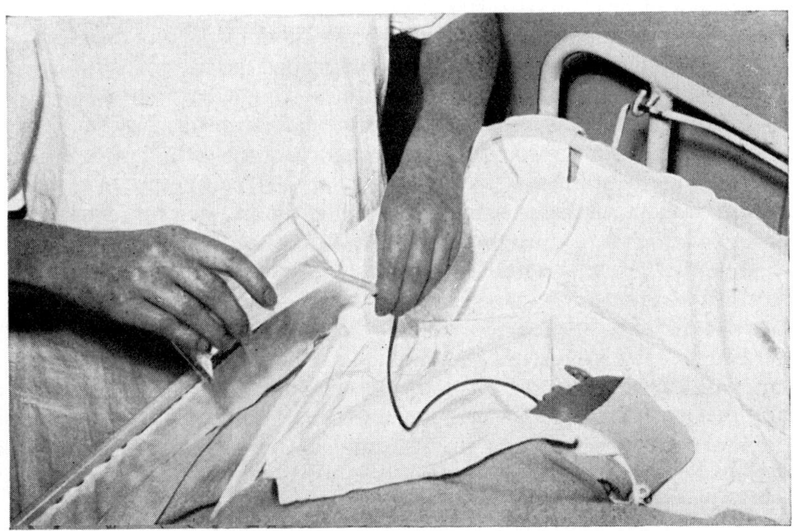

(*Photo by Camera Talks*)

FIG. 31. Catheter feeding. The head end of the cot is raised and the infant lies on its right side. The catheter is passed through the mouth until the mark is on a level with the gums. The rate of flow is controlled by the nurse's fingers on the catheter just below the pipette, and the pipette is filled up as required from the measure glass.

into the larynx. This is specially liable to occur if the catheter is extracted quickly, as this causes the infant to give a deep inspiratory gasp. The correct technique therefore consists of waiting for a full minute after the completion of a feed, pinching the catheter firmly and removing it gently.

If the infant is fit to be handled, it should be supported in the sitting position until the "wind" comes up, then placed on its right side (if clothed and in a cot) or in the prone position (if naked in an incubator). The oesophagus enters the stomach posteriorly and this makes it difficult to bring up wind in the supine position. The head end of the cot, or incubator mattress, should remain up for half an hour after the feed, then can be levelled. If the infant is in a cot, it should be turned on to its left side halfway through the interval between feeds.

If at any time there is marked gaseous distension of the stomach, this should be relieved before giving the next catheter feed. The catheter is passed into the stomach (i.e. a further 1½ in. or 4 cm.) and the air allowed to escape; it is then withdrawn to the cotton mark and the feed given in the usual way.

Indwelling nasogastric catheter feeding. In 1951 Royce *et al.* reported a new method of gavage, using an indwelling polyethylene catheter which was passed through the nose and left *in situ*. This method allows the administration of frequent small feeds without disturbing the infant. Wagner and his co-workers (1954) recommended the use of a softer and more pliable polyvinyl catheter instead of polyethylene.

The infant is measured from the ensiform cartilage to the lobe of the ear and then forward to the nostril, and this length is clearly marked on the catheter (from the tip) with a ball-point pen. The sterilized catheter, which has an atraumatic tip and holes on alternate sides near the tip, is introduced through the nose as far as the mark (the catheter is then in the stomach); a plastic spigot is placed in the open end of the catheter (or into a cannula which fits the end of the catheter) and the catheter is fixed to the infant's face with waterproof or steristrip strapping. After 5 days' use, the catheter is removed, re-sterilized (unless disposable) and inserted through the opposite nostril. To give a feed, the formula is drawn up into a 10–20 ml. syringe, the spigot is removed and the syringe is inserted into the catheter or cannula, and the formula is slowly introduced. The catheter is held up vertically until the formula has all disappeared and then the spigot is replaced in the catheter.

Unfortunately active infants tend to be restless when the nasal catheter is *in situ* and there is no doubt that the nasal mucous membrane is sometimes injured and may become infected. Nevertheless this method of feeding must be considered for the smaller infants who cannot tolerate the frequent passage of a feeding catheter. There is no doubt that this method of feeding is particularly useful in nurseries where there is a shortage of nurses specially trained in the care of low-weight babies, because the catheter can be inserted by a doctor or senior nurse and the feeds given by less experienced staff.

Pipette feeding. In the author's opinion, there are few indications for pipette feeding in a low-weight baby because if the sucking reflex is poor, the swallow reflex is also poor. A pipette may be used for larger infants with a good swallow reflex but difficulty with suction due to such factors as severe cleft palate, severe thrush or facial palsy, but even in these cases a teat with a large hole or a boat-shaped bottle used as described in a previous section usually gives better results.

Before giving a pipette feed the head should be raised. The pipette is placed well back on the tongue and pressure on the tongue will usually stimulate the act of swallowing.

Before leaving the infant, the nurse should always inspect the back of its throat to make certain that all the feed has been swallowed.

Frequency and size of feeds. The first feed may be given as early as 2 hours after birth if the infant is light-for-dates. The timing of the first feed for pre-term infants will depend on the birth weight and condition of the infant, but it is usually given between the ages of 6–12 hours. Some units use 10% dextrose for the first feed, in case the feed is vomited.

If the infant can suck, the best results have been obtained by giving small frequent feeds at the beginning and increasing the interval between feeds as the infant becomes stronger and able to take the larger amounts required. Two-hourly feeds (10 or 11 feeds per day) are given at first to the smallest babies; these being changed to 3-hourly feeds (7 feeds) when a healthy baby reaches the weight of 4½–5 lb. (2,040–2,270 g.). Larger babies are started on 2-hourly feeds (10 feeds) or 3-hourly feeds (7 feeds), according to their general condition and their ability to suck and to swallow. One reason for giving small frequent feeds is that the low-weight infant tires rapidly. It may suck quite vigorously for a few minutes, but then suction becomes feeble and the remainder of the feed may only be taken after another 15–20 minutes. It is a great mistake to persevere too long as the infant becomes so exhausted that it will probably not recover in time to take the following feed. The frequency of the feeds must therefore depend on the amount the infant can take before becoming tired; if only small amounts are taken, then the feeds must be given more frequently in order to ensure that the child receives sufficient for its requirements. With difficult feeders the feed can be divided and given in two portions with a rest of 5–10 minutes between the portions. A second reason for giving small frequent feeds is to reduce the possibility of regurgitation from over-filling the stomach, with the subsequent risk of inhalation.

If the infant cannot suck it is fed by catheter. The smallest infants (those being fed by an indwelling nasogastric catheter) must be given small frequent feeds at first (hourly or 2-hourly); and a continuous drip may be necessary for babies who tend to regurgitate. The intervals between feeds is gradually lengthened as the infant's condition improves.

However small the infant may be, the stomach should be allowed a period of rest during the night, and no feeds should be given between midnight and 4 a.m. even to the smallest infants; as the infant becomes stronger and able to take larger feeds this period should be extended until 6 a.m.

Charts and Records

The following records should be kept:

(1) Kind of food given.
(2) Method of giving feeds.
(3) Frequency of feeding.
(4) Amount taken at each feed.
(5) Total quantity of fluid taken in 24 hours.
(6) Total calories taken in 24 hours.

A feeding chart (such as the chart on p. 103), can be used, on which the kind of food given is entered for each day and the exact amount taken at each feed is recorded under the time of day at which the feed is given. Feeds given by catheter may usefully be marked with the letters CF; and any feed followed by vomiting marked "Vom", with a rough estimate of the amount, e.g. "small" or "large". At the end of each day the total quantity taken is added up, the caloric value calculated and both these totals charted in the columns provided.

The quantities to be recorded on this chart are those *actually taken* by the infant, and not the amount suggested in the feeding instructions. Babies naturally vary from feed to feed in the amount they take, and the feeding instructions can only be an indication of the average quantity required at each feed.

On the chart human milk may be shown in red ink, and cow's milk mixtures in black ink.

Fluids given by other routes, e.g. intravenous, are also charted under the time at which they are given and are included in the daily total of fluids given.

This feeding chart is of great importance, because the instructions for the next few days are based on the results obtained on the fluid and calorie intake of the previous few days, as judged by the progress chart (see Fig. 29, p. 95).

Feeding Chart

Special Baby Care Unit

		A.M.									P.M.													
Date	Diet	4	5	6	7	8	9	10	11	12	1	2	3	4	5	6	7	8	9	10	11	12	Total Fluid	Total Caloric Value

Human Milk Feeding

Importance of human milk. The food of choice for a low-weight baby is still a matter of controversy. Some paediatricians believe that human milk is not ideal because of the low protein and mineral salt content, and the high fat content, and it is likely that the needs of the pre-term infants are different from those of the light-for-dates infants. In any case low-weight babies born after 37 weeks gestation have good powers of digestion and can usually digest cows' milk as well as human milk.

Many paediatricians, including the author, believe that human milk is the best food for pre-term infants, especially those with the lowest gestational age. The retention and utilization of available protein is higher in the pre-term than in the term infant (Grauel and Syllm-Rapoport, 1964), and human milk provides more than enough protein for pre-term infants (Pincus *et al.*, 1962), the relatively high proportion of lactalbumin giving a high ratio of essential amino-acids. The fat of human milk is more easily utilized than cow's milk fat (Gordon and McNamara, 1941; Nicolaj, 1958). The low mineral salt content offers an advantage over cow's milk during the first few weeks of life when excessive electrolytes can lead to oedema; and babies fed on human milk rarely develop neonatal tetany because of the low phosphate content (Oppé and Redstone, 1968; Watney *et al.*, 1971). Gonzaga *et al.* (1963) suggest that human milk can act as an effective agent for the prevention of various types of enteric infection provided that the mother is immune and excretes the respective antibodies in the milk. Smangoen (1957) thought that feeding with cow's milk mixtures predisposed to infection with *E. Coli* and/or salmonellae; and Svirsky-Gross (1958) eliminated *E. Coli* 0.111 from a premature nursery by using human milk, after failing to control a 2-year epidemic with antibiotics or closure of the nursery.

Osborn (1967) correlated the state of coronary arteries of teenagers with early feeding. Those who had no human milk had mainly abnormal arteries while most of those who were breast fed for more than 2 months had normal coronary arteries.

In two feeding experiments in the Sorrento unit, diet appeared to have little effect on babies weighing more than $3\frac{1}{2}$ lb. (1,590 g.) at birth; but below this weight the best all-round results (judged by initial weight loss, time taken to regain birth weight, subsequent rate of weight-gain, serum protein and haemoglobin levels, mortality rates and infection rates) were obtained with human milk, and failing that S-M-A. or half skimmed dried or evaporated cow's milk (2·5% protein). The worst results were obtained with an unskimmed cow's milk mixture (1·7% protein). Human milk was tolerated best during the first few days of life; and those fed on human milk had the lowest incidence of anaemia, infection and mortality (Crosse *et al.*, 1954 and 1960). During the latter investigation (1960) the stools of infants fed on human milk and S-M-A. were acid, while the stools of infants fed on other cow's milk mixtures were alkaline. Cultures from the stools of infants fed on human milk almost invariably showed heavy growths of lactobacilli by the age of 2–3 weeks and coliform bacilli were rare (no pathological coliforms were found). But cultures from the stools of babies fed on cow's milk mixtures (even S-M-A.) usually only showed scanty growths of lactobacilli, whereas coliform bacilli were always present and occasionally these were pathological.

It is important to try to get a low-weight baby feeding from its mother's breasts before it is sent home because breast feeding reduces the death rate during the first year of life. This is particularly important in families with a poor standard of hygiene, i.e. the families from which so many of the low-weight babies come. Wilcox (1936) drew attention to the fact that low-weight infants receiving little or no breast milk after the first 10 days of life showed relatively a greater susceptibility to disease and a higher mortality rate. In a follow-up of 1,377 low-weight babies born in the City of Birmingham during 1 year, the author found the death rate between the ages of 1 month and 6 months to be 1·3% in breast-fed infants and 4·0% in artificially-fed infants. To obtain the maximum reduction of the mortality rate, breast feeding should be continued until the baby reaches the age of 6 months. If this is not possible, human milk should be provided until the infant reaches the weight of at least 4–4½ lb. (1,800–2,040 g.) and this can be achieved in one of two ways:

(1) By maintaining the milk supply of the baby's own mother.
(2) By providing human milk from a human milk bank.

The latter method is both expensive and difficult to organize, and should only be used when every effort to maintain the mother's own supply has failed.

Maintenance of mother's own milk. The mother's own milk supply is difficult to maintain if the powers of suction of her infant are feeble or absent, but it is most important to do so in developing countries, where the death rate is very high in artificially fed infants.

If the baby is strong enough to put to the breast, care must be taken to see that both breasts are used at each feed because frequent reduction of tension is essential for the maintenance of an adequate supply. The breasts should be emptied by an efficient pump or by hand expression after the infant has fed, and the milk obtained in this way used to complement any later feed at which the infant fails to suck sufficient for its needs.

If the baby is too feeble to be put to the breast, the milk must be taken off at regular intervals, at least five or six times daily, both breasts being emptied on each occasion.

The diet of the nursing mother has a very definite effect on her ability to produce milk. Sufficient protein is required and half should be given in the form of "first-class" proteins. The water intake should be increased and extra calories are usually required: the Department of Health and Social Security (1969) and Thomson *et al.* (1970) suggest a supplement of 500 calories daily. Sufficient mineral salts and vitamins should be given. Contrary to the general belief stout has no special value.

Rest, fresh air, suitable exercise and freedom from worry help to promote a plentiful milk supply. It is most important that a mother should have the desire to feed her infant, and this can often be stimulated by explaining the benefit derived by the baby.

Table A gives a summary of the dietary allowances recommended for a lactating woman by the B M A in 1950 (Manual of Nutrition, 1955) and by the U S A Food and Nutrition Board (1963).

TABLE A

	B M A (1950)	U S A Food and Nutrition Board (1963)
Calories	3,000·0	3,100·0
Protein (g.)	111·0	98·0
Calcium	2·0	1·3
Iron (mg.)	15·0	20·0
Vitamin A (i.u.)	8,000·0	8,000·0
Thiamine (mg.)	1·4	1·2
Riboflavine (mg.) ..	2·1	1·9
Nicotinic Acid (mg.) ..	14·0	21·0
Ascorbic Acid (mg.) ..	50·0	100·0
Vitamin D (i.u.) ..	800·0	400·0

Table B shows various diets which have been recommended for nursing mothers.

Human milk banks. A human milk bank or bureau is an organization for the collection and distribution of surplus human milk.

Most maternity hospitals organize their own banks on a small scale, but there is often difficulty in obtaining human milk for large special baby care units, for infants in children's hospitals, and for infants at home if their own mothers are unable to feed them.

The only solution to this difficulty is the setting up of central human milk banks. The first bank to be established in England was at Queen

TABLE B

Food	Quantity per head per week	League of Nations, 1936	Stiebeling, 1939	Tisdall *et al.* 1941
Milk	Pints	12	12	14
Cheese	Ounces	7·4	—	4·25
Butter	Ounces	As needed	8·0	12
Other fats.. ..	Ounces	As needed	12·8	8
Eggs	Number	7	7	3
Meat and Fish ..	Ounces	29·5	41·6	20
Liver	Ounces	Not stated	Not stated	4
Tomatoes and citrus fruits	Ounces	As needed	32·0	64
Potatoes	Ounces	61·5	51·2	56
Dried legumes and nuts	Ounces	2·5	2·2	4
Leafy Greens and yellow vegetables	Ounces	24·6	80·0	32
Other vegetables and fresh fruit..	Ounces	Not stated	121·6	36
Bread and/or flour and cereals ..	Ounces	61·5	51·2	88
Sugar	Ounces	As needed	16·0	16

Charlotte's Hospital, London. Now quite a number of centres, including Birmingham, have such banks.

The organization of a human milk bank or bureau includes:

(1) *A scheme for the notification of mothers who have surplus milk.* Doctors, midwives, maternity hospitals, health visitors, maternity and child welfare centres, and district nurses can be asked to co-operate in the scheme by notifying suitable women. Women should only be used if they are healthy and the home is clean. Their babies must be under 9 months of age, healthy, breast fed and gaining weight satisfactorily.

(2) *Collection of the milk.* A special nurse should visit the mother daily to collect the milk. She must make sure that the home is clean and that the mother and child both remain healthy. The collection of milk should be temporarily discontinued in the case of any illness of mother or child, the mother being advised to take off the surplus milk as usual and to throw it away until the collection can be resumed. Suitable equipment should be lent to the mother, who must be taught how to collect the milk in a clean way. An ice-box should be provided for storage of the milk if there is no refrigerator in the house. The nurse should call daily to collect the milk and to leave clean, sterile bottles and carbon dioxide ice for the ice-box: she can also be responsible for

the weekly payment of the mother (the rate of pay in Birmingham is 2p per oz.). A car should be provided for the use of the nurse.

(3) *Treatment of the milk.* The milk should be strained through sterile gauze, pooled and bottled before pasteurization. After rapid cooling the bottles are stored in a refrigerator at 4·5°C (40°F) until required for use. Milk can be sent by train in bottles packed in carbon dioxide ice.

Milk which will not be required within 48 hours of pasteurization can be preserved more or less indefinitely by freezing in the hardening compartment of an ice cream refrigerator or "deep freeze" at −12° to −14°C (7–10°F). Human milk can also be dried but this method is unsuitable for small quantities.

(4) *Laboratory control.* Tests should be made on a specimen of each new mother's milk before it is used; and on any individual specimen at any time if dilution, substitution by cow's milk or lack of cleanliness is suspected. Every batch of pasteurized pooled milk should be tested before it is used.

Methods of using human milk. If infants are too small and weakly to be put to the breast, expressed milk can be given by bottle, or catheter, according to the condition of the baby.

Human milk should only be given "raw", i.e. not boiled or pasteurized, if it is collected under close supervision and given to the mother's own infant. Any mother's milk which is being given to babies other than her own must be pasteurized or brought to the boil before use. It is also wise to treat milk brought up by mothers from outside in a similar manner, even if it is to be used for their own babies entirely, as the method of collection is seldom above reproach.

It was the custom to dilute human milk at first for the smallest babies, but it is now suggested that undiluted human milk should be used from the beginning (Wilkinson *et al.*, 1962; Smallpeice and Davies, 1964). The immature kidney is known to be deficient in the excretion of water, sodium, chloride and ammonium ions (McCance, 1959) and it is probable that undiluted human milk presents the infant with a combination of protein, carbohydrate, fat, water and minerals in a ratio with which the immature kidney can deal (*Brit. med. J.*, 1965). If there is any intolerance to full strength human milk, it may be diluted with 10% glucose at first, but full strength milk should be given by the end of the first week of life.

Technique of breast feeding. Healthy infants weighing over 5 lb. (2,270 g.) at birth may be put to the breast after the first 4–6 hours of life. Those weighing from 4½–5 lb. (2,040–2,270 g.), with good powers of suction, can commence breast feeding on the fourth or fifth day of life, but until then should be fed with appropriate amounts of expressed colostrum or human milk.

The larger and stronger infants can be breast fed every 3 hours, but small infants should only be put to the breast once during the day to begin with, expressed milk being given by bottle at the other feeds. The number of breast feeds given during the day is gradually increased as the condition of the baby improves, until eventually the baby is feeding from the breast every 3 hours.

The baby should never be allowed to stay at each breast longer than 10 minutes. At first, each feed should take the form of a "test feed" and deficiencies in quantity made up by giving a complement of expressed milk after the infant has been returned to its cot. Such complements should be given by bottle rather than by spoon, because it has been found in practice that the pre-term baby sucks better at the breast as a result of this experience with the bottle.

In special baby care units, breast feeding mothers should be accommodated in single rooms with their infants, whenever possible. If a baby has to be carried to the mother's room, great care must be taken to protect it from loss of heat: it should be carefully wrapped in one or more of its blankets and the mother's room and the communicating passage must be kept warm and free from draughts.

Care must also be taken to prevent cross-infection when taking infants to their mothers. Infants can either be carried individually by a nurse wearing the "cot gown" belonging to the infant concerned, or they can be pushed in their cots. On no account should babies be placed side by side on a communal "carrier", nor should two babies be carried at once.

The mother must wash her hands carefully before receiving the child, and the breasts must be washed before feeding is commenced.

Cow's Milk Feeding

If all attempts to obtain breast milk fail, then a modification of cow's milk will have to be used as a substitute.

Because a pre-term baby may have more difficulty in digesting cow's milk than breast milk, any pre-term infant on cow's milk feeds should be closely watched for signs of digestive disturbance such as vomiting, diarrhoea, constipation, abdominal distension or abnormal stool.

It is most important that the nurse in charge should be able to recognize the earliest signs of disturbance so as to avoid serious developments. When disturbances occur, medical advice should be sought without delay, and until this has been obtained boiled water only should be given to the child.

Because of the difficulty in utilizing the fat in cow's milk, a low-fat, high-protein, high-carbohydrate formula must be given to the smaller infants (under 3½ lb. or 1,590 g.). In a desire to obtain a more rapid gain there is a tendency to overfeed pre-term infants, and it is especially important to avoid this in the case of an infant fed on cow's milk.

Fresh, dried, and evaporated cow's milk can all be modified to meet the requirements of a low-weight baby and for this reason there are many possible methods of feeding such a baby. Some of the methods of feeding are more elaborate than others, and it is worthy of note that the simplest methods have given some of the best results. When midwives and nurses are being trained in the care of the low-weight baby it is important that they should be taught simple methods of feeding; and it is also useful if they can be taught to use foods which are available in their own countries so that what they have learnt can be carried out in their future work, wherever this may be. Good results can be obtained with dried or evaporated milk (half-skimmed and full-cream) and most of these preparations have the advantage of being generally available. These milks can be used for all routine cow's milk feeding of healthy low-weight infants, other types of food only being given for special indications.

A point which requires to be particularly stressed is the importance of avoiding frequent or unnecessary changes in the type of food given, as such changes may be tolerated badly. When possible, any modification required should be obtained by means of increasing or decreasing the dilution, adding more or less sugar, and skimming or changing to a half-cream variety of the same food, rather than changing from one type to another. If at any time, however, it does become necessary, the change-over should be effected gradually. That is to say, on the first day only a small quantity of the new food should be mixed with the old, the quantity being increased daily until finally the new one replaces the old entirely. It is also a good plan to give any new food in such a dilution that the percentages of the food elements are slightly less than those in the mixture previously given. When the change-over is complete and it is certain that the new food is well tolerated, the strength can be increased according to requirements.

Cow's Milk

In the modification of cow's milk to make it suitable for pre-term babies, the main difficulty is in relation to the fat.

Fat. Utilization of cow's milk fat is poor in pre-term babies: the fat is split normally but absorption is poor, especially for saturated fats (Holt, 1961). Few pre-term babies can utilize more than 2·0% fat in a cow's milk formula, and the best way out of the difficulty is to give a feed with a low fat content. In 1941 Gordon and McNamara reported that pre-term babies fed on modifications of cow's milk in which 30–55% of the calories were derived from fat, excreted an excessive amount of faecal fat. If, however, the milk was skimmed so that only

15–20% of the calories were derived from fat, the faecal fat excretion was reduced to the level observed in term infants fed on unskimmed milk.

Restriction of the fat content in a formula to 2·0% or less is not detrimental in any way because the pre-term infant obtains its calories even more exclusively from carbohydrates than the term baby, and its store of body fat is increased mainly by the conversion of carbohydrates into fat.

Protein. Although unmodified cow's milk protein is indigestible it can easily be made digestible by heating: the protein of dried and evaporated milks is very digestible as a result of the process of drying or evaporating.

All low-weight infants have a special need for protein because of their relatively very rapid growth. Luckily they retain and utilize protein better than normal term infants; in fact, the smaller the weight of the infant the better the percentage of utilization of protein.

In the Sorrento feeding experiments already described (p. 104) it was shown that human milk provided sufficient protein for the needs of the pre-term baby but a considerably higher protein content was necessary when a cow's milk mixture was used (except in the case of S-M-A in which the protein had been modified).

Various feeding trials have been undertaken to discover the correct intake of cow's milk protein for low-weight babies (Omans *et al.*, 1961; Davidson *et al.*, 1967; Tachai *et al.*, 1969; Snyderman *et al.*, 1969; Goldman *et al.*, 1969; Babson and Bramhall, 1969). From the results it would appear that more than 2 g./kg./day of cow's milk protein is required to avoid oedema and low serum protein levels; and less than 6 g./kg./day to avoid hyperpyrexia, deficient hydration and unduly high serum protein levels. Babies given high protein feeds are unable to complete the metabolism of aromatic amino-acids if there is a deficiency of vitamin C, thus the administration of relatively large doses of this vitamin (100 mg. daily) become vitally important in such cases (Levine and Gordon, 1942).

It is possible that a very high protein feed should not be given for too long a period. Williams (1963) found that, among babies weighing more than 1,500 g., a protein intake above 5·5 g./kg./day raised the blood urea level above 30 mg./100 ml. (It had no effect on babies smaller than this.) Avery (1964) and Takai *et al.* (1969) found high levels of serum phenylalanine and tyrosine in low-weight babies fed on cow's milk mixtures with high protein levels.

Sugar. A high sugar content is required in order to provide sufficient calories (together with the amount of fat which can be utilized) to cover all requirements except growth. Sugar is well tolerated by low-weight infants. A sugar content of 4–5% is well taken from the beginning, and this can be increased until 10% is being given. As a result of experiments it has been found that cane or beet sugar (sucrose) is tolerated in the highest percentages, and dextrin-maltose (e.g. Daltose, Cow & Gate) in the next highest percentages. It is, however, necessary to exercise care in the administration of lactose and glucose because fermentative stools may occur if either of these sugars is given in too high a percentage.

Balance between food elements. It is necessary to maintain a proper balance between the three main food elements, for an excess of protein causes the stool to become alkaline, offensive and more formed; while an excess of either fat or sugar gives rise to frequent and loose acid stools, i.e. fermentative stools. In the case of the low-weight baby a fermentative stool is practically always due to fat intolerance, the stool containing undigested compressible fat curds; and the condition should be treated by reducing the fat and increasing the sugar in the feed. Because of the necessity for keeping the fat content low, the sugar content must be kept high if the balance is to be kept between the protein on one hand, and the sugar and fat on the other.

Concentration of formula. Pre-term babies will usually gain satisfactorily if they reach a daily intake of 110–130 calories/kg. (50–60 calories/lb.) and a daily fluid intake of 165–200 ml./kg. ($2\frac{1}{2}$–3 oz./lb.) during the second week of life; and these calorie and fluid requirements are met if the formula contains 70 calories to 100 ml. (20 calories to 1 oz.).

When calculating the requirements of light-for-dates babies (malnourished group), the expected weight for their gestational age must be used, to give them the extra calories and fluid that they require.

During recent years there have been several trials with more concentrated formulae. Keitel and Chu (1965) and Frears (1968) obtained faster gains in weight with mixtures containing 30–34 calories/oz.; but other investigators have shown that early feeding with concentrated cow's milk formulae can lead to hypocalcaemia (Pugh, 1968), hypernatraemia (Skinner, 1967) and even to intestinal obstruction with milk curds (Cook and Rickham, 1969). On the other hand, unduly diluted mixtures lead to poor weight gain and hyponatraemia (Skinner, 1967).

Human milk provides 70 calories/100 ml. (20 calories/oz.) and it would seem sensible to use this concentration for cow's milk mixtures unless there is any good reason for reducing or increasing the fluid intake.

Modification of cow's milk. The various modifications of cow's milk are set out and their use discussed in regard to the feeding of low-weight babies. All the mixtures suggested supply more than 2 g. and less than 6 g. of protein/kg./day if 165–200 ml./kg./day ($2\frac{1}{2}$–3 oz/lb./day) of the mixture are given. If necessary the mixtures can be diluted with

10% glucose during the first few days of life, but the full strength mixture should be given by the seventh day in order to supply the necessary calories.

Half-skimmed dried milks. Examples are National half-cream dried milk, and Cow & Gate special half-cream milk food. These milks are useful for routine milk feeding of low-weight babies. Half-skimmed dried milks are available in most countries, and a suitable low-fat, high-protein, high-sugar mixture can be obtained by the simple addition of water and sugar. Dried milk is easy to keep in households with poor facilities for storage and no facilities for refrigeration.

The following table shows a mixture which can be used for low-weight infants if human milk is not available.

	Half-skimmed dried milk powder	10 g. milk powder and 6 g. sugar in 100 ml. water (1 measure powder in 1¼ oz. water and 1 level teaspoon (3·4 g.) sugar to 2 oz. of mixture).
	%	%
Protein	30	3·0
Fat	17	1·7
Carbohydrate ..	44	10·4
Calories/oz. ..	130	20
Calories/100 g. ..	450	70

Half-skimmed evaporated milk. (An example is Regal half-skimmed evaporated milk.) This milk is useful for routine cow's milk

	Undiluted half-skimmed evaporated milk	1 part milk to 1½ parts water (1 in 2½) with 1 level teaspoon (3·4 g.) sugar to 4 oz. mixture (3 g. sugar to 100 ml.)
	%	%
Protein	8·2	3·3
Fat	4·65	1·9
Carbohydrate ..	12·0	7·8
Calories/oz. ..	40	20
Calories/100 g. ..	45	70

feeding of low-weight babies when human milk is not available. For use during travel it is more bulky than the dried half-skimmed milk but, for home use, the evaporated milk has the advantage that a tin of evaporated milk is used more quickly than a packet of dried milk and therefore has less opportunity to become contaminated.

Full-cream dried milks. (Examples are the full-cream varieties of National dried milk, Cow & Gate and Ostermilk No. 2.)

These milks are not so useful during the first few months of life, during which time the low-weight infant requires much protein but can digest only a limited amount of fat. They become useful after the infant's capacity for dealing with fat has improved, and when there is less need for protein. As a general rule low-weight infants should be changed over on to full-cream mixtures at the "corrected age" of 4 weeks (4 weeks after their *expected* date of delivery). By this time, if they have gained well, they should have reached the average weight of a term baby aged 1 month (i.e. 8 lb. or 3,630 g.).

At first, a 1 in 10 dilution (with added sugar) is gradually introduced and later, when the child reaches the "corrected age" of 3 months, a 1 in 8 dilution (reconstituted cow's milk) may be given. The composition of these formulae is shown in the following table.

	Full-cream dried powder	10 g. powder and 4 g. sugar in 100 ml. water. (1 measure powder in 1¼ oz. water and 1 teaspoon sugar to 3 oz. of mixture)	12½ g. powder in 100 ml. water. (1 measure powder in 1 oz. water)
	%	%	%
Protein ..	26	2·6	3·2
Fat	26	2·6	3·2
Carbohydrate	38	7·8	4·8
Calories/oz. ..	146	20	19
Calories/100 g.	520	68	65

When changing from one type of food to another, start by giving three parts of the old food and one of the new on the first day, equal parts on the second day, one part of the old to three of the new on the third day, and entirely the new food on the fourth day. If the new food is not well tolerated, the change-over may have to be accomplished more gradually than this.

Full-cream evaporated milks. (Examples are Regal, Ideal and Carnation full-cream evaporated milks.) These may be used as an alternative to full-cream dried milks, after the first few months of life; a 1 in 3½ mixture being introduced at the "corrected age" of 1 month and a 1 in 2½ mixture at the "corrected age" of 3 months. The following table shows the composition of these formulae.

	Undiluted evaporated milk	1 part milk to 2½ of water (1 in 3½) with 1 teaspoon sugar to 3 oz. mixture (4 g. sugar in 100 ml.)	1 part milk to 1½ parts water (1 in 2½)
	%	%	%
Protein ..	8·2	2·3	3·3
Fat	9·14	2·6	3·6
Carbohydrate	12·0	7·4	6·5
Calories/oz. ..	53	20	21
Calories/100 g.	192	70	77

Full cream dried milk with added lactose. Ostermilk No. 1 is an example. It may be used as an alternative to unmodified full-cream dried milks, but is not recommended for *young* low-weight babies who can only digest limited amount of fat. At the "corrected age" of 1 month, a 1 in 7 mixture may be used, and no additional sugar is required. The table below shows the composition of this formula.

Ostermilk No. 1	Dried powder	14 g. powder in 100 ml. water (2 measure powder in 1¼ oz. water) (1 in 7)
	%	%
Protein	18·1	2·6
Fat	19·0	2·7
Carbohydrates	56·0	8·0
Calories/oz.	134	19
Calories/100 g.	460	66

Dried milks with some reduction of fat. Examples are Trufood half-cream and Cow & Gate half-cream (*not* Cow & Gate *special* half-cream which is half-skimmed milk and is considered in a former section). Both of these milks are badly named because neither is true *half-skimmed* milk.

These milks may be used from the first few days of life for the larger infants who have lower protein requirements (infants over 4 lb. at birth), a 1 in 8 mixture with added sugar being used as a substitute for undiluted breast milk. They are usually more expensive to use than true half-cream milks and have the disadvantage of having a higher fat content in relation to the protein.

	Trufood half-cream		Cow & Gate half-cream	
	Powder	$12\frac{1}{2}$ g. powder to 100 ml. water. (1 oz. powder to 8 oz. water, and 1 teaspoon sugar to 3 oz. of mixture)	Powder	$12\frac{1}{2}$ g. powder to 100 ml. water. (1 oz. powder to 8 oz. water, and 1 teaspoon sugar to 4 oz. of mixture)
	%	%	%	%
Protein ..	21·5	2·7	19·5	2·4
Fat	14·5	1·8	15·5	1·9
Carbohydrate	54·4	10·8	57·0	10·1
Calories/oz. ..	126	21	130	20
Calories/100 g.	444	71	458	69

S-M-A (Scientific Milk Adaptation). This milk contains the same proportions of protein (including sulphur-containing amino-acids essential to growth), fat (saturated and unsaturated), and carbohydrate (lactose only) as in human milk. It is supplied either as a powder or as a liquid.

	Powder		Liquid	
S-M-A		$13\frac{1}{2}$ g. powder to 100 ml. water (1 oz. powder in $7\frac{1}{2}$ oz. water)		Equal parts of liquid S-M-A and water
	%	%	%	%
Protein ..	11·25	1·5	3·0	1·5
Fat	26·25	3·5	7·0	3·5
Carbohydrate	52·25	7·0	14·0	7·0
Calories/oz. ..	150	20	40	20
Calories/100 g.	500	67	134	67

This milk is suitable for feeding low-weight babies when human milk is not available. The following table shows the composition and the mixtures to be used.

Modified dried milks with added fat and lactose. Examples are the "humanized" varieties of Trufood and Cow & Gate.

Both these milks contain protein, fat and carbohydrate in proportions similar to human milk. In humanized Trufood the protein has been modified so as to provide the same proportions of casein and soluble protein as in human milk.

As the fat content in both these milks is high and unmodified (unlike S-M-A.), they should not be used for small pre-term infants during the first few weeks of life. The following table shows the composition of these milks.

	Humanized Trufood		Humanized Cow & Gate	
	Powder	12·5 g. powder in 100 ml. water (1 measure powder in 1 oz. water)	Powder	12·5 g. powder in 100 ml. water (1 measure powder in 1 oz. water)
	%	%	%	%
Protein ..	14·5	1·8 {Casein 0·7; Soluble protein 1·1}	15·5	1·9 (unmodified)
Fat	24·0	3·0	26·0	3·3
Carbohydrate	53·1	6·6	52·0	6·5
Calories/oz. ..	142	18	147	18
Calories/100 g.	500	62·5	510	65

Sweetened condensed milk. This is a full-cream milk and therefore unsuitable for pre-term infants during the early weeks of life. Unfortunately the sugar content is too high to make it a good food even after this age.

Fresh cow's milk. Because the protein of evaporated and dried milks is so much more digestible and, in addition, these milks are so much easier to keep in the average household, the author never recommends fresh milk for the feeding of low-weight babies.

If fresh milk is used it should be half-skimmed; sugar must be added (1 drachm to 2 oz. or 6 g. to 100 ml.) and the mixture heat-treated (boiled or pasteurized). Such a feed is equivalent to a 1 in 8 dilution of half-cream dried milk. At the "corrected age" of 2 months, when fat is tolerated better, a suitable mixture is three parts of whole milk to one part of water, with the addition of 1 drachm of sugar to every 3 oz. of the mixture (4 g. to 100 ml.). This mixture may be replaced by undiluted cow's milk at the "corrected age" of 3 months.

Acidified milks. It has been suggested that acid milk might be the best food for low-weight babies because the acid aids the digestion of casein curd. The low-weight baby digests the curd of heat-treated cow's milk (dried, evaporated, pasteurized or boiled) with such ease that there is no need for acid milks. Goldman *et al.* (1961) fed small pre-term infants (weighing less than 1,800 g.) on lactic acid milk and stated that it was inferior to non-acid milks and caused metabolic acidosis. Ungari *et al.* (1965) also found that acidified milk induced acidosis and had no advantage over non-acidified milk.

Vitamins

Extra vitamins must be given to all low-weight babies, whether they are breast fed or artificially fed, because their requirements are great and their stores low.

Vitamins A and D. The need for vitamin D is especially great (see section on rickets, p. 211). The need for vitamin A is also great, because it affects metabolism, development and maturation of epithelial cells and bone growth. In low-weight babies the liver store of vitamin A is low, low-fat formulae provide little of this vitamin and defective absorption of the fat reduces still further the amount available.

Administration of a water-miscible preparation of vitamins A and D may be started at the age of 1 week (800 i.u. of vitamin D and 4,000 i.u. of vitamin A daily). Oily solutions should be avoided because of the danger of aspiration.

These water miscible vitamins are given immediately before (or in) one of the feeds because of the increased effect of vitamin D when given with milk (Supplee *et al.*, 1936).

Vitamin B. Little is known as regards the requirements of a low-weight baby for the various factors of the vitamin B complex. Litchfield *et al.* (1939), reported an improvement in the rate of gain of weight after the use of vitamin B concentrates. Vitamin B is normally present in both human and cow's milk, but it is likely that some loss occurs during the preparation of the feeds, especially if milk is sterilized by autoclaving.

At least three factors in vitamin B complex are concerned in the metabolism of carbohydrates, and protein combustion probably also requires their presence. The use of a high-carbohydrate low-fat diet may require higher intakes of thiamine. In addition, a deficiency in any single factor may cause failure to grow.

The administration of a vitamin B complex (alone or in combination with other vitamins) should start at the age of 2 weeks and be continued until the weight of 8 lb. (3,640 g.) is reached. The National Academy of Sciences, U.S.A. (1954) recommended the following daily dosage for term infants aged 1–3 months: thiamine 0·3 mg., riboflavine 0·4 mg. and nicotinic acid 3·0 mg. The requirements of a low-weight baby are probably greater than those of a healthy term baby.

Vitamin C. Toverud (1935) showed that the ascorbic acid content of the liver of pre-term infants, at or shortly after birth, was lower than that of term infants. In addition, pre-term infants have a special need for vitamin C in order to complete the metabolism of aromatic amino-acids. The need for vitamin C is also increased during infections, to which all low-weight infants are extremely prone. As vitamin C is not synthesized in the body, it must be supplied in the diet. A daily dose of 40–50 mg. is therefore suggested for an infant fed on breast milk and possibly more if fed on a high-protein mixture.

An ounce of average orange juice is equivalent to approximately 30 mg., and the Government concentrated orange juice contains 60 mg. in 1 oz. (30 ml.). Because of the large quantity involved the total daily dose cannot be given in this form, and synthetic preparations must be employed. The administration of vitamin C should commence at the age of 1 week.

Vitamin E. The requirements of vitamin E are not known but low-weight babies are known to be deficient in this vitamin (Gordon and Nitowsky, 1956). Chadd (1970) found that small pre-term infants were born with low vitamin E levels, and that some developed progressive anaemia, oedema and a typical blood film showing vitamin E deficient erythrocytes. He recommended the administration of vitamin E to all very small pre-term infants.

Vitamin K. The administration of this vitamin is discussed in the section on haemorrhagic disease (p. 181).

Administration of vitamins. All low-weight infants in the care of the author received a small daily dose of Protovite (Roche) from the age of 1 week and the dose was increased each day until they were receiving 0·8 ml. daily from the 14th day of life. This dose supplied 4,000 i.u. vitamin A, 800 i.u. vitamin D, 40 mg. vitamin C, 1·6 mg. thiamine, 0·8 mg. riboflavine, 8·0 mg. nicotinic acid and 2·4 mg. vitamin E. When the child reached the weight of 4½ lb. (2,040 g.), small doses of diluted orange juice were started. Infants were sent home on Protovite and orange juice. On reaching the weight of 8 lb. (3,630 g.) the infant was changed from Protovite to a daily dose of 1 drachm of Government cod liver oil which supplies 700–800 i.u. vitamin D and 3,500–4,000 i.u. vitamin A.

Larger doses of vitamin D are not required (see p. 212) and the possibility of the development of hypercalcaemia from over-dosage is always present. If a dried milk formula is being used, it should be remembered that dried milks usually contain added vitamin D.

Mineral Salts

Iron. Attention should be given to the supply of iron to low-weight babies, because of their deficient stores at birth and their relatively greater growth after birth. The position as regards the prevention of anaemia by the administration of iron is discussed in the section on anaemia (see p. 203). No useful purpose is served by giving iron before the age of 4–6 weeks.

Sodium and chloride. Owing to the low mineral clearance of immature kidneys, especially in regard to sodium and chlorides, great care must be exercised in the administration of saline to pre-term babies (see sections on oedema, p. 228 and infective diarrhoea, p. 156).

Preparation of Formulae

A chapter on the management of feeding would not be complete without some reference to the preparation of the formulae.

Owing to the extreme liability of the low-weight baby to infection, scrupulous care must be taken in the preparation, storage and administration of formulae.

Formulae can be prepared in the central milk kitchen of the hospital to which the special baby care unit is attached or prepared "ready-to-use" sterile feeds (now obtainable from certain firms manufacturing baby foods) may be used; or the formulae can be made up in a special milk-kitchen in the unit itself.

If formulae are prepared in the unit, the nurse preparing the formulae should ideally take no part in the general nursing of the infant. Unfortunately this is rarely possible but it can generally be arranged that the nurse who prepares the formulae does not change napkins. If it is ever necessary for the same nurse to do both, then formulae should be prepared at the beginning of a duty period before the infants are handled.

When preparing formulae the nurse should wear a gown, cap and mask and, if she is also responsible for changing babies, she should wear gloves during the preparation of formulae at all times except at the beginning of a duty period before she has done any changing.

Because of the relatively weak digestive powers of the pre-term baby, it is most essential that formulae should be made up accurately. *Domestic spoons should not be used as fluid measures* because there is no universal standard for these (also one domestic tablespoon contains approximately two "fluid tablespoons" of fluid!). Glass measures and measure jugs should be used for measuring fluids. Sugar should be weighed, and dried milk powder either weighed or measured in the scoops provided by the makers of the dried milk concerned; the powder must be pressed down then levelled off with a knife.

Milk kitchen. The room used for the preparation and storage of formulae must not be used for any other purpose.

If possible the room should be divided into two sections by means of a partition in which there is a sliding window or hatchway. One section (Section A) should be used for the reception and washing of used feeding equipment, and the other (Section B) for the sterilization of utensils and the preparation and storage of formulae. (See Fig. 32.)

The minimum equipment of Section A should be a sink and draining board and cupboards for storage; and that of Section B:

Sink and draining board.
Electric kettle or boiling ring.
Sterilizer.
Pasteurizing and cooling apparatus.
Refrigerator.
Cupboards.
Tables.

If it is not possible to divide the room in this way, the washing

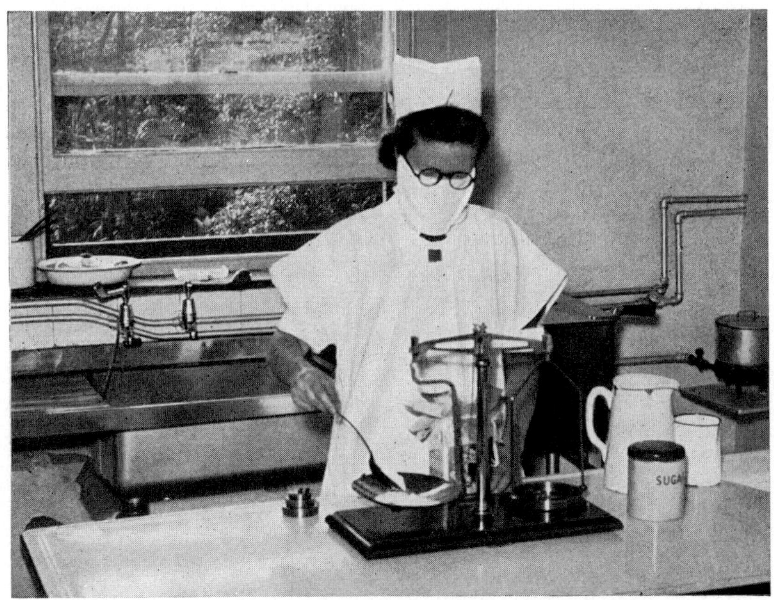

(*Photo by Camera Talks*)

FIG. 32. Milk preparation room Section for milk preparation and storage. The window is protected with fly-proof wire-gauze, and the floor and walls are washable. There are no open shelves. Nurses wear gowns and masks. When preparing formulae for the smaller infants, solids are weighed to ensure accuracy.

of used equipment must be done elsewhere, for example in the ward kitchen, so as to keep the milk kitchen free from contamination.

Nurses working in Section B should wear gown, cap and mask. Any nurse who is changing napkins or looking after infected infants is not allowed to enter this section of the milk kitchen.

Preparation of formulae should be carried out with strict aseptic technique and special precautions are required to avoid contamination of bottle teats. Unless they are sterilized on the bottles with the formulae (terminal sterilization) they must be boiled or autoclaved immediately before use and great care exercised in putting the teats on to the bottles (only the neck of the teat may be touched by the hands). Teats must be protected by sterile caps, cellophane, or gauze before distribution of the formulae.

It has been the practice in many nurseries and homes to use 1 in 80 sodium hypochlorite solution (Milton) for the sterilization of bottles and teats (Cousins, 1947). In 1964 Robson and Anderson suggested that thrush could be spread by teats sterilized with Milton; and recently doubt has been cast on the efficacy of Milton sterilization, after finding *Klebsiella aerogenes, E. Coli and Pseudomonas aeruginosa* in milk feeds and faeces of babies after the use of Milton (Ayliffe *et al.*, 1970). Terminal sterilization or the use of prepared sterile feeds are much safer than the use of Milton.

However, Milton sterilization is still useful in the home if heat sterilization is not possible. Anderson and Gatherer (1970) investigated the standard of home sterilization of bottles and teats, and found that the mothers using the Milton method of sterilization and storage of bottles produced significantly better results than the others.

REFERENCES

ANDERSON, J. A. D. and GATHERER, A. (1970). *Brit. med. J.*, **2,** 20.

ANDERSON, N. A. (1946). "Textbook of Pediatrics", Mitchell-Nelson Saunders, Philadelphia.

AVERY, M. E. (1964). "The Adaptation of the Newborn Infant to Extrauterine Life", p. 60. H. E. Stenfert Kroese. N. V., Leiden.

AYLIFFE, G. A. J., COLLINS, B. J. and PETTIT, F. (1970). *Lancet*, **1,** 559.

BABSON, S. G. and BRAMHALL, J. L. (1969). *J. Pediat.*, **74,** 890.

BARRIE, H. (1968). *Lancet*, **2,** 1158.

BEARD, A. G., PANOS, T. C., MARISIGAN, B. V., EMINIANS, J., KENNEDY, H. F. and LAMB, J. (1966). *J. Pediat.*, **68,** 329.

BLACK, J. (1961). *Arch. Dis. Childh.*, **36,** 633.

Brit. Med. J. (1965), **2,** 6. Leading article.

CHADD, M. A. (1970). Paper presented by title to the 2nd European Congress of Perinatal Medicine. London.

CHURCHILL, J. A. (1963). *Obstet. and Gynec.*, **22,** 601.

COOK, R. C. M. and RICKHAM, P. P. (1969). Paper presented at the 16th International Congress of the British Association of Paediatric Surgeons.

CORNBLATH, M., FORBES, E. A., PILDES, R. S., LUEBBEN, G. and GREENGARD, J. (1966). *Pediatrics*, **38**, 547.
COUSINS, C. M. (1947). *Nursing Mirror*, August 16th.
CROSSE, V. M., HICKMANS, E. M., HOWARTH, B. E. and AUBREY, J. (1954). *Arch. Dis. Childh.*, **29**, 178.
CROSSE, V. M., WALLIS, P. G., LOW, A. and HENLY, A. A. (1960). *Nutrition*, **14**, 65.
DAVIDSON, M., LEVINE, S. Z., BAUER, C. H. and DANN, M. (1967). *J. Pediat.*, **70**, 695.
DAVIES, P. and DAVIS, J. P. (1970). *Lancet*, **2**, 1216.
DEPARTMENT OF HEALTH AND SOCIAL SECURITY (1969). Reports on Public Health and Medical Subjects, No. 120.
DRILLIEN, C. M. (1964). "The Growth and Development of the Prematurely Born Infant". E. and S. Lingstone, Edinburgh.
FREARS, J. F. (1968). *Nutrition*, **22**, 69.
FREEDMAN (1961). New York Premature Study. New York Medical College Department of Psychiatry.
GOLDMAN, H. I., FREUDENTHAL, R., HOLLAND, B. and KARELITZ, S. (1969). *J. Pediat.*, **74**, 881.
GOLDMAN, H. I., KARELITZ, S., SEIFTER, E., ACS. H. and SCHELL, N. B. (1961). *Pediatrics*, **27**, 921.
GONZAGA, A. J., WARREN, R. L. and ROBBINS, F. C. (1963). *Pediatrics*, **32**, 1039.
GORDON, H. H. and MCNAMARA, H. (1941). *Amer. J. Dis. Child.*, **62**, 328.
GORDON, H. H. and NITOWKY, H. M. (1956). *Amer. J. clin. Nutrit.*, **4**, 391.
GRAUEL, E. L. and SYLLM-RAPOPORT, I. (1964). *Ann. Paediat.*, **202**, 332.
HENDRICKS, C. H. (1964). *Obstet. and Gynec.*, **24**, 357.
HESS, J. H. and LUNDEEN, E. C. (1949). "The Premature Infant", 2nd ed., p. 115. Lippincott, Philadelphia.
HOLT, L. E. (1961). "Recent Advances in Human Nutrition". Ed. J. F. Brock. J. & A. Churchill, London.
HOLT, L. E., DAVIES, E. A., HASSELMEYER, E. G. and ADAMS, A. O. (1962). *J. Pediat.*, **61**, 556.
HUBBELL, J. P., DRORBAUGH, J. E., RUDOLPH, A. J., AULD, P. A. M., CHERRY, R. B. and SMITH, I. C. A. (1961). *New Engl. J. Med.*, **265**, 835.
HUGGETT, A. St. G. (1946). *Brit. med. Bull.*, **4**, 196.
KEITEL, H. G. and CHU, E. (1965). *Ped. Clin. N. Amer.*, **12**, 309.
KEITEL, H. G., MENDUKE, H., SMITH, T. and FIORENTINO, T. (1965). *Ped. Clin. N. Amer.*, **12**, 347.
KITCHEN, W. H. (1968). *Aust. paediat. J.*, **4**, 29.
LEAGUE OF NATIONS' TECHNICAL COMMISSION ON NUTRITION (1936).
LEVINE, S. Z. and GORDON, H. H. (1942). *Amer. J. Dis. Child.*, **64**, 297.
LITCHFIELD, H. R., LICHTERMAN, J., KNOLL, J. and KURLAND, I. (1939). *Amer. J. Dis. Child.*, **57**, 546.
LUBCHENCO, L. O., HANSMAN, C., DRESSLER, M. and BOYD, E. (1963). *Pediatrics*, **32**, 793.
MANUAL OF NUTRITION (1955). H.M. Stationery Office, London.
MCCANCE, R. A. (1959). *Arch. Dis. Childh.*, **34**, 361.
NICOLAJ, P. (1958). *Clin. Pediat. Bologna*, **40**, 479.
OMANS, W. B., BARNESS, L. A., ROSE, C. S. and GYÖRGY, P. (1961). *J. Pediat.*, **59**, 951.
OPPÉ, T. E. and REDSTONE, D. (1968). *Lancet*, **1**, 1045.
OSBORN, G. R. (1967). Colloques Internationaux du Centre National de la Recherche Scientifique. No. 169. Paris.

PINCUS, J. B., GITTLEMAN, I. F., SCHMERZLER, E. and BRUNETTI, N. (1962). *Pediatrics*, **39**, 622.

PUGH, R. J. (1968). *Lancet*, **1**, 644.

RABOR, I. F., OH, W., WU, P. Y. K., METCOFF, J., VAUGHAN, M. A. and GABLE, M. (1968). *Pediatrics*, **42**, 261.

ROBSON, A. and ANDERSON, K. (1964). *Med. J. Aust.*, **1**, 519.

ROYCE, S., TEPPER, C., WATSON, W. and DAY, P. (1951). *Pediatrics*, **8**, 79.

SHELLEY, H. J. (1964). *Brit. med. J.*, **1**, 273.

SKINNER, A. L. (1967). *Pediatrics*, **39**, 625.

SMALLPEICE, V. and DAVIES, P. A. (1964). *Proc. roy. Soc. Med.*, **57**, 1173.

SMANGOEN, I. (1957). *J. Trop. Med. Lond.*, **3**, 13.

SNYDERMAN, S. E., BOYER, A., GOGUT, M. D. and HOLT, L. E. Jr. (1969). *J. Pediat.*, **74**, 872.

STIEBELING, H. K. (1939). U.S. Dept. Agric. "Year Book of Agric", 1939, p. 380.

SUPPLEE, G. C., ANSBACHER, S., BENDER, R. C. and FLANIGAN, G. E. (1936). *J. Biol. Chem.*, **114**, 95.

SVIRSKY-GROSS, S. (1958). *Ann. Paediat.*, **190**, 109.

TACKAI, T. and 20 colleagues (1969). *Acta. Paed. Jap. Overseas Ed.*, **11**, 101.

THOMSON, A. M., HYTTEN, F. E. and BILLEWIEZ, W. Z. (1970). *Brit. J. Nutrit.*, **24**, 565.

TISDALL, F. F., WILLARD, A. C. and BELL, M. (Nov., 1941). Mayor's Office, Toronto.

TOVERUD, K. U. (1935). *Arch. Dis. Childh.*, **10**, 313.

UNGARI, S., DONATH, A., ROSSI, E. and MURATT, G. (1965). *Z. Kinderheilk.*, **92**, 55.

U.S.A. NATIONAL ACADEMY OF SCIENCES. National Research Council (1954). Publication 302. Washington, D.C.

USHER, R. and MCLEAN, F. (1969). *J. Pediat.*, **74**, 901.

WAGNER, E. A., KOCH, C. A. and JONES, D. U. (1954). *J. Pediat.*, **45**, 200.

WATNEY, P. J. M., CHANCE, G. W., SCOTT, P. and THOMPSON, J. M. (1971). *Brit. med. J.*, **2**, 432.

WENNBERG, R. P., SCHWARTZ, R. and SWEET, A. Y. (1966). *J. Pediat.*, **68**, 860.

WHARTON, B. A. and BOWER, B. D. (1965). *Lancet*, **2**, 969.

W.H.O. (1968). Technical Report Series, No. 400.

WILCOX, D. A. (1936). *Amer. J. Dis. Child.*, **52**, 848.

WILKINSON, A. W., STEVENS, L. H. and HUGHES, E. A. (1962). *Lancet*, **1**, 983.

WILLIAMS, C. M. (1963). *Med. J. Aust.*, **50**, 698.

WU, P. Y. K., TEILMANN, P., GABLER, M., VAUGHAN, M. and METCOFF, J. (1967). *Pediatrics*, **39**, 733.

CHAPTER 7

COMPLICATIONS LIABLE TO OCCUR IN THE LOW-WEIGHT BABY DURING EARLY LIFE

ANY disorder of early life may occur in the low-weight infant but, because of the physiological and anatomical handicaps associated with early birth and low weight, certain disorders tend to occur more frequently than in the normal term infant. In addition, a pre-term infant is usually more severely affected by any disorder than a term infant.

The following table sets out the chief physiological and anatomical handicaps and the complications to which they predispose. The third column, indicates whether these handicaps are present in pre-term infants or light-for-dates infants or in both.

Handicap	*Possible complication*	*Infants affected*
Respiratory		
Poor lung development Weak respiratory muscles Deficient lung surfactant Decreased lung compliance	Primary and secondary atelectasis, cyanosis and anoxia	Pre-term
Poorly developed respiratory centre	Irregular respiration	Pre-term
Soft thoracic cage	Rib recession	Pre-term
Feeble or absent cough reflex	Aspiration	Pre-term
Cardiac		
Immature conductile tissue	Cardiac irregularity	Pre-term
Digestive		
High requirement of calories, protein, mineral salts and vitamins; and inadequate stores at birth	Liability to deficiency diseases	Both
Poor feeding reflexes	Difficulty in obtaining food	Pre-term
Poor tolerance for fat of cow's milk	Liability to abdominal distension, diarrhoea and vomiting	Pre-term
Poor development of mechanism for closing cardia	Liability to regurgitation	Pre-term
Poor muscular development throughout digestive tract	Liability to abdominal distension and constipation	Pre-term

Cause	Complication	Occurs in
Liver		
Decreased enzyme activity	Poor metabolism of drugs; Hyperbilirubinaemia and kernicterus	Both
Deficient clotting factors	Haemorrhages	Both
Inadequate glycogen stores	Hypoglycaemia	Both
Kidneys		
Poor mineral salt clearance	Oedema	Pre-term
Poor acid-base balance	Acidosis	Pre-term
Poor excretion of drugs	Drug intoxication	Pre-term
Brain		
Poor calcification of skull; Increased capillary fragility	Birth trauma and intracranial haemorrhage	Pre-term
Increased permeability of blood-brain barrier	Kernicterus from jaundice	Pre-term
Eyes		
Immature retina	Retrolental fibroplasia	Pre-term
Regulation of body temperature		
Poor heat production; Excessive heat loss; Poor heat regulating centre	Temperature low and unstable	Pre-term
Inadequate sweating	Easily overheated	Pre-term
Blood		
Immature blood cells; Excess of breakdown over formation of red cells	Anaemia and jaundice	Pre-term
Increased foetal haemoglobin	Poor release of oxygen to tissues	Pre-term
Hypoproteinaemia	Oedema; Kernicterus from unconjugated bilirubin	Pre-term
Antibody formation		
Inadequate transfer of maternal antibodies; Poor manufacture of antibodies; Deficient gamma globulin	Liability to infection	Both
Body water content		
Increased	Dehydration	Pre-term
Subcutaneous fat		
Deficient	Hypothermia	Both
Brown fat		
Deficient	Hypothermia	Pre-term

The greatest causes of early neonatal death among low-weight babies are:

(1) Respiratory distress (primary and secondary atelectasis).
(2) Congenital malformations.
(3) Intracranial birth injury (traumatic and anoxic).
(4) Neonatal infections.

These conditions will be considered first because of their importance.

Respiratory Distress with Atelectasis

The lungs are the least well developed organs in pre-term infants (see p. 4) and respiratory distress has long been recognized as the chief cause of mortality among such babies.

Atelectasis can be divided into:

(1) Primary atelectasis or failure (total or partial) of the lungs to expand after birth.

(2) Secondary (resorption) atelectasis, or collapse after initial expansion.

A certain degree of primary atelectasis is present in all pre-term babies. In the majority, the lungs gradually expand as the condition of the baby improves. As a general rule the lower the gestational age the less readily will the lungs expand. The reasons for this are:

(1) The incomplete development of the lungs.
(2) The weak respiratory muscles and the yielding thoracic cage.
(3) The poorly developed respiratory centre.
(4) The high incidence of damage to the respiratory centre as the result of birth injury or anoxia.

Distress due to primary atelectasis. Severe primary atelectasis is usually due to extreme immaturity of the lungs in infants born before the 28th week and weighing less than 1,000 g.; but it can also occur in conjunction with severe damage to the central nervous system. Infants suffering from severe degrees of primary atelectasis are in poor condition from birth. They lie quietly, making little effort at spontaneous movement; the body temperature tends to be low; the colour is poor; and the cry is feeble. Respirations are rapid, shallow and irregular (unless complicated by cerebral pathology when respirations tend to be slow and gasping); an expiratory grunt is often present and periods of apnoea and cyanosis (grey attacks) are common. The chest movements are feeble; the air entry is poor; and with the occasional deep breath, rib and sternal recession are seen and fine crackling crepitations may be heard at the end of inspiration.

In mild cases, the only sign is shallow breathing, and a mild degree of cyanosis which disappears when the infant cries; but even among such infants cyanotic attacks are easily precipitated by incorrect handling and feeding.

Distress due to secondary (resorption) atelectasis. Atelectasis may be secondary to pulmonary disease, e.g. pneumonia, massive pulmonary haemorrhage, etc.; aspiration of amniotic fluid or meconium; or it may be a complication of such conditions as intracranial oedema or haemorrhage, diaphragmatic hernia or pneumothorax; and in pre-term infants it may be found without any of these complications (idiopathic respiratory distress).

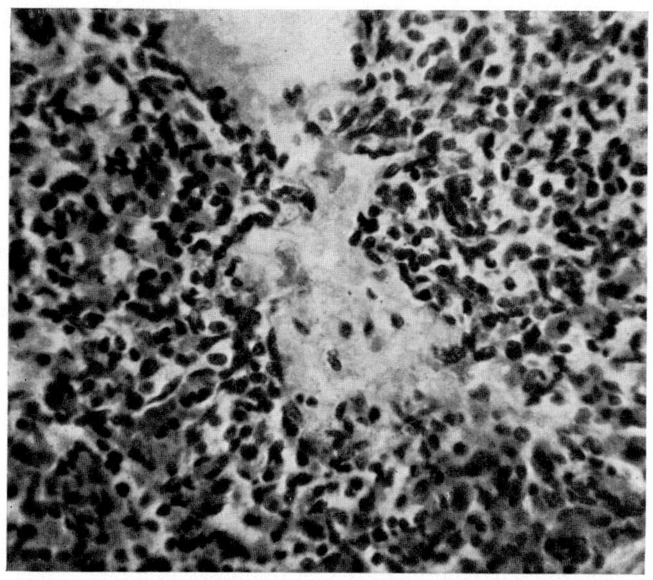

(By courtesy of H. S. Baar)

FIG. 33. Secondary atelectasis with hyaline membranes.

It is often extremely difficult to distinguish between the various causes of secondary atelectasis, especially if the infant is not observed from birth. The difficulties of diagnosis are obvious when one realizes that atelectasis may be secondary to intracranial haemorrhage, and intraventricular haemorrhage is usually the result of anoxia, due to atelectasis; also that pulmonary haemorrhage may be the cause, or the result, of atelectasis.

Conditions requiring surgical treatment such as diaphragmatic hernia and pneumothorax must be excluded by radiological examination. Pneumonia is suspected if there is a history of infected liquor or of a long labour with early rupture of membranes. Meconium aspiration is a possibility if the infant was born in an asphyxiated state, especially if the infant is light-for-dates. Massive pulmonary haemorrhage, which also occurs more often among light-for-dates infants, may be diagnosed if there is bleeding from the respiratory tract. Congenital heart disease can sometimes cause difficulties in diagnosis.

Idiopathic respiratory distress. Because of the difficulty of distinguishing between the various causes of respiratory distress, it was suggested (at the 9th International Paediatric Congress in Montreal, 1959) that the term "idiopathic respiratory distress of the newborn" should be used as a clinical diagnosis to cover respiratory disorders from all causes which cannot be separated off during life.

This condition occurs most frequently among the smallest pre-term infants, the incidence increasing as the gestational age decreases. But it is also seen among larger infants born to mothers suffering from diabetes (Farquhar, 1962) or after maternal antepartum haemorrhage (Cohen *et al.*, 1960; Butler and Alberman, 1969). Infants born by Caesarean section are more prone to this condition (Usher *et al.*, 1964) especially if the section is performed before the onset of labour (Butler and Alberman, 1969).

Some of the infants which develop idiopathic respiratory distress are born with asphyxia; others breathe spontaneously but develop some respiratory distress within a few hours after birth. The first sign is a steadily rising respiration rate with an expiratory grunt (a rate of 65/minute is considered proof of distress). Respirations gradually become more rapid and more laboured with increasing rib and sternal retraction, respiratory flaring of alae nasi and "chin tug": the air entry remains poor in spite of great respiratory effort. At this stage moist sounds are often heard in the lungs and there may be excessive mucus production. Generalized pitting oedema often develops. The baby tends to be restless and often has a whining cry; it becomes progressively more cyanotic as the retraction becomes more severe and periods of apnoea occur. A systolic murmur may be heard, and Burnard (1959) has shown that these babies have an enlargement of the heart which decreases if the baby recovers. The heart rate remains slow in spite of respiratory difficulty; and the blood pressure and body temperature both tend to fall. Signs of cerebral anoxia may develop, the infant becoming quiet, less distressed, hypotonic and unresponsive to stimuli; periods of apnoea become more prolonged and, unless improvement commences, death occurs. The majority of the deaths occur during the first 48 hours of life, and nearly all before 72 hours, unless life has been prolonged artificially by mechanical ventilation.

Signs of improvement are more regular and less laboured breathing with gradual disappearance of cyanosis, an increase in the heart rate and diminution in the size of the heart, an increase in muscle tone and in responsiveness to stimuli, and gradual disappearance of oedema. Recovery is usually complete when it occurs but occasionally, after prolonged use of mechanical ventilation with 80–100% oxygen, the respiratory distress continues for a long time and an autopsy shows a "bronchopulmonary dysplasia" (Northway *et al.*, 1967) which Pusey *et al.* (1969) think is due either to prolonged pressure or oxygen toxicity.

Blystad (1956) and Miller *et al.* (1957) drew attention to the chemical changes in the blood of hypoxic infants i.e., anoxia plus a mixed acidaemia. The pH, arterial Po_2 (Pao_2) and plasma standard bicarbonate levels all fall while the Pco_2 rises. Usher (1961a) found hypoglycaemia and high levels of blood potassium, and noted changes in the E C G when the potassium level rose above 7 mEq./litre. He suggested that distressed infants might die from the side effects of asphyxia rather than from asphyxia itself and thought that correction of the metabolic disturbance could be life-saving in some cases.

The blood pressure is low in infants with respiratory distress, and the heart is enlarged. There is a R → L shunt, largely through the foramen ovale (Stahlman, 1964; Roberton, 1967). The ductus arteriosus plays a minor role in idiopathic respiratory distress (Murdoch *et al.*, 1970), only up to one third of the shunt occurring at this level (Roberton and Dahlenburg, 1969). Chu *et al.* (1967) found a high pulmonary vascular resistance and a low effective pulmonary blood flow.

Measurements of the respiratory function of infants with distress have demonstrated a marked increase in the functional dead space of the lungs and a diminished lung compliance. These conditions increase the work of respiration and death may result from exhaustion and anoxia (Karlberg *et al.*, 1954).

In regard to radiological findings, the lungs have been variously described as having: the appearance of ground glass; miliary mottling; and diffuse reticulogranular images of increased density. The trachea and bronchi are usually clearly outlined giving the effect of an air bronchogram.

In fatal cases of idiopathic respiratory distress, the lungs have a typical microscopic appearance: the bronchioles and alveolar ducts are distended and the alveoli collapsed. Oedema fluid is usually found in the air sacs and intra-alveolar and interstitial haemorrhages are also frequently present. In many cases hyaline membranes are found, i.e. the distended alveolar ducts and bronchioles are irregularly lined with a homogenous eosinophilic material (Fig. 33): but membranes are never found in stillborn infants nor in infants dying under the age of 1 hour.

Pulmonary surfactant (the lipoprotein which normally lines the alveoli and prevents their collapse by reducing surface tension) is deficient or absent (Clements *et al.*, 1958; Avery and Mead, 1959;

Gruenwald, 1964; Adams *et al.*, 1965; Reynolds *et al.*, 1968). Gandi *et al.* (1970) demonstrated the presence of osmophilic granules in the alveolar epithelial cells when surfactant was present but found very few granules in infants dying of idiopathic respiratory distress.

Other lesions, including intraventricular haemorrhage, pulmonary infection, massive pulmonary haemorrhage, cerebral birth trauma and meconium aspiration are often found in association with idiopathic respiratory distress. Fedrick and Butler (1970) found associated lesions in 44% of deaths with hyaline membranes.

Idiopathic respiratory distress is the result of a deficient exchange of gases between the air in the pulmonary alveoli and the arterial blood but the primary cause of this is still unsolved.

The condition is definitely associated with a deficiency of pulmonary surfactant but it is not yet known whether this deficiency is the cause or the result of the disease, or whether the deficiency of surfactant and the disease have a common cause. A deficiency of surfactant leads to alveolar collapse and a high pulmonary resistance and this causes blood to be shunted from the venous to the arterial side (R → L shunt) without passing through aerated alveoli, the major part being shunted through the foramen ovale (Roberton and Dahlenburg, 1969).

Acidosis and anoxia (Chu *et al.*, 1965 and Scarpelli, 1969), also hypothermia (Chu *et al.*, 1965) are all capable of causing vaso-constriction. The local anoxia due to this pulmonary hypo-perfusion may cause direct damage to the alveolar cells which produce the surfactant (Chu *et al.*, 1967), or it can increase the permeability of the pulmonary capillaries, so causing pulmonary oedema which is known to reduce the formation of surfactant (DeSa, 1969). Roberton (1967), stresses the fact the pulmonary surfactant does not appear at a low pH level, i.e. with acidosis.

It is therefore possible that a vicious circle is created, starting with any one of the factors which can cause a high pulmonary resistance and pulmonary hypo-perfusion. Reynolds *et al.* (1968) suggest that idiopathic respiratory distress will arise either because the mechanism for the synthesis of surfactant is too immature to supply the demand for surfactant, or because it has been damaged by asphyxia before, during or immediately after birth, or because of the interaction of these two influences.

Formation of the hyaline membrane is a secondary result of the vascular disturbance. The membrane consists mainly of fibrin (Gitlin and Craig, 1956; Duran-Jorda *et al.*, 1956; Van Breedon *et al.*, 1957; Wade-Evans, 1962; Gajl-Peczalska, 1964) and it is derived from pulmonary oedema fluid which leaks out of the pulmonary capillaries because of pressure changes, or anoxic damage to the capillary walls (Verger *et al.*, 1963). The presence of the membrane reduces still further the exchange of gases. Robertson (1963) found that the membrane increases in thickness until the 3rd or 4th day, while intra-alveolar oedema was marked on the 1st day then decreased. Gandy *et al.* (1970) described an early stage of interstitial oedema and localized areas of necrosis and desquamation of alveolar cells with virtual absence of surfactant granules, then a stage of extensive atelectasis with hyaline membranes in the distended alveolar ducts, and finally repair of the denuded alveolar surface and removal of the membranes.

Studying 923 low-weight babies, the author (Crosse, 1957, 1959a and 1959b) found that the incidence of idiopathic respiratory distress was increased by low birth weight, birth asphyxia and low rectal temperature on admission to the Sorrento unit.

Whatever part other factors play in its causation, idiopathic respiratory distress is closely associated with gestational age, the incidence increasing as the gestational age decreases (Crosse, 1957 and 1959a; Silverman and Silverman, 1958; Avery and Drolette, 1958; Miller, 1962; Dunn, 1965; Miller and Futrakul, 1968; Fedrick and Butler, 1970). This is probably due to certain handicaps due to low gestational age which include the following:

(1) The respiratory handicaps listed at the beginning of this chapter, especially the deficiency of pulmonary surfactant. This first appears in very small amount at about 23 weeks gestation (Reynolds *et al.*, 1965) and the amount increases as the gestational age increases (Reynolds *et al.*, 1968; Gandy *et al.*, 1970).

(2) Increased permeability of the blood capillaries (DeSa, 1967) which increases the liability to pulmonary and generalized oedema.

(3) Poor recovery of plasma proteins by the lymphatics after the normal shift of fluid from the vascular compartment, which may be a factor in causing pulmonary and generalized oedema (Gairdner *et al.*, 1958).

(4) Low serum protein levels (see p. 6) which again increase the liability to oedema.

(5) Inadequate removal of fibrin deposits due to a deficiency of fibrinolysins (Lieberman, 1959; Ambrus *et al.*, 1965).

(6) Greater susceptibility to severe anoxia due to inadequate pulmonary function (Wade-Evans, 1962).

For all these reasons the pre-term infant cannot always cope with the changes which occur after birth. Such complications as birth asphyxia and hypothermia increase the difficulties.

Preventive treatment. Because low gestational age is the greatest cause of both primary atelectasis and idiopathic respiratory distress, preventive treatment consists of reduction in the incidence and degree of curtailed pregnancy (see p. 275). Good prenatal care and care during delivery (see pp. 14 and 16) should also reduce the risk of birth asphyxia which increases the incidence of subsequent respiratory difficulty. Special care must be taken of diabetic mothers, and Caesarean section should never be performed unnecessarily.

Once the baby is born, efficient resuscitation is essential, including aspiration of the stomach in cases likely to develop respiratory trouble, i.e. babies weighing less than 2,000 g. or with a gestational age less than 34 weeks; babies delivered by Caesarean section; and babies of mothers with diabetes or antepartum haemorrhage. Loss of body heat must be avoided.

Curative treatment. In babies with mild degrees of *primary atelectasis* treatment consists of making the baby cry at regular intervals, e.g. by pinching its nose or flicking the soles of its feet.

Severe degrees are treated in the same way as idiopathic respiratory distress.

As *idiopathic respiratory distress* is a self limiting disease, treatment should be aimed at keeping the infant alive until spontaneous recovery occurs; and this is best done by breaking the vicious circle of hypoxia → falling pH → increased pulmonary vascular resistance → increased R to L shunt → increased hypoxia.

Treatment includes:

(1) General measures.
(2) Careful administration of oxygen.
(3) Correction of abnormal biochemistry.
(4) Maintenance of respiration.
(5) Maintenance of circulation.
(6) Prevention and treatment of infection.
(7) Careful feeding.
(8) Other suggested forms of treatment.

General measures. These infants require skilled nursing by specially trained and experienced nurses.

A distressed infant must be kept in thermal balance (see p. 61) in order to minimize its oxygen requirements and also because hypothermia increases hypoperfusion of the lungs by causing vasoconstriction (Chu *et al.*, 1965). Unless the infant's temperature can be monitored, a relatively high humidity helps to keep the infant warm. The infant should be nursed naked in an incubator if possible because clothing hampers respiration and also prevents good observation of the respiratory movements.

In many cases the infant improves if placed in the prone position for regular periods, especially if much mucus is being produced. Kravitz *et al.* (1958) and Bruns *et al.* (1961) reported higher respiration rates and less periodic breathing in the prone position; and Bruns and his collaborators found an increased ventilation among distressed babies nursed in the prone position. When nursed on the back, Rossier (1953) suggested that the chest should be raised by placing a folded towel under the shoulders: this allows drainage of mucus and also leaves the abdomen at a lower level than the chest, thus avoiding pressure on the diaphragm.

Apart from any necessary changes in position the infant should be disturbed as little as possible and all unnecessary nursing procedures should be avoided.

Because many infants with idiopathic respiratory distress die of intraventricular haemorrhage, the coagulation status should be assessed by means of the Thrombotest. If this is less than 10%, and the administration of 1 mg. vitamin K_1 fails to correct this deficiency, fresh frozen plasma can be tried (Gray *et al.*, 1968).

A radiological examination can be made in the incubator, with a portable apparatus with minimal time exposure. A distressed infant should not be taken out of its incubator for this examination. A radiological examination will help in prognosis (see later) as well as excluding conditions requiring surgical treatment.

Careful administration of oxygen. Sufficient oxygen must be given to prevent cerebral damage from hypoxia, but an excess of oxygen given to a baby with a gestational age less than 34 weeks can cause retrolental fibroplasia (R L F) and possibly broncho-pulmonary dysplasia. There is no reliable clinical guide to hypoxia as cyanosis only appears when the Pao_2 is unsatisfactorily low, especially in the smaller pre-term babies with a high proportion of foetal haemoglobin. Small babies have thin skins and may appear to be better oxygenated that they are, when nursed in a high oxygen environment. There is also no clinical method of determining an excessively high Pao_2.

Pure oxygen can be safely used for short periods to resuscitate infants from cyanotic attacks, provided the concentration is reduced immediately to 30%, or less, on their recovery. If more than 30% is required for a long period for infants with a gestational age less than 34 weeks, special precautions must be taken to avoid R L F (see p. 206).

Direct measurement of the Pao_2 is the most reliable guide to the safe administration of oxygen. The environmental concentration of oxygen must be noted at the time of taking the blood, to enable the concentration of the inspired oxygen to be suitably adjusted. The Pao_2 should be kept at 90–100 mm. Hg which is approximately the maximum level found in the newborn (Gupta, 1965). The temporal, radial, brachial or tibial arteries can be used for blood sampling, but if the infant is seriously ill it is probably better to introduce an indwelling catheter into the umbilical artery so that frequent blood samples can be obtained without undue disturbance of the infant. After recutting and sterilizing the umbilical stump a FG5 polyvinyl catheter is inserted into one of the umbilical arteries, up to the depth of about 10 cms. (slightly less in a very small baby) and tied in place with catgut. At the same time a similar catheter is inserted into the umbilical vein for the administration of intravenous fluids (see correction of abnormal biochemistry). The passage of an umbilical arterial catheter requires skill and experience because it can cause a reflex arterial spasm, or lodge in a small artery, causing blanching of the leg with diminished pulses. If this occurs, or if no blood can be withdrawn, the catheter must be removed at once. Thrombi may form but are less likely if a smooth tipped catheter, with a hole at the end only, is used and if the catheter is flushed through with heparinized saline (10 units/ml.) each time it is used. In addition the arterial catheter should be removed as soon as possible after 48 hours. Haemorrhage may occur after removal of the arterial catheter, so it should not be removed for 6 hours after heparin has been used and, before removal, a purse-string suture should be inserted round the catheter. This suture can be pulled tight as the catheter comes out.

If catheterization of the umbilical artery fails, it may be possible to catheterize the radial artery, or to advance the umbilical venous catheter into the right or left atrium (Roberton, 1967).

These methods of control of oxygen can usually only be achieved in an Intensive Care Unit with an adequate number of highly trained nursing and medical staff, available day and night. A unit with no facilities for blood sampling will have to use less precise methods of control, such as finding the minimum percentage of oxygen required to eliminate cyanosis, then adding 25% more if distress is still present, e.g. if cyanosis is eliminated with 60% oxygen, give 75% (Gairdner, 1965). There is, of course, still some risk of hypoxia or hyperoxaemia.

Estimations of the oxygen concentration, near the baby's face, must be made at regular intervals and nurses must be taught to estimate and record the concentration being inspired by the baby and not just the flow in litres per minute; and they should *never* use more than 30% oxygen continuously without medical advice. A simple chemical oxygen analyser is shown in Fig. 34, but the more accurate (and expensive) paramagnetic analysers should be provided in Intensive Care Units. To avoid infection with the squeeze-bulb variety, each incubator should have its own tube for use with the analyser. Some analysers (Fig. 35) are now being provided with a sensor probe to eliminate the squeeze-bulb technique which may be inaccurate if the apparatus is not airtight (Tizard, 1971).

It is difficult to obtain a continuous high concentration of oxygen in an incubator unless a very high flow rate is used, and Gairdner (1965) suggested that the oxygen should be delivered into a transparent

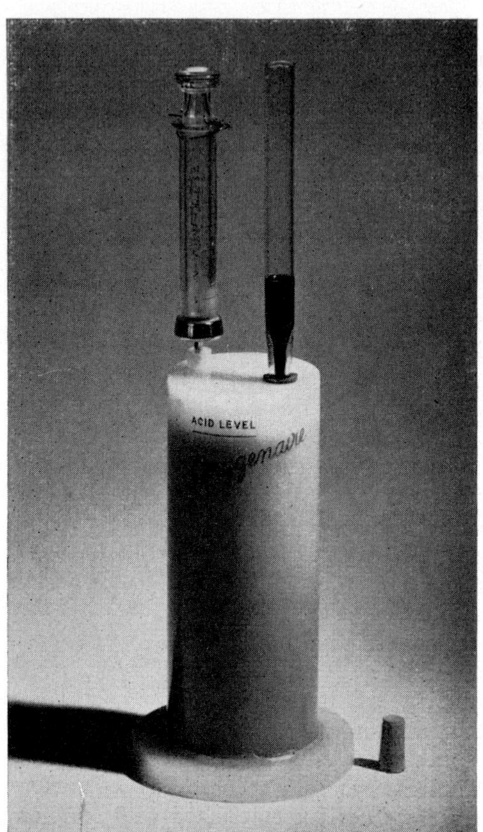

FIG. 34. *Chemical Oxygen Analyser.*

plastic box (Gairdner head box) placed over the head of the infant (Fig. 36). This allows a high concentration to be given with a relatively low flow rate. A short period of 100% oxygen (e.g. to resuscitate a baby with a cyanotic attack) is best given by means of a small soft rubber face mask. The rubber face mask or the Gairdner head box can also be used for giving oxygen to infants nursed in cots.

Oxygen must always be warmed and humidified before administration by face mask or head box and this is most simply done by passing the oxygen through a Wolff's bottle containing sterile hot water.

Correction of abnormal biochemistry. Usher (1959) first suggested the use of intravenous sodium bicarbonate and glucose for correction of the acidosis which usually occurs with respiratory distress, and the principle

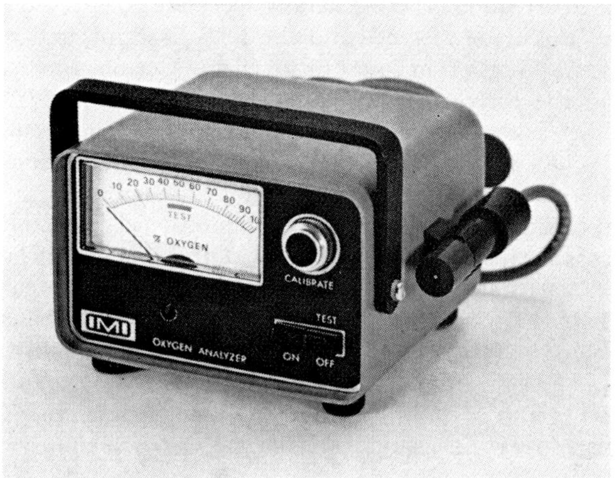

(*Photograph by courtesy of Becton, Dickinson U.K. Ltd.*)

FIG. 35. *Portable Oxygen Analyser*. An immediate reading is obtained by placing the sensor probe in the environment to be tested.

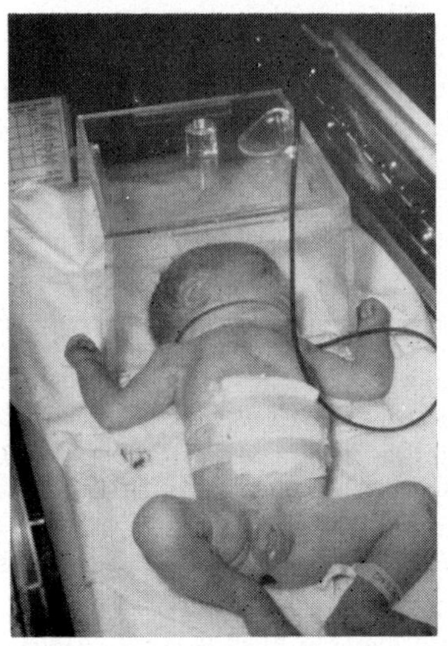

(*Photograph by courtesy of Dr Douglas Gairdner*)

FIG. 36. *The Gairdner Head Box.*

of acid-base correction is now generally accepted. Alkalis can reduce the pulmonary vascular resistance and the R → L shunt, and so increase the Pa_{O_2} level (Gupta *et al.*, 1967; Russell and Cotton, 1968), especially if given in the early stages of the disease (Usher, 1963). There is evidence that a low pH inhibits the production of surfactant and that untreated acidosis leads to hyperkalaemia. The administration of glucose reduces the risk of brain damage from hypoglycaemia.

Arterial blood is obtained from the umbilical arterial catheter, if one has been passed for estimating the Pa_{O_2}. Otherwise it can be obtained from the radial, brachial or tibial artery at the same time as taking blood for the Pa_{O_2}. The pH, P_{CO_2}, plasma standard bicarbonate, blood glucose, blood potassium and blood calcium levels should all be estimated. The first three can be rapidly measured with an Astrup micro-apparatus (Astrup *et al.*, 1960), and the blood sugar with Dextrostix enzyme test strips. As a guide, the normal values for pre-term infants should be approximately: pH 7·3–7·4; P_{CO_2} 15–30 mm. Hg. (Gupta, 1965); bicarbonate level 19 mEq/litre or more; blood glucose level 20–30 mg./100 ml. (Schiff, 1967) and serum potassium level 4–5 mEq/litre.

If the pH is less than 7·3, the P_{CO_2} is above 70 mm. Hg. and the plasma bicarbonate is less than 18 mEq/litre, treatment is definitely indicated. Sodium bicarbonate is most generally used to correct the acidosis and the amount given depends on the level of the pH. Scopes (1970) suggests the following dosage based on pH findings:

pH finding	Dose of sodium bicarbonate
Less than 7·0	8 mEq/kg. as an 8·4% solution (1 mEq in 1 ml.)
7·0–7·1	6 "
7·1–7·2	4 "
7·2–7·3	2 "

Usually half the dose of bicarbonate is given into the umbilical vein fairly rapidly, and the rest is given in a glucose drip (10% glucose in water) into the umbilical vein at the rate of 65 ml./kg./24 hours. The use of the umbilical vein carries very little risk and causes the least disturbance to the infant. In severe cases, further doses of bicarbonate may be necessary (controlled by frequent estimations of the pH and blood gases). A large dose of alkali can cause quite dramatic changes in the shunt and in the Pa_{O_2} level so it is important to monitor the blood gases in addition to the pH in order that the oxygen concentration can be reduced as the condition of the infant improves and the Pa_{O_2} rises.

At first frequent blood sampling may be necessary but, after the pH has risen to 7·25–7·35 and the Pa_{O_2} to 80–100 mm. Hg., and the P_{CO_2} has come down to a reasonably normal level (15–30 mm. Hg.) and all these levels have remained steady for 24–48 hours, sampling may be less frequent and its purpose is then mainly to allow adjustment of the oxygen concentration so as to avoid an excessive administration as the infant's condition improves.

All this blood sampling will exsanguinate the infant unless accurate ultramicro-methods are used and Schiff (1967) suggests the use of an accurate non-wettable plastic semi-automatic pipette by Sanz (1957) and a Beckman Spinco Spectrophotometer to achieve this. The amount of blood taken must be carefully recorded and if a total of more than 1% of the infant's body weight in blood is removed (i.e. more than 20 ml. from a 2,000 g. infant) a top-up transfusion should be given (Roberton, 1967).

Some paediatricians prefer to use THAM (Tris-hydroxy-methyl-aminomethane) in severe cases because of its greater alkalinity and ability to lower the P_{CO_2}. Behrman (1970) recommends the use of THAM (0·3 M. in 5% glucose) if the pH is less than 7·1, then bicarbonate when the pH reaches 7·15. Gupta *et al.* (1967) consider THAM particularly useful if given at an early stage in a severe case. Because THAM is strongly alkaline, an unbuffered solution cannot be given into a small peripheral vein. It sometimes induces apnoea and, in addition, the calculation of the amount required is difficult. So far THAM has failed to show sufficient advantage over bicarbonate to justify the extra risks from its use.

If severe hyperkalaemia is present before treatment has commenced (e.g. in a baby admitted in the later stages of the disease) 20% glucose with one unit of insulin to every 3 g. of glucose (Usher, 1961b) or 20% fructose (Hutchison *et al.*, 1964) should be given before starting the administration of alkalis. Fructose is non-irritating to veins and can be metabolized independently of insulin so replenishing glycogen stores rapidly (Stuhlfauth, 1958). Hypocalcaemia must be treated when present.

Nurseries unable to carry out these specialized therapeutic and laboratory techniques can use heparinized capillary blood from a heel stab for measurement of the pH if they have an Astrup apparatus (Fig. 37). Severe cases of respiratory distress should be transferred to an Intensive Care Unit but mild cases can be treated with sodium bicarbonate, the dose being calculated from the pH finding (see Scopes' table, p. 138). This can be given over a period of several hours in a 10% glucose drip into the umbilical vein. The pH must be checked regularly and treatment continued until the pH has risen to 7·3 and remained constant for 24 hours. If the condition deteriorates, the infant should be transferred.

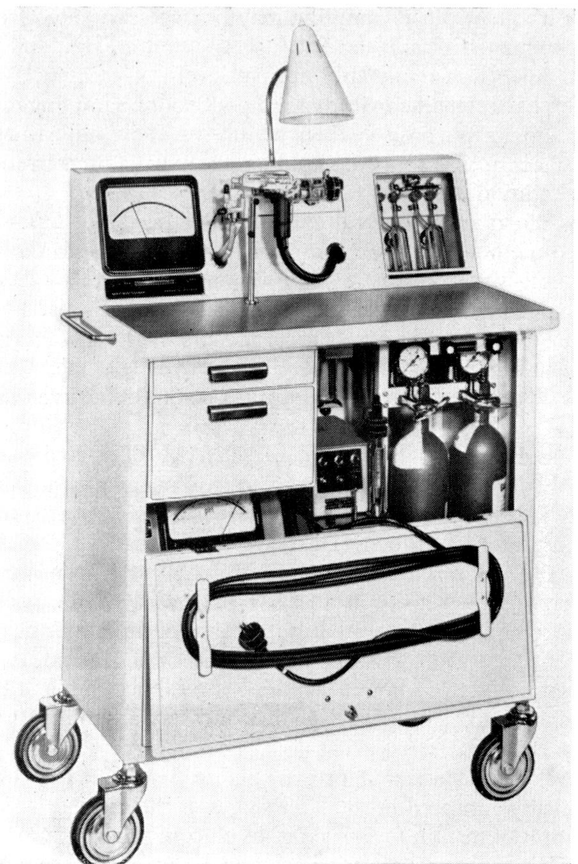

(Photograph by courtesy of Radiometer A/S)

FIG. 37. *Astrup Micro-apparatus.*

Maintenance of respiration. The most important treatment is to keep the airway clear. Infants with respiratory distress are liable to have apnoeic attacks. For this reason it is useful to monitor their respiration. An apnoea monitor warns the nurses when an apnoeic period is sufficiently prolonged to require attention. The monitor can take several forms: the infant may be attached to the control unit by skin electrodes or it may lie on a special mattress (Fig. 38) which is connected to the control unit (Lewin, 1969). More complicated and expensive instruments are available which can monitor the heart rate, and skin or rectal temperature as well as the respiration rate; with warning alarms for apnoea, unduly high or low heart rates and unduly high or low temperatures, e.g. Beckman's Vital Signs Monitor (Fig. 39).

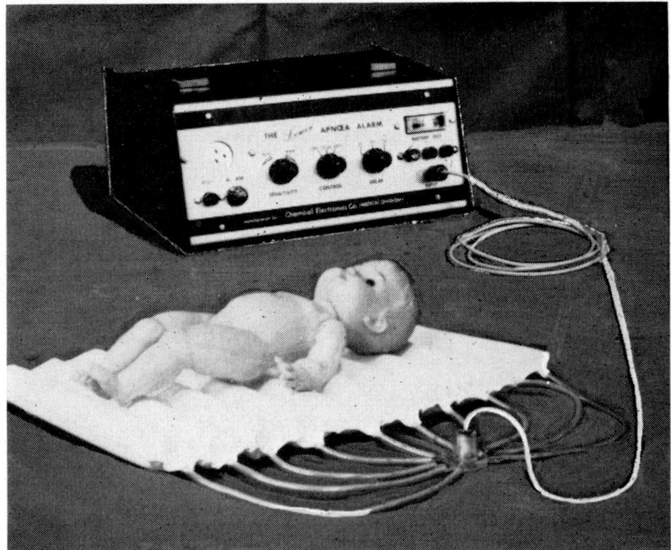

(Photograph by courtesy of Chemical Electronics Co.)

FIG. 38. *Apnoea Mattress.* If the infant stops breathing, the movement of air in the mattress ceases and, after a pre-set time, an alarm is sounded.

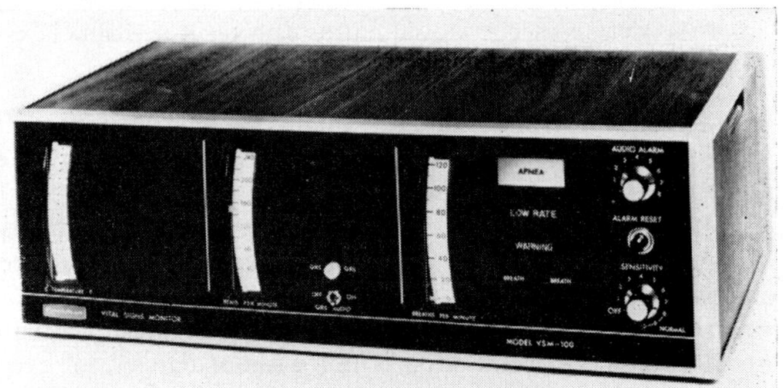

(Photograph by courtesy of Beckman Instruments Ltd.)

FIG. 39. *Beckman Vital Signs Monitor.* This monitors and displays heart rate, temperature and respiration rate; and operates alarms when pre-set limits are exceeded.

In mild cases, during apnoeic periods, respiration can often be recommenced by the simple procedure of bumping the incubator or by clearing the airway with a mucus extractor. If this fails, the chest can be gently arched forward (by a hand placed under the infant's back at chest level) until the spine is well extended. This procedure often provokes an inspiratory effort (see Figs. 40 and 41).

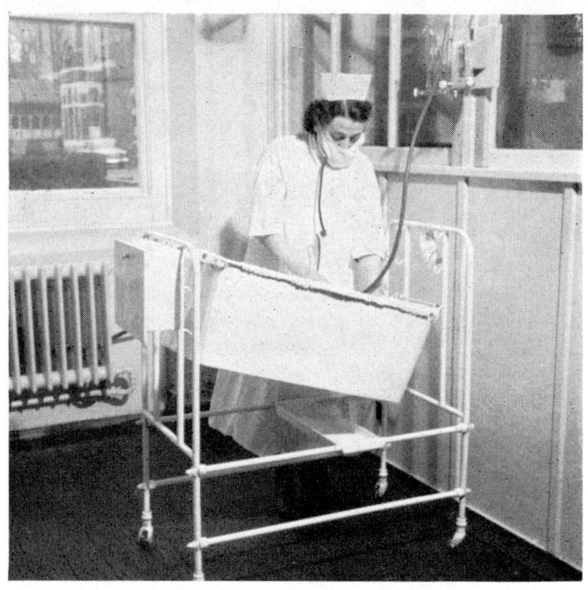

FIG. 40. Resuscitation I. The air passages are cleared with a mucus catheter and oxygen is given by face mask. The head end of the cot is lowered to facilitate clearing of the air passages. A second mucus catheter is available in case the first one becomes blocked.

If these simple methods fail, the infant may be resuscitated with intermittent mask and bag therapy (Gruber and Klaus, 1970) or endotracheal tube and bag ventilation (see p. 25). Facilities for these procedures should always be readily available. A rate of ventilation of about 30–35 per minute, at a pressure of 25–56 cms. H_2O, is recommended with an oxygen flow of 5–8 litres per minute.

If the infant still fails to breathe naturally, mechanical ventilation is indicated. Mechanical ventilation is not without danger so, except in an emergency, no infant should be submitted to this treatment until all other methods have failed. The main indication for its use is severe asphyxia (apnoea, cyanosis, slow heart, loss of tone and reflexes) either (1) on admission or (2) after correcting metabolic acidosis, hypoglycaemia, hypothermia and giving 100% oxygen and, in both cases,

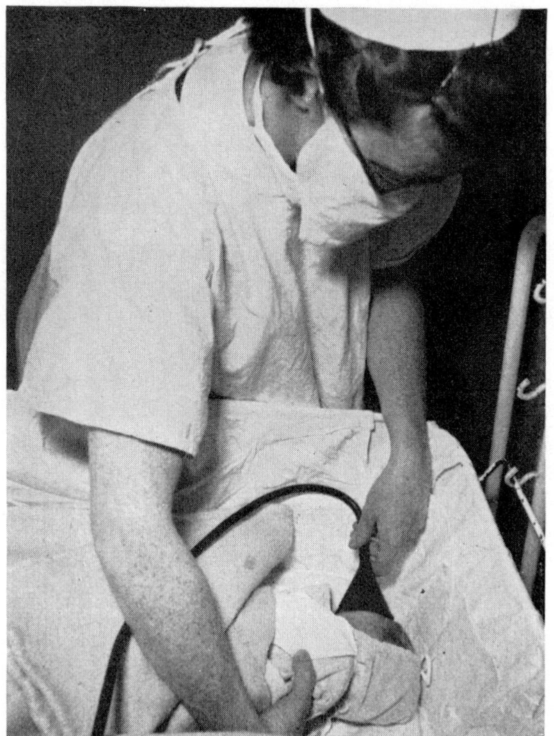

FIG. 41. Resuscitation II. Stimulation of respiration by back-lifting.

after failure to respond to mask and bag ventilation or endotracheal tube and bag ventilation. In such a situation mechanical ventilation may save life. Another indication might be a Pa_{O_2} level less than 70 mm. Hg despite all other efforts: in this case mechanical ventilation might reduce the risk of cerebral damage. An example of a ventilator suitable for low-weight babies is shown in Fig. 42.

The advantages of ventilation are:

(1) Reduction of the Pa_{CO_2} level.
(2) Reduction of the R $\rightarrow$ L shunt (Sinclair *et al.*, 1968).
(3) Increase in pulmonary inflation, blood flow and Pa_{O_2} level.
(4) Sparing the exhausted infant from making further respiratory efforts.

The disadvantages are:

(1) The possibility of infection.
(2) Exsanguination of the infant by frequent blood sampling.

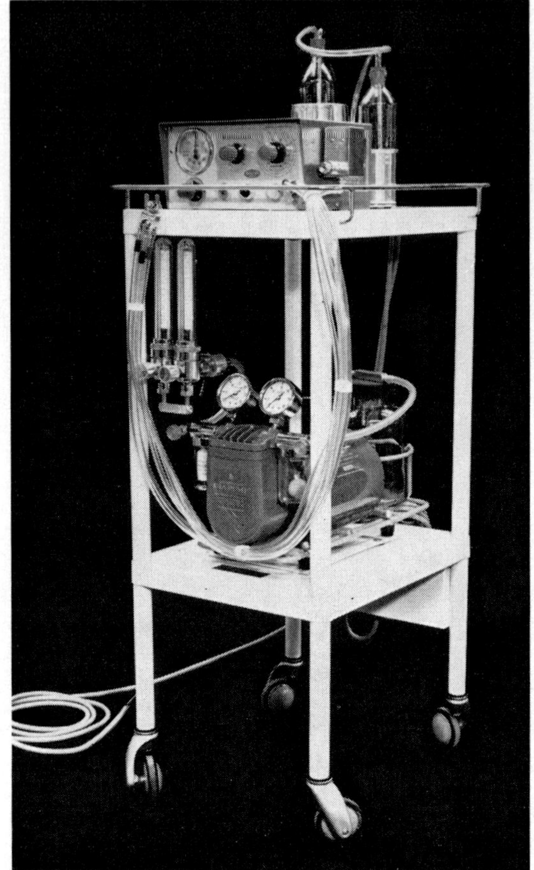

(Photograph by courtesy of Air-Shields (U.K.) Ltd.)

FIG. 42. *Amsterdam Infant Ventilator (G. L. Loos & Co.)*. A ventilator suitable for use with low-weight infants.

(3) Toxic effects of oxygen on the retina (R L F) and on the lungs (broncho-pulmonary dysplasia).

(4) Rupture of the lungs due to the high pressure sometimes required to achieve adequate gas exchange.

(5) The possibilities of cardiac arrest during the introduction of an endotracheal tube, of injury to the trachea by the tube, and of blockage or dislodgment of the tube.

(6) Danger to the eyes and facial skin if a face mask is used.

(7) The equipment is expensive and requires specially trained and experienced nurses to use it.

Both intermittent positive pressure ventilation (Tunstall *et al.*, 1968) and intermittent negative pressure ventilation (Silverman *et al.*, 1967) have been used. Intermittent negative pressure ventilation (I N P V) has less danger than intermittent positive pressure ventilation (I P P V) because neither mask nor endotracheal tube is required. In addition its use so far has been free from injury to the lungs but, unfortunately, these ventilators are difficult to regulate.

At present I P P V is more commonly used and Tunstall *et al.* (1968) and Adamson *et al.* (1968) give good descriptions of the technique of prolonged mechanical ventilation, using a Warne No. 12 endotracheal tube introduced through the nose. Some paediatricians prefer to use an orotracheal tube rather than a nasotracheal one because oral intubation is more easily carried out by the nursing staff who may have to replace tubes when they become blocked or dislodged (Reynolds, 1968; Stoneman and Orme, 1969). Helmrath *et al.* (1970) suggest the use of a face mask instead of an endotracheal tube with I P P V; the advantage being that less secretions are produced, there is no injury to the trachea and a less skilled staff is required. But care must be taken to avoid injury to the eyes and facial skin, and a nasogastric tube is necessary to decompress the stomach.

Whichever method is used, the concentration of oxygen administered must be controlled by the Pao_2 level (regularly monitored) and the oxygen must be warmed and humidified. The airway must be kept clear by suction and, when necessary, bronchial lavage must be performed (with 0·5–1·0 ml. of distilled water). To prevent infection antibiotics should be given (see later). Control of metabolic acidosis, hypoglycaemia and electrolytic disturbances (by intravenous infusions) must be continued. The heart rate and rhythm should be monitored, and it is useful to measure the systolic blood pressure from time to time (see later). Above all, it is extremely important to keep the infant warm and to wean it from the ventilator as soon as possible.

Nurseries without facilities for intensive care should have the necessary equipment for short periods of ventilation by mask and bag, or by endotracheal tube and bag, in case of emergency; but should transfer any baby requiring continuous ventilation to the nearest Intensive Care Unit.

Maintenance of circulation. Anoxia, a low pH and hyperkalaemia can all depress cardiac function. In severe cases of respiratory distress the heart rate and rhythm should be monitored, if possible with an electrocardiographic monitor. The systolic blood pressure is another indication of the condition of the circulation and can be measured with a modification of the two-cuff method (Ashworth *et al.*, 1959).

There is usually no evidence of heart failure until the terminal stages (Keith *et al.*, 1961). If signs of heart failure develop immediate action must be taken. The best cardiac stimulant is respiration, so respiration must be assisted (see previous section). If necessary, external cardiac massage can be used. Compression of the middle portion of the sternum will massage the heart as it rests on the vertebral column (Thaler and Stobre, 1963). If combined with I P P V, pressure over the heart must coincide with expiration; or massage can be alternated with ventilation. Adrenalin may be given intravenously, using 0·5–2 ml. of an adrenalin solution (1 ml. of 1:1,000 adrenalin in 10 ml. normal saline or 10% glucose). As a last resort, an intracardiac injection of 0·2 ml. of 1 in 1,000 solution of adrenalin in 2 ml. normal saline may be given through the fourth intercostal space.

Feeding. It is important to feed the infant as soon as possible in order to reduce the risk of hypoglycaemia, hyperkalaemia and hyperbilirubinaemia. Nasogastric or intravenous feeding is usually necessary. Opinions differ as to the best of these two methods; some believe that the need is for milk and give small frequent feeds (to avoid the risk of vomiting and inhalation) through a fine indwelling nasogastric catheter, while others prefer to give only intravenous glucose during the worst stages of distress, progressing to nasogastric feeding as soon as possible.

Thomas *et al.* (1965) and Jones and Reid (1966) suggest that a gastrostomy might be necessary for babies on I P P V for more than 24 hours, but this has not usually been found necessary.

Prevention and treatment of infection. Because infection may be superimposed on idiopathic respiratory distress, some paediatricians give routine prophylatic antibiotic cover (see p. 176 for antibiotics and dosage). Others prefer to make frequent cultures from blood, nasopharynx, etc., and only treat if infection occurs.

A baby being treated with I P P V is very liable to become infected, so prophylactic antibiotics are usually given in this case, both systemically and into the endotracheal tube. If cultures from the tube show the presence of a resistant organism, the antibiotic is changed to a more suitable one.

Other suggested forms of treatment. Suggested forms of treatment now believed to be of no value include gastric oxygen, hyperbaric oxygen, antihistamines, noradrenalin, acetylcholine, nebulized "Alevaire" and hypothermia.

Further research is required into the use of rocking and electrophrenic stimulation for apnoea; stabilization of the thoracic cage for marked recession; the relative merits of intragastric and intravenous bicarbonate; the effect of early or late tying of the cord on idiopathic respiratory disease; and partial heart-lung by-pass with oxygenated blood.

Records. It is important to keep full records of respiration and heart rates, body temperature, oedema, colour and degree of retraction.

Silverman and Anderson (1956) suggested a method of scoring retraction based on:

(1) Synchronization of respiratory movements of chest and abdomen.
(2) Retraction of lower chest.
(3) Xiphoid retraction.
(4) Dilatation of nares.
(5) Expiratory grunt.

Grade 0 means no difficulty, grade 1 moderate difficulty, and grade 2 maximum difficulty. The retraction score is a sum of these values; thus a total score of 0 indicates no difficulty and 10 maximum difficulty.

The blood chemistry findings must be recorded, with full details of treatment given to correct abnormalities.

The temperature and humidity in the incubator must be recorded; also the percentage of oxygen given, with the length of administration.

Full particulars of the feeding and any other treatment given must be recorded.

Intensive Care Units may also be able to make electrocardiographic records and also records of the systolic blood pressure.

Prognosis. The incidence and mortality decrease with increasing gestational age, and are both slightly less in a female than a male infant of the same gestational age.

Signs of a good prognosis are a high respiratory rate (Roberton *et al.*, 1967; Stoneman and Orme, 1969; Scopes, 1970), moderate recession, limited biochemical changes, little or no cyanosis, and a chest X-ray showing no lung changes or only local changes.

Signs of a bad prognosis are generalized radiological lung changes, cyanosis which cannot be abolished in 30% oxygen, marked biochemical changes, and a slow respiratory rate.

Stoneman and Orme (1969) use the following respiratory efficiency score for assessing the prognosis:

	Score		
	0	1	2
Respiratory rate	0–39	40–89	90+
Colour	Cyanosed in over 80% oxygen	Cyanosed in less than 80% oxygen or not cyanosed in over 80% oxygen	Not cyanosed in less than 80% oxygen
Grunting	Continuous	Intermittent	Absent

The maximum score is 6, and the infants are divided into 3 prognostic groups: 5–6 good prognosis, 3–4 uncertain prognosis and 0–2 bad prognosis.

The Silverman and Anderson retraction score (already mentioned) can also be used for prognostic purposes, the prognosis becoming worse as the score rises.

Roberton (1967) uses the level of the Pa_{O_2}, after breathing 100% oxygen for 15 minutes, as a prognostic index. He states that infants with a level above 100 mm. Hg. have a 10–15% mortality, while those unable to reach this level have a mortality rate of about 80%.

The place of care has a marked effect on the mortality of infants with idiopathic respiratory distress. The best results are obtained in units with Intensive Care Nurseries specially staffed and equipped to undertake the highly specialized treatment required. Usher (1970) has shown that neonatal intensive care for pre-term babies is very effective if begun at birth in a maternity hospital with an Intensive Care Nursery; and not very effective after transfer from another hospital (see p. 36). For this reason every effort must be made to secure delivery of small pre-term infants in maternity hospitals, or departments, with Intensive Care Nurseries.

In regard to late prognosis, there is always a danger of bronchopulmonary dysplasia occurring if an infant has been submitted to prolonged intermittent positive pressure ventilation (see p. 130). Another possibility is neonatal necotizing enterocolitis (see p. 218).

The Late Respiratory Distress Syndrome of Wilson and Mikity

Wilson and Mikity first described this syndrome in 1960. Nearly all the infants affected have weighed less than 1,500 g. and had a gestational age less than 32 weeks (Grossman *et al.*, 1965). Cyanosis and rapid respiration with retraction develop insidiously any time during the first month of life. A chest X-ray shows bilateral interstitial infiltrates and small cyst-like structures giving a honeycomb appearance. Pathological examination shows areas of emphysema and collapse, and interstitial thickening.

If the infant survives, the signs gradually disappear; and Grossman and his colleagues think that the condition is solely due to immaturity, i.e. unduly soft chest wall and air passages.

Congenital Malformations

This is the second greatest cause of early neonatal death among low-weight babies (Butler and Bonham, 1963). The death rate from congenital malformations increases as the gestational age and birth weight decrease, and many of the malformed babies are light-for-dates.

About half of all infants with major malformations are low-weight babies (Potter, 1961; Colman and Rienzo, 1962); and the incidence of chromosomal abnormalities is three or four times higher among light-for-dates babies than among all newborn babies (Sergovich and Leong, 1970). According to Drillien (1970) the incidence of congenital abnormalities increases as the weight for gestational age decreases.

There is evidence of a relationship between maternal diet and malformation (Burke *et al.*, 1943) and the incidence of malformation is influenced by maternal age (greatest over 35), birth order (greatest among first babies) and socio-economic status (greatest among the poorest).

Congenital defects may be inherited by gene transmission (dominant or recessive and sometimes sex-linked); they may be due to chromosomal abnormalities; or they may be caused by prenatal environmental factors. Sometimes there is a combination of causes. Prenatal environmental factors include radiation of the mother with X-rays or radium; virus infections in early pregnancy such as rubella, cytomegalic inclusion disease, etc.; other maternal infections and complications such as toxoplasmosis, antepartum haemorrhage and endocrine disorders; and drugs given to the mother including androgens, thalidomide, anti-folic and anticancer drugs, thiouracil, iodine and iodides, streptomycin, quinine, etc.

Several defects are often present in the same infant, especially if they are the result of prenatal environment.

Prevention. A reduction in congenital malformation would lead to a reduction in the number of low-weight babies, especially those which are light-for-dates.

The prevention of rubella is discussed on p. 176. Vaccination against smallpox during early pregnancy should be avoided unless the mother has been in contact with this disease and is unprotected. Pregnant women should not be exposed to radiation unless absolutely necessary, especially during the first 3 months of pregnancy. An adequate diet (avoiding an excess of any one food) should be ensured. Steroids, hormones and drugs known (or suspected) to be dangerous to the foetus, and all proprietary drugs, should be avoided. Until more is known, it must be assumed that any drug given to a pregnant woman, especially during the first 3 months, may expose the foetus to risk. Careful records should be kept of any drug prescribed, and all malformations reported.

Where there is a family history of congenital malformation, genetic counselling should be available. The prognosis for future babies is worse if the abnormality was genetic in origin than if it was due to prenatal environmental factors.

Diagnosis. Early diagnosis is particularly important for conditions amenable to surgery e.g., tracheo-oesophageal fistula, atresia of the digestive tract and diaphragmatic hernia.

Because low-weight babies are more likely to suffer from congenital defects, they should be examined particularly carefully for such defects as soon as possible after birth; especially if the mother is a diabetic, if there is a family history of malformation, or a history of illness or haemorrhage during early pregnancy, or of hydramnios later. The umbilical cord should be examined carefully at birth, especially in twins (Strong and Corney, 1967), because the presence of only one umbilical artery is frequently associated with congenital malformation. Approximately one-third of infants with one umbilical artery have malformations which are often multiple and severe (Froehlich and Fugikura, 1966; Ainsworth and Davies, 1969). If one defect is found, a careful search must be made to exclude others.

Diaphragmatic hernia should always be considered as a possible cause of asphyxia or dyspnoea at birth, especially if the heart is found on the right side. All babies who continue to be "bubbly" after the first hour (after mucus extraction) should be suspected of having a tracheo-oesophageal fistula until this has been disproved. The passage of catheters into the various orifices can exclude choanal, oesophageal and anal atresias. Intestinal atresia must be excluded (by radiological examination) in all babies who vomit bile. The eyes of all low-weight babies should be examined for cataract before discharge, especially if other defects are present.

Treatment. Curative treatment of malformations is the same for low-weight babies as for babies weighing more than 2,500 g. All babies requiring operative treatment should be dealt with by surgeons who are specially skilled in neonatal surgery, and the babies should continue to be under expert paediatric care.

The need for neonatal surgical units with facilities for intensive care, and the medical and nursing staff requirements for such a unit are set out in "Surgery for the Newborn" (1968), a report from the Ministry of Health and the Scottish Home and Health Department.

Intracranial Birth Injury (Traumatic and Anoxic)

There is a much higher incidence of neonatal death from birth injury and asphyxia among low-weight babies than among babies weighing more than 2,500 g.; and this is the third greatest cause of early death among the low-weight babies (Butler and Bonham, 1963).

Intracranial birth injury and asphyxia associated with intracranial symptoms should be regarded as one syndrome to which prematurity is often a predisposing cause (Parsons, 1944). It is probable that all severe cases of intracranial haemorrhage are fatal, and that the majority of babies who have shown signs of cerebral disturbance and survived have suffered from cerebral anoxia or cerebral oedema.

Intracranial haemorrhage can sometimes be due to haemorrhagic disease, but it is more likely that the presence of this disease only influences the extent of an existing haemorrhage (see p. 181).

Intracranial haemorrhage is a frequent post-mortem finding among low-weight babies: the lower the birth weight the more frequently does intracranial haemorrhage occur.

Subarachnoid and intraventricular haemorrhages occur more frequently in pre-term babies, while subdural haemorrhages and haemorrhages into the brain substance are more common among term and post-term infants. In low-weight infants, intracranial haemorrhages are more often due to asphyxia than trauma. Intraventricular haemorrhage is almost certianly due to asphyxia (either *in utero* or during the neonatal period), the bleeding occurring from the subependymal vessels on the surface of the thalamus and the blood then tracking through to the subarachnoid space and ventricles. Intraventricular and subarachnoid haemorrhages are frequently found in association with pulmonary disease, especially idiopathic respiratory distress (Ahvenainen, 1965; Minkowski, 1965; Butler and Alberman, 1969).

The reasons why pre-term infants are particularly prone to intracranial haemorrhages are:

(1) The fragility of the vascular system, including the intracranial vessels.

(2) Their relatively greater deficiency in blood clotting mechanisms.

(3) Their increased risk of birth trauma: the head is more compressible, and precipitate labour and breech presentations are more frequent in premature labours.

(4) The frequent presence of anoxia due to pulmonary complications.

An infant suffering from severe intracranial injury may be stillborn or born in a state of severe asphyxia from which it never recovers; or respiration is established with difficulty but remains shallow, irregular and slow, or respiratory distress develops. Cyanosis may be constant but more usually it occurs intermittently during periods of apnoea. At first the most severely affected babies are flaccid and apathetic; they make little effort at spontaneous movement; they may be unable to suck; and they have a diminished, or absent, Moro reflex. Less severely affected babies (also the severely affected ones as they show improvement) tend to be wakeful and restless, and to have an anxious expression; their fists tend to be clenched, with the thumbs tucked into the palms of their hands; their legs may be extended with the toes acutely flexed; the neck and spine may be stiff and their general tone increased; and in many cases the Moro reflex is increased. The cry may be feeble and moaning but often the characteristic high-pitched "cranial" cry occurs. The fontanelle may be tense but is rarely bulging (subdural haemorrhage should be suspected if the fontanelle feels unduly full). The pupils may be unequal or fail to react to light, and nystagmus may be present. Localized twitching may occur and sometimes these become generalized. Feeds are taken badly owing to poor powers of suction and swallowing, and vomiting may occur. The body temperature is variable.

These signs of intracranial pressure may develop slowly if caused by haemorrhage from anoxia or to cerebral oedema.

Because intracranial haemorrhage and idiopathic respiratory distress can each lead to the other, and the two conditions are frequently present together, differential diagnosis is often extremely difficult, especially among the smaller infants; but the history of the delivery may be helpful. Babies with congenital cerebral defects add to the difficulties of diagnosis. In addition, when symptoms develop gradually, the condition must be differentiated from meningitis, kernicterus, haemorrhagic disease, hypocalcaemia and hypoglycaemia; and, in light-for-dates babies, from hypernatraemia (Minkowski, 1965).

Preventive treatment. Hypoxia, acidosis and hypothermia all increase the risk of haemorrhage. Special precautions must be taken during labour to prevent birth trauma and asphyxia in low-weight babies (see Chapter 2). After delivery the infant must be kept warm, vitamin K_1 (1 mg.), should be given and anoxia and acidosis must be treated if present. Any coagulation defect not responding to vitamin K_1 should be treated with fresh frozen plasma.

Curative treatment. The infant must be kept in a thermoneutral environment and disturbed as little as possible. The air passages must be kept clear and oxygen should be administered if cyanosis is present. If apnoea occurs, intermittent positive pressure ventilation may be necessary (see p. 142), and if acidosis develops this must be treated. The head of the cot (or head end of the mattress of the incubator) should be raised in order to reduce the intracranial pressure, and sedatives given to reduce the blood pressure generally. Chloral hydrate has proved one of the most useful sedatives in this condition and can be given orally in large doses (1 grain or 60 mg. hourly) if the infant is closely watched for signs of overdosage. If oral administration is contraindicated, soluble phenobarbitone ($\frac{1}{8}$–$\frac{1}{4}$ grain or $7\frac{1}{2}$–15 mg.) may be given by intramuscular injection, this being repeated as often as necessary. Prophylactic antibiotics should be given because pneumonia tends to supervene. Catheter feeding may be required.

Vitamin K_1 (1 mg.) should be repeated if 24 or more hours have elapsed since the dose given at birth and fresh frozen plasma given if the clotting time is still prolonged. By improving clotting ability vitamin

K_1 may control the degree of haemorrhage if only small vessels are involved.

Lumbar puncture has a very limited place in the early treatment of intracranial birth injury. In the author's opinion it may do more harm than good by increasing the infant's blood pressure with the handling entailed, and by reducing the intracranial pressure and allowing the haemorrhage to continue or recommence: however, occasionally it may be a life saving measure by relieving excessive intracranial pressure. After the first few days of life, a lumbar puncture will exclude meningitis and may identify a gross subarachnoid haemorrhage. A considerable number of crenated red blood cells and a marked xanthochromia should be found in the cerebrospinal fluid before a diagnosis of intracranial haemorrhage can be made. If these are found, a short course of prednisone (1 mg./lb./day or 2 mg./Kg./day, with antibiotic cover) may prevent fibrin formation with possible interference with the normal flow of cerebrospinal fluid, leading to hydrocephaly. The head circumference should be watched for some weeks.

Subdural haemorrhage is not frequent among pre-term babies, but if it is suspected, subdural taps should be performed.

Prognosis. Disabilities following birth injury or asphyxia include hydrocephalus, cerebral palsy, convulsions and mental retardation.

Apgar's scoring system (especially the 5 minute score, see p. 23) is usually of prognostic value to later morbidity. Drage and Berendes (1966) found that small infants with low scores had the worst prognosis.

Saint-Anne Dargassies (1962) has developed an elaborate neurological examination for early detection of sequelae; and Tibbles and Pritchard (1965) consider the electro-encephalogram to be of prognostic value.

Prognosis should certainly be guarded at first because it is likely that slight damage may not become evident for some time.

Neonatal Infections

The pre-term baby is more prone to infection than the term baby because of incomplete placental transference of immune bodies (Vahlquist, 1960) and impaired capacity to manufacture them. The low serum globulin level may contribute to the poor response of pre-term babies to infection since globulin contains antibodies. The low-weight baby (pre-term or light-for-dates) is not only more prone to infection but also reacts badly to it. Infection is the fourth greatest cause of early death among low-weight babies (Butler and Bonham, 1963).

Infection may occur before, during, or after birth. Infection before birth (transplacental infection) is relatively rare and includes toxoplasmosis, syphilis, listeriosis and a number of virus infections (see p. 173). Infections during birth may follow early rupture of the membranes, manipulations during delivery or a long labour, or passage through an infected birth canal, e.g. gonorrhoea or herpes simplex. Postnatal infection may occur in the delivery room or in the nursery.

Infection may enter through the umbilicus, the skin or a mucous membrane (gastro-intestinal tract, respiratory tract or eyes) and owing to the lack of immunity local infections rapidly develop into septicaemia or pyaemia. The chief organisms causing early infection are *E. Coli*, *Klebsiella-Aerobacter* and enterococci, and those causing later infections include the *Pseudomonas*, *Proteus*, *Klebsiella-Aerobacter* and *Staphylococcus aureus*. Infection by *Pseudomonas* has become more common since the hexachlorophane soaps and detergents have reduced the population of Gram positive organisms.

In many cases infection is preventable and its occurrence indicates a defect in technique. The prevention of infection during birth has been discussed (p. 19) and the prevention of infection after birth is one of the chief problems of both hospital and domiciliary care. In hospital practice, the danger of cross-infection is well known. In domiciliary practice the advantage gained from less exposure to cross-infection is nullified by the extra risks of respiratory infections (Crosse and Mackintosh, 1953). Williams (1961) could find no difference between hospital-born and home-born infants in regard to contamination with staphylococci.

Prevention of postnatal infection is extremely important. Sources of infection must be eliminated; measures must be taken to prevent spread of infection by droplet, dust and contact (including fly control); and possible sites of entry for infection must be protected. Experiments in the Sorrento unit (Crosse *et al.*, 1954 and 1960) have shown that low-weight babies fed on human milk have not only the lowest incidence of infection but also the lowest mortality due to this complication. Feeding from the breast eliminates the risk of infection from the use of bottles, and this is of the greatest importance when the babies belong to families with a low standard of hygiene.

Early diagnosis of infection is often difficult but if the increased risk of infection among low-weight babies is borne in mind, this will lead to full investigation and earlier diagnosis and treatment and so to a lower mortality from this cause.

As the subject of infection is of great importance in the low-weight baby the more common forms will be discussed in detail.

Oral Thrush (Moniliasis)

White patches are seen on the mucous membrane of the mouth, which bleed if an attempt is made to wipe them off. This condition is due to infection with the fungus *Monilia albicans*. It is particularly liable to occur in low-weight infants and may run a prolonged course in spite of treatment. If the infant is healthy it remains localized to the buccal mucous membrane, but in debilitated infants it may spread and involve the oesophagus and gastro-intestinal tract; and occasionally the lungs, presumably from aspiration after birth (Linhartova and Chung, 1963). The skin of the napkin area may become infected and occasionally there is a generalized papulovesicular scaling rash. Thrush may occur in epidemic form and may even prove fatal (Ludlam and Henderson, 1942). The administration of oral antibiotics predisposes infants to thrush and severe generalized infections are often complicated by thrush.

Infection normally occurs during birth, from a maternal vaginal infection; but it can also occur after birth through contact with infected infants, contaminated bottle-teats, or contaminated hands of those caring for the infants, or by air-borne infection with dust.

Preventive treatment. This includes prenatal treatment of vaginal thrush in the mother, care of the infant's mouth (see pp. 30 and 67), sterilization of feeding equipment, control of dust and flies, and careful barrier nursing. Apparently healthy infants of mothers who have vaginal thrush should be isolated until proved free from infection.

Curative treatment. As the condition is most easily cured in the early stages, every infant's mouth should be inspected frequently (preferably before every feed) and treatment commenced at the earliest sign.

Good results are obtained by painting the affected area with a saturated aqueous solution of gentian violet. The applicator should be *rolled* over the surface; no attempt should be made to remove the patches as this causes trauma and prolongs the disease. The application can be made twice daily after feeds for as long as necessary. An alternative form of treatment is amphotericin (100 mg.) given orally every 6 hours. Any treatment should be continued for 1 week after the disappearance of the last visible lesion.

Skin lesions can be treated with gentian violet in spirit, nystatin cream, amphotericin cream, or 1% tinture of iodine.

An infant with thrush is liable to refuse feeds, and care must be taken to ensure that sufficient food is taken. In severe cases, thrush oesophagitis may cause inco-ordination of swallowing and aspiration pneumonia. This may be treated with intravenous hydroxystilbamidine (5 mg./kg. in 0·75 ml. water) and if necessary with additional antibiotic treatment for secondary bacterial invasion (Wolff *et al.*, 1955).

In order to prevent spread of infection to other babies any case occurring in a nursery must be isolated and provided with separate equipment. Soiled napkins and linen must be placed in disinfectant immediately, because the organisms are excreted in the stools up to 3 weeks after the buccal lesion has cleared (Ludlam and Henderson, 1942).

Mothers of infected infants should be examined and treated if they are also infected.

Infective Diarrhoea

In this section, only the more serious epidemic or infective diarrhoea will be dealt with, other types (parenteral and dietetic) being considered in the section on diarrhoea later in the chapter. Sporadic cases may occur but epidemics are more usual.

Epidemic diarrhoea is most frequently due to the enteropathogenic serotypes of *Escherichia coli* (Bray, 1945; Rogers *et al.*, 1949; Taylor *et al.*, 1949; Stulberg and Zuelzer, 1956; Lapatsanis and Irving, 1963; Laboratory Reports, 1969). The commonest of these are the serotypes 0·111, 0·55, 0·128 and 0·127; less frequently, epidemics have been caused by 0·126 and 0·119. The incidence of each type seems to vary from place to place and from year to year. Epidemics due to Shigellae are rare but Salmonellae have caused epidemics among the newborn (Murray and Walker, 1958) and in addition to the classical signs of septicemia and gastro-enteritis, these babies have developed meningitis. It is possible that viruses may have caused some of the epidemics in which no bacterial pathogen could be identified because Rosen *et al.* (1964) definitely incriminated some of the ECHO viruses.

The incubation period of true epidemic diarrhoea varies from 4–10 days. The onset may be acute but usually it is insidious with loss of appetite, loss of weight, listlessness and possibly a low grade fever (i.e. very difficult to diagnose from any other infection); the stools become loose and vomiting may occur. Except in infections with the Salmonella-Shigella group, there is no pus, blood or mucus in the stool. Acidosis, dehydration and oliguria develop as the result of loss of fluid and electrolytes. Loss of potassium leads to lethargy, hypotonia and abdominal distension. In severe cases the infant becomes comatose and ashen grey, the cry becomes feeble and whining, the skin inelastic and the eyes and fontanelle sunken; and death may be sudden. In mild cases the condition may improve rapidly or run a more chronic course before improvement occurs.

Possible complications are otitis media, pneumonia, meningitis, septicaemia, etc.

Preventive treatment is of great importance and includes all the general suggestions for the prevention of infection made in Chapter 3 (p. 53) in addition to a careful technique in the preparation and administration of feeds (see p. 120).

Feeding with human milk is an important factor in the prevention of this disease. Smangoen (1957) suggested that feeding with cow's milk mixtures predisposed to infection with *E. coli* and/or Salmonellae; and Svirsky-Gross (1958) eliminated *E. coli* 0.111 from a premature baby nursery by using human milk, after failure to control a 2-year epidemic of diarrhoea with antibiotics or closure of the nursery. In the author's experience, pathological types of *E. coli* have never been found in the stools of infants fed on human milk.

Any potentially infected baby, a sick baby, or any baby admitted from its home or another hospital more than a few hours after birth, must be isolated in an isolation nursery until proved to be free from infection. In suspicious cases investigations should include a stool culture and, in vomiting babies, a culture from the vomitus; Rogers (1951a) has shown that early cases of gastro-enteritis due to *E. coli* may have the organism in the vomitus before the diarrhoea commences.

Because of the risk of introduction of *E. coli* into a special baby care unit, babies transferred to an infants' ward of a children's hospital for surgical or other treatment should never be re-admitted to a special baby care unit.

Early diagnosis of gastro-enteritis is essential in order to ensure early isolation. To enable an early diagnosis to be made, the nursing staff must report any abnormal stool immediately. In addition there should be a good liaison with the Public Health Department so that cases of diarrhoea developing after discharge from the unit are immediately notified to the doctor responsible for the unit.

Cases due to Salmonellae or Shigellae can be safely barrier-nursed in isolation nurseries; but any case due to *E. coli*, mild or severe, should be completely removed from a special baby care unit, because of the impossibility of preventing spread of infection by this organism, even in a well-organized cubicled unit (Rogers, 1951b). The baby's mother must be investigated, and isolated and treated if infected.

Contact babies must remain in the same nursery with the same nursery staff. They should be given prophylactic drugs and their stools must be cultured daily to detect spread of infection. All clinical cases and carriers so discovered must be isolated (or removed from the unit if due to *E. coli*). The stools of all adults working in the unit should be examined and carriers treated and excluded from the unit until free from infection.

New babies may be admitted to a clean empty nursery only if they can be looked after by nurses who are not in contact with the infected baby or the contact babies. Regular stool cultures must be taken and if a case appears in this clean nursery, the whole unit must be closed.

No new baby can be admitted to any nursery where there has been a clinical case, or a carrier until:

(1) All remaining healthy contact babies (free from infection for at least 10 days after removal of the last case or carrier) have been disinfected and moved to a clean nursery.

(2) The nursery has been thoroughly cleaned and fumigated with formalin. This includes all furnishings and equipment; antibiotics can

sterilize the stools but they cannot eliminate the organisms from the dust and furnishings.

If all these precautions are taken (particularly those in relation to the admission of potentially infected babies) outbreaks of epidemic gastro-enteritis should be extremely rare in a special baby care unit. If one occurs, all techniques must be overhauled in order to discover the source.

Curative treatment. The baby must be isolated immediately. Cultures of stool, vomitus and blood must be taken and blood sent for chemical analysis.

Treatment must be instituted at the first sign of illness and the standard of nursing must be of a high order. The most important single factor in treatment is the prevention and relief of dehydration and acidosis.

General treatment includes keeping the infant in thermal balance, avoiding unnecessary handling, and giving oxygen and stimulants when required.

Antibiotics may be given before the causative organism or the sensitivity are known but when the report on the cultures has been received, the drug must be changed if the organism is insensitive to the drug being used, or if improvement is not taking place. Until 1962, neomycin was the drug of choice for *E. coli* enteritis (Stulberg *et al.*, 1955) but since then some epidemics have been caused by neomycin-resistant organisms; and it is now very important to ascertain the sensitivity of the organism if an epidemic is to be controlled. Once the sensitivity to neomycin has been proved, neomycin can also be used for the contacts. As neomycin is badly absorbed from the gut, any parenteral infection must be treated with another antibiotic. The doses of all drugs which can be used are given at the end of this section on neonatal infections.

Milk feeding should be stopped at once. During the acute stage of the disease the administration of vitamins A and D should be suspended but vitamins B and C may be continued orally. If intravenous therapy is prolonged, a small dose of vitamin K_1 (1 mg.) may be indicated. The mouth should be kept moist with normal saline.

The treatment of dehydration is a medical emergency, and the two important points in assessing relief of dehydration are gain in weight and free secretion of urine. The methods of relieving dehydration are discussed under the following headings:

(a) Restoration of body fluid.
(b) Restoration of electrolyte and water balance, and preservation of acid-base balance.
(c) Methods of administration of water, electrolytes and glucose.

Restoration of body fluid. The daily maintenance requirements (2 oz./lb./day or 130 ml./kg./day if age of 7 days or more) must be given as usual and, in addition, extra fluid to correct any dehydration present, i.e. equal to the amount of weight lost. If dehydration is severe, at least 10% of the normal weight is lost, i.e. 1½ oz./lb. or 100 g./kg.: with moderate dehydration this loss is halved. In all calculations the body weight to be used is the weight of the infant before dehydration occurred.

Restoration of salt and water balance and prevention of acidosis. In hospitals with facilities for chemical analysis of the blood, replacement therapy is controlled by studies of the blood before and during treatment. Blood studies include blood group, haemoglobin, haemocrit, pH, Pco_2 and standard bicarbonate (Astrup micro-methods are useful for the last three of these estimations) also sodium and potassium levels. If facilities for these examinations are not available, severe cases of dehydration should be transferred, if possible, to a unit with a 24-hour laboratory service. Whether, or not, such services are available, the following principles must be borne in mind:

(1) It is essential to give the correct amount of sodium salts to replace extra-cellular deficits. The administration of too small an amount will not relieve the condition, while too large an amount will lead to serious complications. The powers of concentration of the kidneys in the pre-term baby are poor, and become worse when the flow of urine is diminished, as in dehydration. Salt retention leads to water retention, oedema and uraemia. In a *severe* case of dehydration (with a loss of 10% weight) the infant will require during the 24 hours:

(a) At least 2 oz./lb. (130 ml./kg.) of one-fifth physiological saline to cover the maintenance requirements (less before the 7th day of life).

(b) An additional 1½ oz./lb. (100 ml./kg.) of physiological saline to repair severe dehydration. The correct amount of salt and water to correct severe dehydration will therefore be provided if 3½ oz./lb. (230 ml./kg.) of half strength physiological saline is given per 24 hours until the infant is rehydrated.

(2) The need for potassium for the repair of intracellular deficits must also be recognized. Darrow and Govan (1946) drew attention to the loss of potassium that occurs with dehydration and reported striking results from replacement of potassium in cases of severe diarrhoea. The danger to be avoided is overdosage because this may cause heart block. Milk contains potassium and infants able to tolerate early milk feeding do not become depleted of potassium, but infants who are intolerant of food and require prolonged intraveneous therapy must be protected from this deficiency. Signs of potassium deficiency are weakness, anorexia, abdominal distension, cardiac and liver enlargement, cyanosis and respiratory difficulties. Potassium must be

given to all serious cases once the oliguria has been overcome. and Darrow's solution (parenteral) may be used for this purpose.

(3) Sufficient glucose must be given to prevent acidosis, but large quantities should be avoided. If given by the mouth large quantities cause fermentative diarrhoea, and if given intravenously diuresis may occur, increasing the dehydration instead of relieving it. Glucose may be given as a 5% solution (this is isotonic) either by mouth or intravenously. Acidosis (or alkalosis if there is excessive vomiting) is normally corrected if adequate amounts of fluid and electrolytes are given. However, if acidosis is not overcome by a free flow of urine, part of the saline solution can be replaced by M/6 sodium lactate.

Working on these principles, early treatment should consist of intravenous administration of equal parts of normal saline and 5% glucose (3½ oz./lb. or 230 ml./kg. in 24 hours for severe dehydration, and less if not so severe) until the result of the chemical examination of the blood is received; the fluid and electrolyte therapy can then be re-assessed. In the absence of full chemical control, when the infant is passing urine freely, two parts of Darrow's solution and three parts of 5% glucose (2½–3 oz./lb./day or 160–200 ml./kg./day) may be substituted. When the dehydration has been relieved one part of Darrow's solution and two parts of 5% glucose are continued until oral feeding is fully established, the volume given intravenously being reduced as the volume taken orally is increased. When using Darrow's solution intravenously, the rate of flow must be very carefully controlled to avoid a sudden excess of potassium, and the urinary output must be watched. The flow of urine must be maintained by increasing the intake of the glucose solution if necessary. (See Fig. 43 for electronically controlled drip apparatus.)

Oral feeding should be commenced as soon as this is tolerated and if the infant continues to be intolerant of oral feeding and requires prolonged intravenous therapy, serial estimations of the serum electrolytes will be necessary to ensure correct treatment.

In severe or prolonged cases of diarrhoea a blood transfusion may be beneficial.

Methods of administration of water, electrolytes and glucose. These include the following:

Oral administration. In the absence of vomiting, the oral route should be used. Frequent small quantities are most likely to be retained, and a continuous gastric drip (given by an indwelling feeding catheter) may be retained even if vomiting tends to occur with small feeds. If vomiting is present then the water, electrolytes and glucose must be administered intravenously.

Intravenous administration. This is the best method for rapid relief of dehydration, but the fluid and electrolyte requirements must be extremely carefully calculated and administered, in order to avoid water retention with oedema and anuria. Frequent observations must be made of the rate of flow and quantities given. Isotonic fluids must be used and the correct solution for each case can be obtained by using suitable mixtures of the isotonic fluids already mentioned, i.e. normal saline, Darrow's solution and 5% glucose solution.

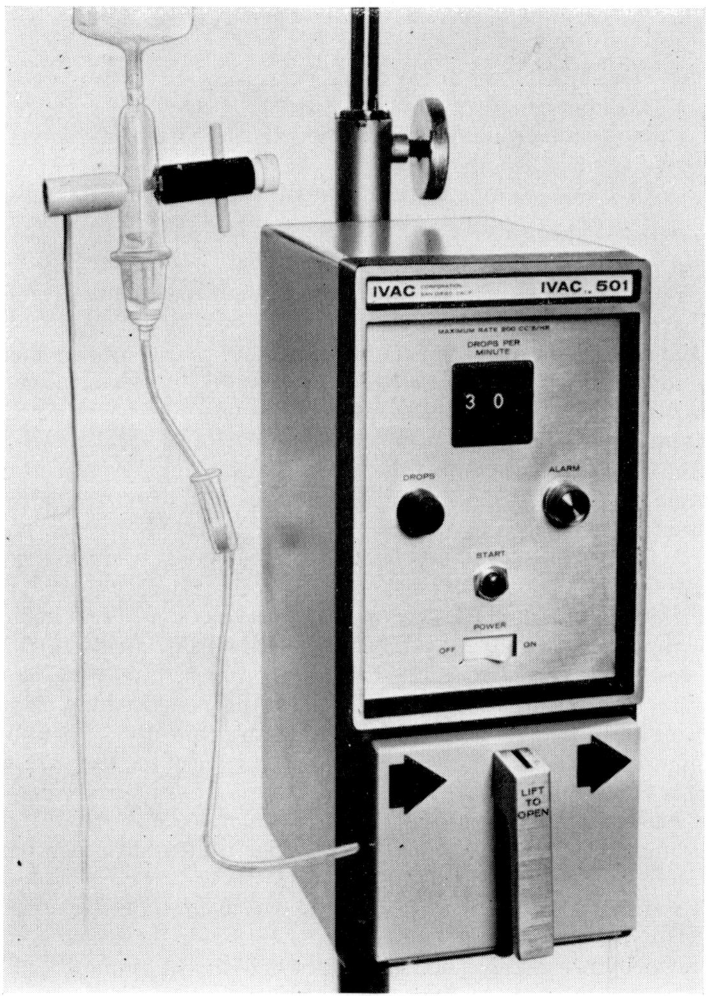

(Photograph by courtesy of Tekmar Medical Ltd.)

FIG. 43. *Ivac Infusion Pump.* An electronically controlled infusion pump which can deliver a slow drip (down to 1 ml. per hour).

In every case of dehydration, the following details should be recorded accurately each day:

(1) Weight of infant.
(2) Fluid intake during the 24 hours.
 (a) Solutions given.
 (b) Quantity given.
 (c) Route given.
(3) Fluid loss during the 24 hours.
 (a) Stools (number and consistency).
 (b) Vomits (numbers and approximate size, i.e. "large" or "small").
 (c) Urine (oliguria or freely passed).
(4) Blood chemistry.

From these records it is possible to make a rough estimate of the requirements for the next 24 hours.

Later treatment. When the diarrhoea has ceased or after marked improvement has occurred, dilute milk feeds may be commenced.

After diarrhoea, tolerance to all food elements is poor, especially to fat, and sometimes there is also a disaccharide intolerance (Lloyd-Still, 1969) so an easily digestible low-fat, low sugar, high-protein formula should be given. Skimmed human milk is excellent but, failing this, a diluted half-skimmed cow's milk (dried or evaporated) mixture may be used. One of these may be given in small amounts every 3–4 hours, suitable mixtures of glucose and saline being given between these milk feeds to make up the necessary fluid and electrolyte requirements. The size and strength of the milk feeds are gradually increased, and the glucose saline decreased, until about 30–40 calories/lb. (66–88 calories/kg.) are being given during the 24 hours. If this is sufficient to maintain weight no further increase need be made for a few days. Then, if the condition of the child allows, the strength and size of the feeds are again increased until 50–60 calories/lb. (110–132 calories/kg.) are being given daily and the infant is gaining weight. Human milk can then be given unskimmed, but it is wise to keep the fat content of a cow's milk mixture low for some time.

Prognosis. Because of their low resistance to infection, the prognosis used to be very poor if babies with a birth weight below 2,500 g. developed this disease; but antibiotics and the appreciation of the importance of replacing fluid and electrolyte losses have improved the prognosis. In addition, the virulence of the specific serological types of *E. coli* appears to have waned (Rogers, 1963). However deaths can still occur unless continuous precautions are taken.

Nasal Discharge

This condition should be treated as a serious one, because of the possibility of spread to the lungs and ears, and its frequent association with diarrhoea and vomiting. Babies are nose-breathers and nasal obstruction leads to respiratory and feeding difficulties.

Preventive treatment. This includes routine care of the nose (see p. 67) and careful use of all catheters, endotracheal tubes, etc., introduced through the nose in order to minimize possible trauma.

Curative treatment. Cultures should be taken from the nose. The infant may be nursed in the prone position, or supine with the head raised, and must be watched carefully for signs of spread to the lungs or ears. If there is much nasal discharge mild antiseptic drops should be used to clear the nose by making the infant sneeze, but no attempt should be made to clear the obstruction by insertion of twisted cotton wool into the nostrils. Ephedrine drops (1–2 drops of 0·5% ephedrine in saline) are useful to clear the nose before feeding. Oily drops must never be used because of the danger of lipoid pneumonia; and any bottle containing nose drops should only be used for *one* baby during *one* infection to prevent the bottle from becoming a source of infection. Antibiotics should be given if a pathogen is isolated, and complications must be suitably treated as they arise.

Any case occurring in a nursery should be isolated at once.

Otitis Media

Infection of the ears occurs readily because the Eustachian tube is short and wide, and the infant is often in the supine position. Infection may spread from the nose; and it can lead to meningitis. The ears must be carefully examined if an infant loses weight or develops pyrexia, anorexia, fretfulness, vomiting or relaxed stools.

Preventive treatment. Clothed infants should be turned regularly from side to side, and infants in incubators should be placed in the prone position at intervals. The head should always be raised during a feed.

Curative treatment. Any discharge should be cultured (cultures can be taken from the nose and throat if no discharge). Prompt treatment is necessary and full doses of antibiotics must be given for 5–8 days if complications are to be avoided (see p. 176 for antibiotics and dosage). Antibiotic ear drops are indicated if the discharge persists.

If the condition is associated with diarrhoea or vomiting these must be suitably treated.

Pneumonia

Pneumonia is the greatest cause of death from infection among low-weight babies; and, compared with babies weighing over 2,500 g. at birth, low-weight babies are more prone to death from pneumonia.

Infection of the lungs may occur as a primary condition; it may be part of a generalized infection, or it may be the result of direct spread from the upper respiratory passages. It may be secondary to inhalation during or after birth, intracranial birth injury, idiopathic respiratory distress or, occasionally, secondary to serious congenital malformation, e.g. tracheo-oesophageal fistula, etc. If it occurs during the first few days of life, it is usually due to aspiration during birth.

The organisms most commonly found in early infections in low-weight babies are the *E. coli* and staphylococci; *Pseudomonas*, *Proteus* and *Klebsiella* are also commonly found. Virus pneumonia usually occurs after the first few weeks of life.

Diagnosis is particularly difficult during the first 48 hours of life when so many conditions may cause respiratory distress (see p. 128), especially as pneumonia may complicate any of these conditions.

A careful study of the history from birth is essential and the time of onset is of great importance. The onset is often insidious and cough is absent in all except the largest infants. Pyrexia is frequently absent; indeed many of the infants become hypothermic. The infants are usually reluctant to take feeds and a nasal discharge may be present in the early stages. The larger infants may become restless but the smaller ones usually become less active. The respiratory rate usually rises and the rise is often out of proportion to the heart rate; cyanosis may develop; laboured breathing with dilatation of the alae nasi and recession of the lower intercostal spaces is generally, but not always, present. Physical signs in the lungs may appear to be absent but the breath sounds tend to be high-pitched and the air entry diminished, and râles can usually be heard at the end of a deep respiration, i.e. with crying. A loss of weight usually occurs; the stools may be green and undigested; and the abdomen may become distended. Radiological examination of the chest is usually helpful.

Preventive treatment. Prevention of infection during labour includes prevention of hypoxia during labour, the prophylactic administration of antibiotics to the mother during labour if the membranes are ruptured and labour prolonged (see p. 19), and effective clearing of the air passages at birth. Prevention of postnatal infection includes provision of adequate air space and good ventilation, control of dust, the use of masks when indicated (see p. 59), isolation of infected babies (especially those with staphylococcal pneumonia and *E. coli* infections), exclusion of attendants with colds and other infections, as well as good barrier nursing. Good general management (e.g. disturbing procedures, such as lumbar puncture, should not be done until at least 2 hours after a feed), and correct methods of feeding should reduce the risk of regurgitation and inhalation. Oily vitamin preparations should never be given orally in case they are regurgitated and inhaled and cause lipoid pneumonia; and oily nose drops must be avoided for the same reason.

Pneumonia of postnatal origin should occur very rarely in a well run nursery unless the infant has been infected before admission.

Curative treatment. Cultures must be taken from the pharynx and blood; and the infant must be isolated.

The treatment is the same as that of idiopathic respiratory distress, with the addition of the administration of antibiotics to control the infection. The antibiotic should be specific if possible but, until the organism and its sensitivity is known, various combinations of drugs may be used. For the indications for the use of each drug, the dosage and the method of administration, see p. 176.

The feeding is of great importance, and sufficient fluid and calories must be ensured. Extra fluids should be given if there is any pyrexia, and fluid lost by diarrhoea or vomiting must be replaced with suitable repair solutions (see p. 159). If sufficient fluid cannot be given by means of small frequent feeds, these should be supplemented with catheter feeds as required. Large feeds should be avoided as they distend the stomach and embarrass the lungs.

Interstitial Plasma Cell Pneumonia

This condition occurs among low-weight or debilitated babies between the ages of 4 weeks and 6 months. It has been reported mainly from European countries. Mickailov (1959) reported two epidemics in premature baby units in Russia; Martoni *et al.* (1965) studied 81 cases in Italy; Stenbäck *et al.* (1968) followed up 17 cases in Finland but cases have also been reported from Canada (Berdinoff, 1958) and other parts of the world. The cause was believed to be the protozoon *Pneumocystis carinii* (Vanek *et al.*, 1953) but Stenbäck and his colleagues think the "protozoon" is an alveolar mass derived from the septal cells and that the cause is still in doubt.

The onset is insidious, with apathy, anorexia and failure to gain weight. The respiration rate then increases and dyspnoea and cyanosis develop; at this stage lung signs may include fine scattered râles and slight impairment of resonance. Fever is often absent and cough is variable. The white cell count is not characteristic. A hypogammaglobulinaemia is often found (McKay and Richardson, 1959). Radiological examination shows diffuse opacity of the lung fields.

The course is prolonged and relapses occur. The case fatality rate is high, but those which recover are physically and mentally normal (Stenbäck *et al.*, 1968).

The diagnosis is confirmed post-mortem by finding a diffuse interstitial pulmonary infiltration by mononuclear cells which resemble plasma cells, and hyaline-like alveolar exudate.

There is no known specific treatment; but hydroxystilbamidine has been tried. Good nursing, careful feeding and supportive treatment with oxygen and high humidity are important.

Cases should be removed immediately from a special baby care unit and all contacts must be isolated until discharged. New admissions should only be accepted if they can be put into clean wards where they will be nursed by a separate staff.

Urinary Infections

The occurrence of pyuria in the newly born is more frequent than is generally believed, and often may pass unrecognized. The urine should always be tested for pus and bacteria in fretful infants; in infants with pyrexia, anorexia, rash in the napkin area, or loose stools; and in those failing to thrive or febrile for no apparent reason. In addition, any urine with a suspicious smell should be investigated. Vomiting may be associated with this condition, but does not seem to be a frequent feature in the low-weight baby. Parenteral diarrhoea is a more frequent complication. Conversely, pyuria may be a complication of an alimentary infection or one aspect of a generalized infection.

The organism responsible is usually *E. coli* but other organisms are sometimes found.

Treatment. Cultures should be taken to determine the infecting organism and its sensitivity to drugs, and a suitable antibiotic should be given. Antibacterial therapy should be continued until two sterile urine cultures have been obtained (with an interval of 3 days between them), and the urine should be re-examined a few weeks later to detect any recurrence. If the condition fails to respond, or if relapses occur, then congenital malformation of the urinary tract should be suspected, especially in male infants.

It is important to maintain the fluid and nutritional requirements. Extra fluids should be given if there is any pyrexia and fluid lost by diarrhoea must be replaced by repair fluids.

Meningitis

Meningitis may be the result of local spread from an upper respiratory or ear infection, or from an infected meningocele or cephalhaematoma; or it may be part of a general septicaemia.

During the first 2 weeks of life, *E. Coli* is still the commonest organism found but *Pseudomonas* infections are increasing. Gram positive cocci infections occur during the 3rd and 4th week of life.

Meningitis is not a common infection among low-weight babies but when it occurs it is often difficult to recognize because the early signs are common to all infections, e.g. irritability or apathy, cyanotic episodes and anorexia; and possibly pyrexia, vomiting and diarrhoea.

Localizing signs are a tense fontanelle, perhaps slight head retraction or stiffness of the back, and nystagmus. Kernig's sign is generally absent. Late signs are twitching (or even convulsions), vomiting, a tense fontanelle, and neck and spinal rigidity. A lumbar puncture with examination and culture of the fluid will differentiate meningitis from intracranial birth injury, congenital defects of the brain, kernicterus and other causes of convulsions (see p. 232). A lumbar puncture should be done in any infant who is doing badly for no obvious reason.

Preventive treatment. This includes early diagnosis and treatment of all infections which, by local or generalized spread, may lead to meningitis; and isolation of any clinical case.

Curative treatment. The final choice of drug must be determined by the organism cultured. Until this is known, a combination of suitable antibacterial agents can be used. Steroids may be useful in the acute phase.

Supportive treatment includes maintenance of body temperature, careful feeding, sedation if necessary, oxygen to relieve cyanosis, and artificial ventilation for apnoea. If biochemical abnormalities develop these must be corrected.

Prognosis. Early treatment is particularly important in low-weight babies if the result is to be good. In any case, prognosis should be guarded for several years. Possible sequelae include hydrocephaly, cerebral palsy, mental retardation, convulsions and loss of hearing.

Septicaemia

Before the days of antibiotics this condition used to occur relatively frequently and cause a high mortality among low-weight infants, owing to their poor powers of resistance to infection; but early treatment of localized infections with modern drugs has dramatically reduced both the incidence of and the mortality due to this complication.

The onset may be insidious, spreading from a localized infection; but it may be sudden, the local infection having passed unrecognized. The larger babies tend to be fretful and restless, but the smaller babies become comatose: the appetite is lost and there is usually some degree of diarrhoea. Rapid dehydration and loss of weight may occur. The colour becomes poor and fever may or may not be present. The spleen is usually enlarged and leucocytosis may be present (the polymorphonuclear leucocytosis persists or returns after the first week of life); the blood culture may be positive. Jaundice, abdominal distension and vomiting are late and serious signs. Haemorrhages tend to occur from the umbilicus and mucous membranes during the later stages of the disease. Signs of inflammation may occur in any part of the body (meningitis, peritonitis, bronchopneumonia, pericarditis) and abscess formation may also occur.

The organisms most commonly found in septicaemia are *E. coli*, Gram positive cocci and *Pseudomonas*.

Preventive treatment. This includes obstetric asepsis and the prophylactic administration of antibiotics to the mother if the membranes are ruptured and labour is prolonged, followed by cultures of cord blood and cultures from the infant's nose and pharynx (so that the infant can be treated with suitable antibiotics if the cultures are positive); a careful technique in the management of the infant after birth, the use of human milk, and immediate recognition and treatment of local sepsis. Any case of septicaemia should be regarded as a failure of technique, and the cause found and corrected.

Curative treatment. Cultures and sensitivity tests should be made from the nose, pharynx, umbilicus, skin, rectum, urine and blood. The cerebrospinal fluid should be examined and cultured and a differential white blood cell count made. Isolation is essential.

The infant must be kept warm (in a thermoneutral environment) and should be disturbed as little as possible. Respiration and circulation must be maintained (see pp. 140 and 145). Nutrition must also be maintained, and sufficient fluid and electrolytes must be given to replace fluids lost by vomiting and diarrhoea (see p. 158), also any biochemical abnormality of the blood must be corrected (see p. 136). Oxygen and stimulants should be given as required and antibiotics used to control the infection (see p. 176).

Blood transfusions are of considerable value if there is a tendency to haemorrhage or anaemia and sedatives may be necessary to control restlessness or convulsions. Abscesses may require surgical treatment.

Skin Infections

Owing to the delicate nature of the skin of a low-weight baby it is particularly liable to infection.

Moniliasis of skin. This has already been discussed in the section on oral thrush (p. 154).

Staphylococcal infections of skin. These vary from mild septic spots which have an indurated base and remain unruptured for some time (pustular dermatitis) and paronychia (infections developing at the edge of the nail beds) to the more severe neonatal impetigo.

Neonatal impetigo. This usually develops during the first week of life, but some infants are infected *in utero* and are born with the disease. The lesions are found first on moist or opposing surfaces, such as neck folds, axillae and groins. Any part of the skin may be affected, but the soles of the feet and palms of the hands are generally free even in severe cases. The vesicles are superficial and soon rupture leaving a raw area on an otherwise normal skin.

In mild cases small vesicles or pustules appear but clear rapidly and have little or no effect on the general condition of the infant. In serious cases, multiple superficial bullous lesions occur (pemphigus), or more rarely, exfoliative dermatitis (Ritter's disease) develops, with general intoxication and possibly death. Congenital syphilis and epidermolysis bullosa must be excluded.

Even the mild form is extremely important from the epidemiological point of view. It may spread rapidly in the nursery, particularly in the presence of overcrowding or understaffing. Concurrently, the staphylococci may cause other infections, such as umbilical sepsis, ophthalmia neonatorum, paronychia and maternal mastitis. Occasionally more severe staphylococcal infections occur, e.g. pneumonia, enteritis, osteomyelitis, meningitis and septicaemia.

There was a great increase in the incidence of staphylococcal infections after 1954 due to the development of an increasing number of antibiotic-resistant strains. Many epidemics were reported from maternity nurseries, affecting the skin, cord and eyes of the baby and the breasts of the mother. During the last 10 years, staphylococcal infections have been greatly reduced by the use of hexachlorophane soaps and detergents, but sporadic cases of mild staphylococcal infection still occur in special baby care units and the possibility of more severe infections, and even of an epidemic, must always be borne in mind. The original source of infection is probably an adult who may be a nasal carrier, a non-nasal carrier (Hare and Ridley, 1958) or a clinically infected case. Selbie (1953) found that staphylococci from clinically infected cases were, on the whole, more active than those from nasal carriers but there were strains of high and low activity in both groups. It is probable that an open lesion is a more dangerous source of infection than a carrier but the potential danger of carriers cannot be ignored. Once the infection is in the nursery, both infants and staff can become carriers and infection is spread from one infant to another, mainly by the hands (Wolinsky *et al.*, 1960; Rammelkamp *et al.*, 1964).

The main reservoir for the staphylococci is the umbilicus and the surrounding skin (Forfar *et al.*, 1953; Jellard, 1957; Pollard and Perry, 1959; Simpson *et al.*, 1960; Simon *et al.*, 1965; Baber *et al.*, 1967). The infants' noses are colonized later (Barber *et al.*, 1953; Cook *et al.*, 1958; Simon *et al.*, 1965; Baber *et al.*, 1967); and the mothers' breasts are infected from the noses of their babies (Duncan and Walker, 1942; Cook *et al.*, 1958; Baber *et al.*, 1967). The more rapidly an infant becomes a nasal carrier, the more liable is that baby to develop pyodermia (Baber *et al.*, 1967). Barrie (1966) has shown that the rectum can also be colonized by staphylococci.

Preventive treatment. This includes:

(1) Removal of all possible sources and reservoirs of infection.

(2) Blockage of routes of spread.
(3) Protection of all possible sites of entry of infection.

Possible sources of infection are reduced by admission of potentially infected babies (babies more than a few hours old "on admission") to special nurseries; exclusion of infected staff and carriers; prompt isolation of infected babies; careful observation of contacts; admission of new babies to clean nurseries only (until all contacts have been discharged and the affected nurseries have been disinfected); and careful screening of visitors.

Indirect contact by handling is the usual method of spread of staphylococcal infection, so all unnecessary handling must be eliminated and a sufficient number of nurses must be provided to allow time for careful barrier nursing (see p. 55). Airborne infections can be reduced by good dust control (see p. 54), good ventilation and natural lighting, and also by small nursery units with good cot spacing or partitions between cots.

Possible sites of entry are the umbilicus, moist skin (especially round the umbilicus, perineum and axillae), the nose and the eyes; and the local care of these sites is given on pp. 66–68. Gluck and Wood (1961), Gezon *et al.* (1964), Simon *et al.* (1965) and Light *et al.* (1968) all reduced umbilical and nasal staphylococcal colonization by using hexachlorophane for skin care, and there is good evidence that the incidence of infection falls when colonization is reduced (Gillespie *et al.*, 1958).

Unfortunately, as staphylococcal infections are being controlled by hexachlorophane, an increase in colonization and infection by Gram negative bacilli (*E. coli*, *Proteus* and *Klebsiella-Aerobacter*) and *Pseudomonas* have been reported by Light *et al.* (1968) and Forfar *et al.* (1968).

To avoid an epidemic, constant vigilance is necessary. All cases of infection must be reported and recorded. Because some babies may develop clinical signs after discharge from hospital, a close liaison with the local public health department is essential.

Curative treatment. All cases of infection of the skin must be submitted to full bacterial investigation including sensitivity to antibiotics and phage-typing.

Mild staphylococcal skin infections usually clear rapidly with hexachlorophane baths (see p. 67) and some simple local application such as surgical spirit (except near the eyes), a saturated aqueous solution of gentian violet, calamine lotion, or 1% chlorhexidine cream (Hibitane). Generally speaking, local treatment with sulphonamides or antibiotics should be avoided because of the risks of sensitization of the baby and the development of bacterial resistance to these drugs. Exceptions to this rule are neomycin, polymyxin and bacitracin because such complications are less likely with these drugs.

In more severe cases, systemic therapy is indicated and the antibiotic to be used is the one proved (by sensitivity tests) to be effective against the particular organism involved. The baby's general condition can be improved by suitable feeding, sufficient warmth and the administration of stimulants and oxygen when necessary.

Direct spread of infection between opposing surfaces may be prevented by nursing the infant naked and restraining the ankles and wrists.

If an abscess develops it must be incised and drained.

Strict isolation is essential, and any nurse looking after a true case of pemphigus should not be allowed to come in contact with nurses caring for healthy babies. During her attendance on the infant the nurse should wear gloves in order to prevent contamination of her own hands. All clothing, bedding and equipment (if not disposable) must be disinfected after use: infected linen or clothing must not be sent to the laundry without preliminary disinfection. The same precautions must be taken with the clothing and bedding used by the mother of an infected infant.

If an epidemic develops an analysis of the records kept (name of infant, date and type of infection, nursery and incubator concerned, phage-type and antibiotic sensitivity of organism, contacts, etc.) may suggest possible sources and methods of spread of the organism. In addition, a search must be made for infections among the staff (doctors, nurses, technicians, cleaners, etc.).

All clinical cases must be isolated. All contact infants must be fully investigated (swabs from skin, cord, nose and eyes); and carriers must be isolated and given suitable local treatment. The noses of all contact staff must be similarly investigated and carriers treated. The noses of carriers (staff and infants) may be treated with 2% hexachlorophane cream twice daily for 7 days, and adults should also use 2% hexachlorophane soap (Noone *et al.*, 1970).

No new cases should be admitted to any nursery until all infected babies and their contacts have been discharged, the nurseries and equipment have been cleaned, the preventive technique has been overhauled and the staff is free from carriers. Members of the staff who continue to carry staphylococci in the nose after all babies have been free from infection for at least 1 week (or after having had a week's holiday) must be regarded as carriers and be excluded from the nurseries until cured.

Light *et al.* (1967) have colonized infants (umbilicus and nose) with a non-pathological coagulase-positive staphylococcus (502A strain) to control nursery outbreaks of pathological staphylococci.

Umbilical Infection

Infection may cause a sero-purulent discharge associated with delay in healing, moist granulations, redness and induration round the umbilicus, or abscess formation; in some cases the umbilicus is apparently healthy. The chief danger is that of spread along the umbilical vein, resulting in hepatitis, peritonitis, pyaemia or septicaemia. The infant may appear normal, or be fretful and fail to thrive.

Preventive treatment. The essential points in prophylaxis are strict asepsis when dividing the cord and the subsequent use of a suitable technique for the protection of the cord (see p. 68).

Curative treatment. Any discharge must be cultured to determine the infecting organism and its sensitivity to antibiotics. The area may be cleaned with surgical spirit and dressed with hexachlorophane powder, chlorhexidine cream, or with powder or creams containing neomycin, polymyxin or bacitracin. Granulations may be treated with silver nitrate stick or "blue stone". Systemic antibacterial therapy should be prompt if there are signs of spread of infection or if the infant appears to be ill. Incision and drainage becomes necessary if an abscess forms.

The strength of the infant must be supported by correct feeding and sufficient warmth; and the infant must be isolated to prevent spread of infection.

Tetanus. This is still a problem in developing countries. Infection gains entry by the umbilical cord which may be cut with an infected instrument or have an infected dressing applied.

The infant becomes restless, hypertonic, and unable to feed; and finally develops trismus and repeated muscular spasms with opisthotonus. The earlier the onset, the worse is the prognosis.

Prevention consists of immunization of the mother with tetanus toxoid during the first 6 months of pregnancy, and ensuring correct care of the umbilical stump.

Treatment includes sedatives and relaxants (e.g. curare) to control the spasms, administration of tetanus antitoxic and antibiotics, the administration of oxygen, and mechanical ventilation when necessary.

Ophthalmia Neonatorum

This condition occurs readily among low-weight babies and the organisms most frequently found are the Gram positive cocci and *E. coli.* Cases with sterile cultures are probably due to virus infections and can be diagnosed by finding inclusion bodies in conjunctival smears. Virus infections do not develop until the 5th or 6th day. The possibility of a gonococcal infection should not be forgotten, as the incidence of this disease has increased recently.

Low-weight infants may have a reaction to prophylactic drops and these should not be used as a routine measure. Reactions usually occur during the first 6–12 hours after treatment.

Preventive treatment. Any abnormal vaginal discharge in the mother must be treated. Prophylactic eye drops should be used at birth if there is any suspicion of vaginal infection in the mother.

Curative treatment. The infant must be isolated and strict precautions taken to prevent any spread of infection. Cultures must be taken to determine the organism and its sensitivity to antibiotics.

The condition usually clears rapidly with an intensive course of chloramphenicol drops (0·5%) or neomycin sulphate (0·5%). Eye drops must be kept separately for each infant, and discarded after 3 days use. Another possible treatment is to bathe the eye with normal saline and apply Neobacrin or neomycin ointment until the result of the culture is known.

For severe infections (those with copious discharge and a velvety red palpebral conjunctiva) systemic antibiotic therapy is required in addition to local treatment. The cornea must be watched carefully for ulceration.

When an infection persists in spite of appropriate treatment, blocking of the lacrimal duct should be suspected and pressure on the lacrimal sac will establish the diagnosis and may also re-establish drainage.

The strength of the infant must be maintained by correct feeding and sufficient warmth.

Transplacental Infections

These include congenital syphilis, congenital toxoplasmosis, congenital listeriosis and various congenital virus infections such as rubella and cytomegalic inclusion body disease.

Because most of these infections result in low-weight babies (often both pre-term and light-for-dates) they should be remembered in the differential diagnosis of generalized infection of the newly born low-weight infant, especially in the presence of hepatosplenomegaly and petechiae or jaundice. Although these infections occur relatively rarely, they are being more often recognized and it is probable that mild forms are more common than is generally accepted.

Congenital Syphilis

This condition (due to the *Spirachaeta pallida*) should be rare if the disease is recognized and the mother is treated during pregnancy. In untreated cases, a curtailed pregnancy is common (McCord, 1935).

Suspicious early signs include "snuffles", pemphigoid or pleomorphic rash (face, buttocks, soles and palms), hepatosplenomegaly and jaundice; and the condition is confirmed by serological tests on the mother and child.

If a mother has had no prenatal care, cord blood should always be tested for syphilis.

Preventive treatment. This consists of immediate treatment of any expectant mother who has a positive Wasserman test.

Curative treatment. Penicillin is the treatment of choice.

Congenital Toxoplasmosis

This condition, which can lead to pre-term birth, is caused by the *Toxoplasma gondii*, from an unrecognized maternal infection during pregnancy. The foetus may be stillborn, born prematurely or at term. Feldman (1959) found 31·0% of affected live born babies were born prematurely, and Sever (1968) reported both low birthweight and curtailed pregnancy as the results of toxoplasmosis.

Toxoplasma gondii was formerly believed to be a protozoon, but Hutchison *et al.* (1970) now believe it to be a coccidian parasite closely related to the genus *Isospora.*

Signs may be present at birth or develop later. The infant may be born with hydrocephaly or microcephaly, and choroido-retinitis. More commonly, an acute meningo-encephalitis develops during the neonatal period, with enlargement of the lymphatic glands, liver and spleen and perhaps with a maculo-papular rash. Choroido-retinitis and cerebral calcification may develop later. In the acute stage the cerebrospinal fluid contains an increased amount of protein and cells; and the organism may be found in smears from the sediment.

Although the encephalitic form is the more common one, there is also a visceral form of this disease. The baby is born with a haemolytic anaemia, a thrombocytopenic purpura, and a large liver and spleen. Jaundice develops early.

In both forms, the Sabin-Feldman dye test for antibodies becomes positive early, with a rising titre for some time. The mother also has a strongly positive dye test, but with a falling titre.

Treatment. Pyrimethamine (1 mg./kg./day) is usually combined with sulphonamides (see p. 177 for dosage of sulphonamides). Since pyrimethamine is an antifolic agent, folic acid should also be given and frequent leucocyte counts must be made during treatment. Prednisone has also been used (Agers, 1964).

Prognosis. Many die in early infancy. Feldman (1959) found that 27·0% of the pre-term affected infants died, compared with 12·0% of infected infants born at term. Those that survive are usually left with some permanent damage, e.g. hydrocephaly, mental deficiency, blindness, cerebral palsy, etc. Vivell and Maas (1962) suggested that 20% of early brain disorders should be considered as due to toxoplasmosis.

It is extremely important that all infants who are born with hydrocephaly without other congenital malformations, or who develop neurological signs and choroido-retinitis, should be investigated at once for toxoplasmosis and treated immediately if positive.

Listeriosis

This condition can also lead to a pre-term birth, but was rare in Britain until 1961 (Barber and Okubadejo, 1965). It is caused by a pleomorphic Gram positive rod, *Listeria monocytogenes.* Usually the foetus is infected transplacentally, the mother having a mild pyrexial illness resembling a cold (rhinitis, sore throat and stiff neck) during the last weeks of pregnancy; but neonatal infection from infected sibs has also been reported. The infected foetus may be aborted, be stillborn (with miliary granulomatosis) or be born alive prematurely, or at term. The liquor amnii often has a brownish-green discoloration (Freyre and Kennedy, 1963). Out of 63 well documented cases in the United States and Canada, 15 were born prematurely (Ray and Wedgwood, 1964).

Signs may develop soon after birth or within the next few weeks; the earlier the onset, the more severe the disease. Those with an early onset usually have signs of cardiorespiratory distress. Other signs include vomiting, loose foamy stools, fever, petechial rash, jaundice, irritability and convulsions. Those with a later onset may start with anorexia, fever, rhinitis and lethargy; then develop the signs already described. Purulent meningitis is common, also generalized granulomatosis (on oropharynx and skin, and in organs). The organism is difficult to identify and isolate but may be found in cultures from the cerebrospinal fluid, nose, throat, and urine; it may also be found in cultures from the blood and genital tract of the mother. Hoeprich (1958) identified the organism in the stool by Gram staining.

Treatment. Many antibiotics have been used but penicillin and ampicillin are probably the best. Tetracyclines (advocated by Ray and Wedgwood, 1964) must be avoided in pre-term infants (see p. 180).

Prognosis. The mortality is high, especially if the onset is less than 4 days after birth. It can be improved with early diagnosis and prompt treatment.

Virus Infections

Rubella. This is the most important of these infections because it causes retardation of foetal growth and a high incidence of congenital malformations which vary according to the time of infection of the mother.

The infant may also have enlargement of the liver and spleen, jaundice, thrombocytic purpura, encephalitis and bone lesions.

The virus can be isolated from the infant at birth and for some months after birth (Alford *et al.*, 1964; Rubella Symposium, 1965) and antibodies can be found in the mother and baby.

Preventive treatment. Mass vaccination of all girls between the ages of 11 and 14 years with rubella vaccine is the ideal method. Until this has been achieved, older girls and women can be vaccinated if they undertake not to become pregnant during the following 2 months. It is possible that susceptible women accidentally exposed to rubella during the first 16 weeks of pregnancy may be protected by high-titre immunoglobulin, if given early enough and in sufficient amounts, but the Public Health Laboratory Service (1970) reported that immunoglobulin did not protect to any appreciable extent. Pregnant women should not be allowed to come in contact with an affected infant during its first year of life when it is still excreting the virus.

Cytomegalovirus Disease (Inclusion body disease). This disease is another cause of low birth weight (Weller and Hanshaw, 1962) and curtailed pregnancy (Medearis, 1957). It is still rare but is becoming increasingly recognized. Mortality is high in recognized cases (second only to rubella in regard to mortality due to virus diseases) but there is probably a relatively high incidence of sub-clinical cases.

If infection occurs during early pregnancy it leads to extensive brain damage with areas of calcification and cerebral malformation (Elliott and Elliott, 1962).

Severe cases have enlargement of the liver and spleen at birth, usually also jaundice and thrombocytopenic purpura, and often respiratory distress. Inclusion bodies can be found in cells in the urine and in many organs. Antibodies can be detected in the blood of both mother and infant; and the virus can be isolated from the cord, placenta, infant's urine, etc. Neurological sequelae and mental retardation are common.

Treatment. Corticosteroids and gamma globulin have been used.

Drugs Used for Control of Infection

Great care must be exercised when giving drugs to pre-term babies. Many drugs are metabolized through the action of enzymes in the liver and these enzymes are deficient in pre-term infants (Kempe, 1958). Drugs are also often protein-bound and these may compete with unconjugated bilirubin for the relatively small amount of serum albumin in the pre-term baby, thus predisposing to kernicterus. Finally, the pre-term baby has a poor renal excretion and drugs may accumulate until they reach toxic levels.

The following drugs should not be given to pre-term infants unless absolutely necessary: sulphonamides, chloramphenicol, tetracyclines, novobiocin and streptomycin. The reasons are given later, in the section on each drug.

The organisms most frequently found in a special baby care unit are coliforms and staphylococci. These organisms are gradually becoming resistant to more antibiotics. The incidence of resistance is directly related to the amount of antibiotic used, so antibiotics must never be used unnecessarily.

Staphylococci have been known to become sensitive again on withdrawal of the antibiotic to which they were resistant: this has occurred with chloramphenicol (Kirby and Ahern, 1953), the tetracyclines (Lowbury and Thompson, 1956) and erythromycin (Lepper *et al.*, 1954). It is therefore a good practice to change the antibiotics in general use every 6–12 months.

Infection with *Pseudomonas* is becoming more frequent among low-weight babies, and the infections it causes can be very serious. The use of broad spectrum antibiotics favours infection with *Pseudomonas* (Forkner *et al.*, 1958; Williams *et al.*, 1960) so these antibiotics must be avoided if there have been any infections in the unit due to this organism.

Double chemotherapy has been recommended to prevent the emergence of drug resistant organisms. This applies specially to drugs given while awaiting the results of sensitivity tests but, as a general principle, this is potentially dangerous since it means an increase in the use of many antibiotics. After the laboratory results have been received the most suitable single antibiotic should be chosen.

Antibiotics in routine use for systemic treatment should not be used for local applications. Various combinations of neomycin, bacitracin, polymyxin and chlorhexidine are more suitable for local application.

Antibiotics must, of course, be used freely for the treatment of infection, but they must be controlled by sensitivity tests. Until the laboratory findings are known, the choice of the antibiotic will depend on the resistance of the prevailing organism in the unit. Whenever possible the drug to be finally used should be one to which the organism concerned does not readily develop resistance, and one with a narrow antibacterial spectrum, e.g. for staphylococci the choice is benzyl penicillin if the strain is sensitive to this.

As many antibiotics as possible should be kept in reserve, for use only with organisms resistant to the drugs in routine use.

If non-absorbable sulphonamides or broad spectrum antibiotics are used orally for more than a few days, vitamins B and K should be given.

Drugs should only be given for definite indications and not as a routine treatment.

Sulphonamides. These drugs have a wide spectrum of activity, but resistance is developed fairly rapidly. For two reasons it is unwise to give sulphonamides during the first week of life: firstly because of the relatively poor kidney function in the pre-term baby combined with the small fluid intake during this period, and secondly because they are protein bound.

After the first week of life Fichter and Curtis (1955) found that pre-term babies maintained a significant level for 12 hours after one dose of 100 mg./kg. given orally (triple sulphonamide suspension) or subcutaneously (sulphadiazine) followed by 50 mg./kg. 12-hourly. With these doses neither crystalluria nor haematuria was seen, but a good fluid intake must be ensured.

Penicillin G. (Benzyl penicillin) has a limited spectrum covering chiefly Gram positive organisms and Gram negative cocci. Many strains of staphylococci are now resistant but when the organism is sensitive, penicillin G is the treatment of choice. It must be given parenterally because it is not acid resistant. Adequate blood levels are obtained with 25,000 units/kg./day, divided into two 12-hourly doses.

Penicillin V. This is an acid resistant penicillin and can therefore be given orally but many staphylococci are resistant. Usually 62·5 mg. are given 6-hourly by mouth, immediately before a feed. Larger doses can be given when indicated because toxic reactions are rare.

Methicillin (Celbenin) is a penicillinase-resistant penicillin and is therefore effective against many resistant staphylococci. It is not acid resistant, so must be injected. At first no strains of staphylococci were resistant to methicillin but unfortunately some have now emerged (Barber and Waterworth, 1962; Stewart and Holt, 1963; Parker and Hewitt, 1970). It should only be used for babies with serious staphylococcal infections resistant to penicillin G. The dosage is 100 mg./kg./day divided into four 6-hourly doses, given intramuscularly.

Cloxacillin (Orbenin), oxacillin, and other isoxazolylpenicillins. These are penicillinase resistant; also acid resistant, so can be used orally. They are irregularly absorbed, especially after food but cloxacillin is better absorbed than oxacillin, and they can be given parenterally. So far no strains of staphylococci have been reported as resistant to these drugs, but there is a cross resistance between methicillin and these isoxazolylpenicillins. Unfortunately they are extensively protein bound, and should be avoided during the first week of life. They should be reserved for staphylococci resistant to other drugs. The dosage is 50–100 mg./kg./day divided into four 6-hourly doses.

Ampicillin (Penbritin) has a far wider spectrum than other penicillins and includes *E. coli* and *Proteus*. It is acid resistant, but not penicillinase resistant, and organisms (including *E. coli*) easily become resistant. The dosage is 50–100 mg./kg./day divided into two 12-hourly doses for the first 5 days of life; and into three 8-hourly doses for older babies when excretion becomes more rapid.

Erythromycin, spiramycin and oleandomycin all have a range of activity similar to penicillin. Resistance develops quickly and there is a considerable degree of cross resistance within this group; but there are strains of staphylococci which are resistant to some members of the group and not to others. Erythromycin is the most active of this group.

It should be reserved for penicillin resistant organisms. The oral dose is 25–50 mg./kg./day divided into four 6-hourly doses. If given intravenously, this dosage is halved and given in two 12-hourly doses.

Novobiocin (Albamycin) has a spectrum like that of penicillin except that it is less active against streptococci. Unfortunately this drug is protein bound and interferes with the conjugation of bilirubin, and it can also cause agranulocytosis. In addition resistance develops easily. For all these reasons, this drug should only be used for organisms resistant to all safer drugs. It should be given orally only and the dose is 20–40 mg./kg./day, divided into four 6-hourly doses.

Streptomycin has a limited spectrum, its chief action being on Gram negative bacilli. In large doses it can cause deafness and it is nephrotoxic if given intravenously. Resistance develops rapidly. Streptomycin should not be used unless all safer drugs fail. The dosage is 25 mg./kg./day, divided into two 12-hourly doses, given intramuscularly. Kanamycin has largely replaced streptomycin in early therapy, before laboratory results are known.

Neomycin has a fairly wide spectrum but there is some risk of development of resistance. It has little toxic effect if given orally but parental administration may cause deafness and kidney damage. Its use is usually confined to oral administration for gastro-enteritis due to *E. coli*, and to local applications. The oral dose is 50 mg./kg./day in four 6-hourly doses. Because it is poorly absorbed from the gut, it must be combined with other antibiotics if parenteral infection is also present; and vitamin K should be given if this drug is used for more than a few days.

Kanamycin has a wide spectrum including staphylococci, *E. coli*, some *Proteus* and *Pseudomonas*. In large doses it can cause deafness and kidney damage, and resistance can develop. Before results of laboratory tests are known, kanamycin is often given with an antibiotic known to be effective against the staphylococci prevalent in the unit concerned. With a dosage of 15 mg./kg./day divided into two doses, given intramuscularly, toxicity is not a problem.

Kanamycin, like neomycin, can be given orally for gastro-enteritis due to *E. coli*. It can also be given intrathecally in meningitis if there is still a positive culture of a sensitive organism after 24 hours intramuscular treatment. The dose is 1 mg. in 1 ml. saline daily until the culture is negative.

Polymyxin B and Polymyxin E (Colistin). The action of these antibiotics is limited to Gram negative bacilli (except *Proteus*) and to *Pseudomonas*. They are nephrotoxic and neurotoxic when used systemically and are not absorbed from the gut. They are the drugs of choice for the increasing number of serious infections due to *Pseudomonas*, but otherwise they should only be used orally for sensitive organisms in the gut which are resistant to all safer drugs or as local applications for short periods for infections due to *Pseudomonas*, e.g. eye and skin infections.

The intramuscular dose is 3–5 mg./kg./day for Polymyxin B and 6–8 mg./kg./day for Polymyxin E: these should be divided into four 6-hourly doses because these drugs are excreted fairly rapidly. The oral dosage is 1 mg./kg./day, divided into four 6-hourly doses.

Polymyxin B can be used intrathecally for meningitis if there is still a positive culture of a sensitive organism after 24 hours intramuscular treatment. The dose is 1 mg. in 1 ml. saline daily until the culture is negative.

Gentamycin sulphate and Carbenicillin. These are two new antibiotics with promising activity against *Pseudomonas*. Carbenicillin is a semi-synthetic penicillin with a moderate activity against *Pseudomonas* while gentamycin sulphate is a wide spectrum antibiotic with good activity against *Pseudomonas*. These have not yet been proved safe for use in pre-term infants.

Bacitracin. This drug has a very wide spectrum, including fungi. It is nephrotoxic when used parenterally and is badly absorbed from the gut. Resistance develops very slowly, so it is generally used for local application and is often combined with neomycin or polymyxin. It may be used orally for enteritis due to organisms resistant to all safer antibiotics, but the fluid intake and output must be carefully watched during its use. The oral dosage is 500 units/kg./day, divided into four 6-hourly doses.

Tetracyclines, i.e. chlortetracycline (Aureomycin), oxytetracycline (Terramycin), tetracycline (Achromycin or Tetracyn) and dimethylchlortetracycline (Ledermycin). These antibiotics have a very broad spectrum of activity. Development of resistance is not common. They are usually given by mouth in a dosage of 20 mg./kg./day divided into four 6-hourly doses. Absorption is improved by giving 1 ml. of fluid per mg. of drug. Reverin is the form for parenteral administration and is given in a dosage of 10–15 mg./kg./day divided into two 12-hourly doses.

During administration of these drugs an overgrowth of non-sensitive organisms may occur (e.g. resistant staphylococci or monilia) and stomatitis, and diarrhoea with excoriation of the perianal region may develop. These complications are reduced by giving vitamin B complex if tetracyclines are given for more than a few days. Dowling (1957) pointed out that the routine addition of an anti-monilial agent (nystatin) only led to the development of a nystatin-resistant monilia which could be very serious among low-weight babies. Witkop and Wolf (1963) observed yellow staining of the first teeth following tetracycline therapy and Cohlan *et al.* (1959) stated that tetracyclines were deposited in growing epiphyses and inhibited linear growth. These drugs should be avoided if possible and, if used, given for the shortest time possible.

Chloramphenicol (Chloromycetin). This is also a broad spectrum antibiotic to which resistance is slow to develop. Because it competes with bilirubin for glucuronyl conjugation it should not be used during the first week of life. Even after this age its use should be limited to 5 days because of the danger of suppression of bone marrow. Low-weight babies have died from high dosage (the grey syndrome) and the blood level should be watched carefully (levels over 100 mg./ml. are toxic in low-weight babies; Lambdin *et al.*, 1960). The oral dose is 25 mg./kg/day divided into four 6-hourly doses. Chloramphenicol succinate is available for parenteral therapy and can be used in a dosage of 15 mg./kg/day in divided doses. As with tetracycline, it is advisable to give vitamin B complex if chloromycetin is used for more than a few days. This antibiotic should only be used as a last resort, after all safer ones have failed.

Haemorrhagic Disease of the Newborn

Haemorrhage in the newborn may be the result of infection, anoxia or trauma; hormonal in origin; due to some defect in the blood clotting mechanism (haemorrhagic disease of the newborn); or a combination of any of these causes.

Haemorrhages due to haemorrhagic disease of the newborn may occur in any part of the body but the most common are intracranial haemorrhage (usually intraventricular), massive pulmonary haemorrhage, melaena and haematemesis. Haemorrhages can occur in otherwise normal infants but are much more likely if the infant has suffered from hypoxia, acidosis or hypothermia (Gray *et al.*, 1968).

The primary cause of intracranial haemorrhage is not necessarily haemorrhagic disease; the increased tendency to bleed may just increase the degree of haemorrhage. But a definite relationship has been found between intracranial haemorrhage and coagulation deficiencies (Gray *et al.*, 1968; Cade *et al.*, 1969).

The administration of certain drugs to expectant mothers, e.g. dicoumarol or soluble phenobarbitone, increases the risk of haemorrhage in the infant.

Bleeding from the vagina is hormonal in origin and not due to haemorrhagic disease. Haemorrhages due to infections or severe obstructive jaundice can be differentiated by the presence of the signs of the causative disease. Melaena or haematemesis due to swallowed maternal blood (from the birth canal or from the nipple) can be differentiated by Apt's test (Apt and Downey, 1953), i.e. mix with water to obtain a pink-red supernatant haemoglobin solution, centrifuge and decant the supernatant fluid. To five parts of this fluid add one part of 1% sodium hydroxide. If a yellow-brown colour develops the blood is maternal in origin; a red colour shows that the blood is from the infant (*Note:* the stool or vomit should be red and not tarry). This test depends on the greater stability of foetal haemoglobin in the presence of alkali.

All newborn infants have a slight coagulation deficiency at birth. Among low-weight babies (both pre-term and light-for-dates) this deficiency is more marked, and increases as the gestational age and the birth weight decrease, especially in regard to factors V, VII and X (Cade *et al.*, 1969). These deficiencies are accentuated during the first week of life, due to a fall in the level of prothrombin, especially among infants who have suffered from intrauterine hypoxia, i.e. many light-for-dates babies. According to Van Creveld (1959), Aballi and De Lamerens (1962), Hardisty and Ingram (1965) and Oski and Naiman (1966) this fall is due to either:

(1) A deficiency of vitamin K (either from inadequate formation and absorption or by abnormal utilization), or

(2) Immaturity of liver function. A number of coagulation factors are synthesized in the liver and are dependent on vitamin K for normal production, i.e. factors II, VII, X and probably IX. Vitamin K is not stored and the newborn infant must depend on ingested vitamin K until it produces its own supply by bacterial synthesis.

The increased liability of low-weight babies to develop this disease, and the increased severity of the disease when it occurs, are due to:

(1) Inadequate hepatic function.
(2) A deficiency of certain coagulation factors.
(3) The greater fragility of blood vessel walls in the pre-term infant.
(4) A greater risk of hypothermia, anoxia and acidosis.
(5) Inadequate production of vitamin K if feeding is delayed for any reason.

Preventive treatment. Although the coagulation defect in low-weight infants is relatively unresponsive to vitamin K (due to their immature or depressed liver function) vitamin K_1 (1 mg.) is usually given to all low-weight babies at birth.

Cade *et al.* (1969) suggest that screening tests such as the prothrombin and partial thromboplastin times should be included in the early assessment of all low-weight babies, while Gray *et al.* (1968) suggest using the Thrombotest (Owren, 1959) during the first day of life. If the Thrombotest is less than 10% another dose of vitamin K_1 may be given and the test repeated after 4 hours. If there is no response to vitamin K_1, correction may be achieved by the administration of small amounts of fresh frozen plasma (Cade *et al.*, 1969).

Preventive treatment also includes the prevention and treatment of hypothermia, anoxia and acidosis, as well as early feeding.

Curative treatment. In all cases of haemorrhage, the blood must be examined (blood group, haemoglobin and film) and the coagulation status assessed.

In addition to correction of any coagulation defect, the general treatment of the infant depends on the site of the haemorrhage. The treatment of massive pulmonary haemorrhage (most common among the light-for-dates babies) is the same as that for idiopathic respiratory distress (see p. 133); and the treatment of intracranial haemorrhage is that set out on p. 152.

If haemorrhage occurs in an infant to whom vitamin K_1 has not been given, 1 mg. should be administered at once. If the haemorrhage is severe a blood transfusion should also be given: this not only replaces the blood lost but also provides sufficient prothrombin to tide the infant over until the level has been raised by the vitamin. Fresh blood should be used because although prothrombin does not diminish with storage, other factors do (e.g. factors V and VII). The amount of blood given depends on the amount lost (see p. 201 for calculation of blood required). The blood must be compatible with the infant's blood in regard to both the ABO and Rh groups.

Haemorrhage in an infant already given an adequate prophylactic dose of vitamin K will be due either to deficiencies of coagulant factors not associated with vitamin K, or to immaturity of the liver. Thus fresh frozen plasma or a blood transfusion (fresh) should be given to supply the deficient factors.

The infant must be kept warm, undue handling avoided, and sufficient fluid ensured. Milk feeds need only be interrupted in severe cases of haematemesis and they should be recommenced as soon as possible in order to increase the natural synthesis of vitamin K in the bowel.

Congenital Thrombocytopenic Purpura

This condition may be confused with haemorrhagic disease. Bleeding occurs into the skin, and this may be followed by other haemorrhages especially melaena. The blood must be examined for platelets (see p. 6 for normal platelet counts) and the bleeding and clotting times investigated. These infants are usually born to mothers with thrombocytopenia or to mothers who have been sensitized to platelet antigens by a previous pregnancy or transfusion. Thrombocytopenia has also been reported in infants of mothers treated prenatally with thiazide drugs. (Rodriguez *et al.*, 1964).

The haemorrhages must be differentiated from the widespread subcutaneous ecchymoses often seen in low-weight babies immediately after birth (which are probably due to fragility of the superficial blood vessels or anoxia and not to any defect of coagulation) and also from generalized petechiae due to infection. The diagnosis depends on the finding of a thrombocytopenia in the baby, and platelet agglutinins or a thrombocytopenia in the mother.

No treatment is necessary unless serious haemorrhage occurs (when a fresh blood transfusion may be required) because the infant's platelet count will usually return to normal within a short period. In severe cases, cortisone may be helpful and a platelet transfusion may be necessary.

Hyperbilirubinaemia associated with Low Birth Weight

This is a diagnosis which must be made by exclusion of all other possible causes of jaundice in babies with low birth weight (see p. 230).

The jaundice usually appears after the first 24 hours of life in an otherwise healthy infant; and the serum bilirubin level rises to 15 mg./100 ml. or more, during the first 7–10 days of life (below this level the jaundice can be regarded as "physiological", see p. 231). The importance of this condition is the potential danger of brain damage (kernicterus) which can occur if the serum bilirubin rises excessively.

Formerly kernicterus was most commonly associated with haemolytic disease of the new-born, but with the introduction of adequate exchange transfusions this complication of haemolytic disease has been virtually eliminated. Among babies suffering from haemolytic disease, it has always been recognized that babies with low birth weight were more liable to develop kernicterus than babies over 2,500 g.; and in 1950, two groups of workers (Aidin *et al.*, 1950; Zuelzer and Mudgett, 1950) independently drew attention to the fact that kernicterus could occur in low-weight babies who were not suffering from haemolytic disease.

Kernicterus associated with low birth weight gives the same clinical picture as that of kernicterus associated with haemolytic disease except that the onset is usually later; the neuropathology of the two conditions appears to be the same (Aidin *et al.*, 1950; Govan and Scott, 1953); and Gerrard (1952) and Plum (1965) have shown that the subsequent development of the survivors is the same in both groups.

Untreated infants develop a well-marked jaundice but appear to make fairly good progress until the second half of the first week. Signs of kernicterus usually develop between the 4th and 8th day of life, with the maximum incidence on the 6th day; the onset tends to be later as the birth weight increases (Crosse *et al.*, 1955). The early signs of kernicterus include lethargy, a disinclination for food, hypotonia, vomiting, cyanotic attacks, a high-pitched cry, restlessness, an expressionless face and eye rolling (particularly downwards, giving a "setting sun" appearance). Later signs are head retraction and alterations in muscle tone (opisthotonus with extended and pronated arms and clenched fists; or generalized hypotonia) and often pyrexia (Fig. 44). Mild cases may easily be overlooked if they show only a transient lethargy, reluctance to feed or occasional rolling of the eyes. Stern and Denton (1965) reported kernicterus in 4 very small infants with respiratory distress who showed no classical signs but died in unexpected apnoea. Because of the plethoric colour of some pre-term infants a marked icterus may be missed unless it is carefully looked for in daylight (or with a daylight lamp at night) by stretching, or pressing on, the skin.

Kernicterus carries a high mortality rate. When death supervenes it occurs 12–48 hours after the onset of signs. Blood-stained mucus may be vomited a few hours before death, and intense jaundice (with a fall in the serum biluribin level) may develop as a terminal event.

Infants who survive improve fairly rapidly. The stiff ones get less stiff and many become hypotonic for a while; they may continue to have spasms of opisthotonos on handling, but after a few weeks they appear to be quite normal. Subsequent development is, however, very disappointing. The most severely affected babies soon develop a generalized "lead-pipe" rigidity, often also convulsions and bouts of pyrexia, and these babies usually die during the first year of life. The subsequent development of less severely affected cases varies tremendously; they may be irritable and jumpy, cry a great deal, feed and sleep badly, and continue to have attacks of opisthotonos and eye rolling. Affected babies

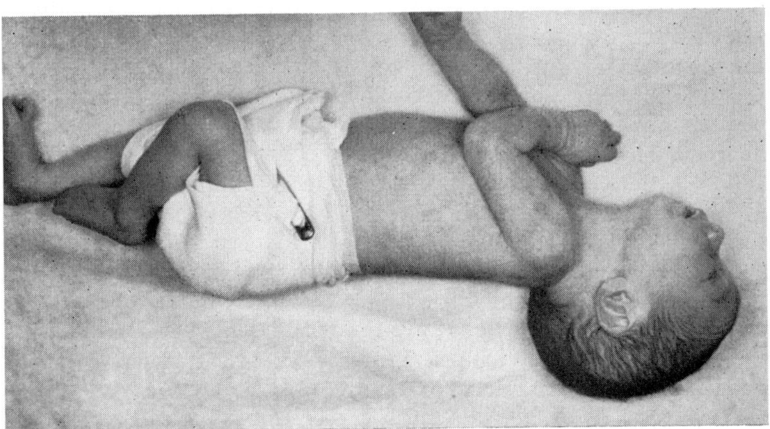

FIG. 44. Baby with kernicterus. This photograph shows the head retraction and the expressionless face. The child also has increased muscle tone with clenched fists and flexed toes.

are usually late in reaching their milestones (head control, etc.) and tend to retain infantile reflexes longer than usual. Residual damage to the central nervous system includes varying degrees of one or more of the following: rigidity, choreo-athetosis, deafness, emotional instability, and mental retardation. Some cases appear to be developing reasonably normally until they begin to walk, and athetoid movements are not as a rule fully developed before the age of 3–5 years (Gerrard, 1952). Evans and Polani (1950) state that 80% of their older survivors showed athetosis, choreo-athetosis or chorea, and that the majority had mental impairment. Gerrard (1952) found perceptive deafness in 80% of his older survivors.

The cause of kernicterus is now well known. Bilirubin is formed from the breakdown of the red blood cells which normally occurs after birth: this is indirect-acting bilirubin which gives an indirect van den Bergh reaction. It is not water-soluble so cannot be excreted in bile or urine. Before it can be excreted it must be conjugated with glucuronic acid by means of a liver enzyme (glucuronyl transferase) to form conjugated, or direct-acting, bilirubin which is water-soluble. The indirect-acting bilirubin is transported in the blood, bound to the plasma proteins (especially albumin). If it is displaced from this binding site it diffuses into extravascular compartments, including the cerebrospinal fluid because the blood-brain barrier is permeable to indirect-acting bilirubin during the first few days of life. Indirect-acting bilirubin has an affinity for lipids so it may be taken up by the brain cells, to which it is toxic. Exposure of the brain cells to high concentrations of bilirubin reduces their oxygen uptake and this is probably the cause of the cell damage (Kuster and Krings, 1950; Day, 1954; Ernster *et al.*, 1957). Babies dying from kernicterus show yellow staining of the brain, most intense in the basal nuclei, with increased vascularity and death of nerve cells in Ammon's horn, globus pallidus and sub-thalamic nuclei and occasionally in the olives (Corner, 1955). Late findings are loss of neurones and gliosis.

The gestational age has a great influence on the bilirubin level. Hsia *et al.* (1953) observed that the serum bilirubin levels in pre-term infants reached higher levels than in term babies and, since then, other investigators have shown that the rise in the level of serum bilirubin increases as the birth-weight decreases (Billing *et al.*, 1954; Crosse *et al.*, 1955; Meyer, 1956). Pre-term infants have an increased rate of haemolysis after birth, an immature liver enzyme system, a poor binding capacity for bilirubin (low serum albumin level), a more permeable blood-brain barrier (Nasralla *et al.*, 1958), and less subcutaneous fat to attract the fat-soluble unconjugated bilirubin from cerebral fat (Zuelzer, 1960). Light-for-dates babies also have poor liver function and little subcutaneous fat.

The incidence of hyperbilirubinaemia varies from centre to centre, and even from time to time in any one centre. This may be due to many factors. Different methods of estimating the serum bilirubin levels can account for variations up to $\pm 3{\cdot}6$ mg./100 ml. (Westphal *et al.*, 1962); and perhaps also the absence of sufficient protection of the blood samples from the effects of light until they can be examined (Lucey, 1960). Other possibilities are the degree of illumination in the nurseries; feeding policies, i.e. infants fed early or late; and drugs used.

The main factors influencing the incidence of hyperbilirubinaemia may be divided into prenatal, natal and postnatal. Prenatal factors include drugs taken by the mother, e.g. long-acting sulphonamides (Silverman *et al.*, 1956) and salicylates (Black, 1962). If sulphonamides are given to the mother shortly before delivery they pass across the placenta easily but are only excreted slowly by a low-weight infant, so that appreciable serum levels can be found for as long as 4 days after birth (Sparr and Pritchard, 1958). Both sulphonamides and salicylates increase the risk of hyperbilirubinaemia in the infant by competing with the free unconjugated bilirubin for albumin binding and glucuronyl conjugation.

At birth, asphyxia is an important factor (Govan and Scott, 1953; Crosse *et al.*, 1955; Brown and Zuelzer, 1957; Crosse, 1959c). Anoxia may act by depressing liver function (oxygen is required for bilirubin conjugation; Dutton, 1959), or by increasing the permeability of the nerve cells. The time of tying the cord may have some effect on hyperbilirubinaemia. Usher *et al.* (1963) and Taylor *et al.* (1963) thought that the level of serum bilirubin was higher when the cord was tied late, but Lanzkowsky (1960) did not find this. However it would seem sensible not to increase the number of red blood cells unduly when the immature liver may have difficulty in dealing with the resulting excess of bilirubin.

After birth, any condition increasing haemolysis (see Jaundice, p. 230) will increase the bilirubin load with which the liver has to deal. Respiratory distress also increases the incidence of hyperbilirubinaemia (Aiden *et al.*, 1950; Crosse *et al.*, 1955; Miller and Reed, 1958; Stern and Denton, 1965) and this may be due to reduction of liver enzyme activity by anoxia or acidosis. Odell (1964) has shown that a low extracellular fluid pH favours intracellular diffusion of free bilirubin (by displacement of bilirubin from albumin by fatty acids) and this can increase the risk of kernicterus.

The author and her co-workers found a definite association between early hypothermia (rectal temperature less than 92°F, or 33·3°C, on admission) and the level of serum bilirubin; the colder the baby the higher the level of bilirubin (Crosse *et al.*, 1955; Crosse, 1959c) and this was believed to be due to depression of liver function.

The administration of certain drugs to the infant during the first week of life increases the posssibility of hyperbilirubinaemia and kernicterus. Vitamin K is one example (Allison, 1955; Laurance, 1955; Crosse *et al.*, 1955; Meyer and Angus, 1956; Bound and Telfer, 1956). Vitamin K may act by increasing haemolysis (Zinkham and Childs, 1927; Vest, 1958); it may be hepatotoxic (Lucey and Dolan, 1959) or it may inhibit bilirubin conjugation (Waters *et al.*, 1958). Other drugs and antibiotics compete with bilirubin for albumin binding and glucuronyl conjugation, e.g. sulphonamides (Silverman *et al.*, 1956; Johnson *et al.*, 1959; Odell, 1959; Donald, 1964; Lewis, 1964); caffeine sodium benzoate (Odell, 1959); novobiocin (Hargraves and Holton, 1962) and chloramphenicol. Drugs which compete for albumin binding may reduce the bilirubin level in the blood but increase the risk of kernicterus by driving the free bilirubin into the interstitial fluid and tissue cells.

Haemoconcentration from excessive weight loss, either from late feeding (Laurance and Smith, 1962; Smallpeice and Davies, 1964; Wharton and Bower, 1965) or from diarrhoea (Shnier and Levin, 1959) can result in high serum bilirubin levels. It is possible that hypoglycaemia is also a factor, because glucose is required for conjugation (Dutton, 1959; Hsia *et al.*, 1959; Zinkham, 1959; and Rozdilsky, 1959). Smallpeice and Davies claim that feeding commenced within 2 hours after birth reduced the incidence of both hypoglycaemia and hyperbilirubinaemia.

Septicaemia is known to predispose to kernicterus (Kleinschmidt, 1930; Zimmerman and Yannet, 1933; Biemond and van Creveld, 1937), presumably by interfering with liver function or by haemolysis.

As in haemolytic disease, the incidence of kernicterus is related to the level of serum bilirubin (Crosse *et al.*, 1955; Koch *et al.*, 1959; Hugh Jones *et al.*, 1960). These investigators have reported an incidence of kernicterus varying from 8–19% with serum bilirubin levels between 20 and 30 mg./100 ml.; and from 30–65% with levels above 30 mg./100 ml. In these three reports there were no cases of kernicterus among infants with bilirubin levels below 20 mg./100 ml. However, cases can occur below this level when drugs are given which compete for albumin binding, or in very small babies with respiratory distress (Stern and Denton, 1965). The serum bilirubin level falls in a dying baby, so if the first estimation is made on a baby dying of kernicterus, the level may be low (Crosse *et al.*, 1955; Harris *et al.*, 1958).

Preventive treatment. The best preventive treatment would be to reduce the incidence of curtailed pregnancy and low birth-weight (see p. 273) and this is difficult. Good prenatal care and care during delivery should reduce the risk of birth asphyxia. The administration of sulphonamides (especially the long-acting varieties) to the mother must be avoided during labour. Good facilities must be available for resuscitation of the infant.

After birth, the dose of vitamin K to the infant must be small. Asteriadou-Samartzis and Leiken (1958) showed that vitamin K_1 had little effect on the serum bilirubin level, neither did the water-soluble analogue (Synkavit) when given in correct therapeutic dosage (0·5–1·0 mg.). Synthetic vitamin K should never be given to any baby belonging to an ethnic group in which there is a possibility of G-6-PD deficiency, e.g. Indian, Greek, Italian etc. (Knutsen and Brewer, 1966).

Hypothermia, infection and dehydration must be avoided, so must drugs which compete with bilirubin for albumin binding and glucuronyl conjugation. The first feed should not be unduly delayed. If the infant develops respiratory distress, anoxia and acidosis must be treated.

All babies with low birth weight must be carefully watched for jaundice and, if any more than a slight degree develops, regular serum bilirubin estimations must be made (daily or more frequently if necessary). For nurseries with poor laboratory facilities, Gossett (1960) has produced a perspex icterometer for quick estimation of the depth of jaundice without taking a blood specimen (Fig. 45). This instrument is pressed against the infant's nose, the colour of which is matched against five yellow strips of different shades numbered 1–5. When the reading is more than 3 an accurate laboratory estimation is required. It should be remembered, however, that the skin colour lags behind the serum bilirubin level when the level is rising rapidly so it is dangerous to depend on the icterometer if babies develop jaundice within 36 hours of birth: on the other hand, when the level is falling it may be lower

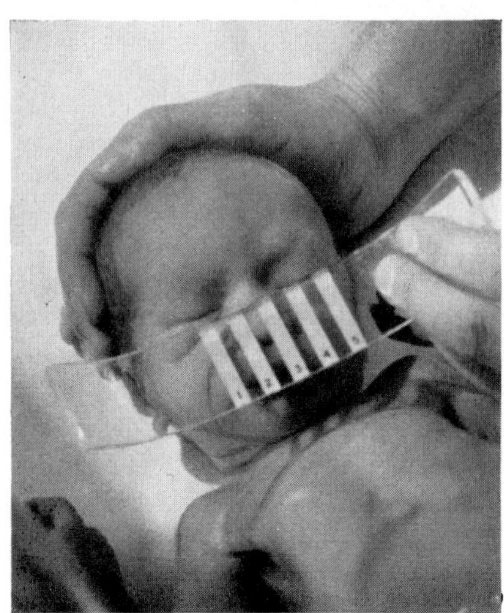

FIG. 45. Icterometer
(Photo by Eothen Films Ltd.)

than the colour of the skin suggests. Daylight is required for matching the colours and a daylight lamp should be provided for use at night.

Curative treatment. This entails keeping the serum bilirubin at a safe level (a level at which kernicterus cannot develop) until such time as the conjugation mechanism has matured, i.e. for the first 7–10 days after birth.

If the level rises to 15 mg./100 ml., the reserve serum binding capacity should be measured because this is a better indicator of the risk of kernicterus than the serum bilirubin level (Odell *et al.*, 1969). At present the most reliable treatment for hyperbilirubinaemia is an exchange transfusion. This removes bilirubin and adds albumin. The bilirubin level at which an exchange is recommended varies from 18–25 mg./100 ml. (the lower level being suggested for very small babies with respiratory distress. Stern and Denton, 1965). In the author's experience, no infant has developed kernicterus with a bilirubin level less than 22 mg./100 ml., thus exchange was undertaken at the level of 20 mg./100 ml. Now that the infant's binding capacity can be estimated (Waters, 1967; Muto, 1969; Odell *et al.*, 1969) it may be safe to delay an exchange if the infant's clinical condition is good and the binding capacity remains adequate (Waters, 1967).

The best route for an exchange transfusion is the umbilical vein (Diamond *et al.*, 1951). The blood used must be compatible with the infant's blood as well as with the mother's serum. The blood should be as fresh as possible (never more than 3 days old for fear of dangerous levels of potassium and a low pH value) and it must be warmed (Hey *et al.*, 1969). Citrated blood is preferred to heparinized blood because the latter has to be freshly collected to avoid haemolysis; also heparin may uncouple bilirubin from albumin by activating the clearing factor and increasing the level of non-esterified fatty acid in the blood (Novak *et al.*, 1962) and increase the risk of kernicterus. Citrated blood should have a PCV of about 40% (obtained by halving the volume of the citrate-dextrose used as an anticoagulant, thus also preventing serious dilution of the albumin fraction). At least 80 ml./lb. (180 ml./kg.) should be exchanged; but only 10 cc. being withdrawn and replaced at a time. The whole procedure should be sufficiently slow to allow the bilirubin to move from the intersitial fluid into the plasma. (This equilibrium is probably complete in 1 hour, but equilibrium with tissue bilirubin takes several days.) Valaes (1963) has found that the optimum length of time for an exchange is about 1 hour. To avoid toxic effects from the citrate, 0·5 ml. of 10% calcium gluconate should be injected after the exchange of each 100 ml. of half citrated blood. Careful records must be kept of the amounts of blood given and removed.

Because the risk of kernicterus is related to the availability of binding sites on the serum albumin (Odell, 1959), the addition of salt-free human albumin to the donor's blood was advocated by Kitchen *et al.* (1960) and Odell *et al.* (1962). Ruys and Gelderen (1962) pointed out the risks of the temporary increase in blood volume, and Usher and Carrier (1961) stated that this might be dangerous in anaemic babies. However, Comley and Wood (1968) have given human albumin safely to non-anaemic babies at three different stages, i.e. before the exchange, during the exchange, and after the exchange. Given before an exchange it protects the infant while it awaits transfusion by providing more binding sites; and given after the exchange it acts in the same way during the rebound period and may save a repeat transfusion. Human albumin is probably only needed if the bilirubin level is rising rapidly and the reserve binding capacity is inadequate (Waters and Porter, 1964).

When hyperbilirubinaemia is associated with idiopathic respiratory distress, the Pao_2, pH, blood sugar level, etc., must be carefully monitored and the necessary treatment given.

During the transfusion the infant must be kept warm and its colour, heart rate and respiration must be carefully monitored. If signs of distress develop the exchange must be stopped temporarily to allow resuscitation of the infant. After a transfusion, antibiotics (known not to be excreted as a glucuronide or as an albumin bound complex) should be given.

In some cases, several exchanges may be necessary to keep the bilirubin below dangerous levels and regular bilirubin estimations must be continued until it is certain that the level is falling. Repeat exchanges can usually still be given through the umbilical vein, especially if a plastic obturator has been left *in situ* to keep the vein patent. In the author's experience this has never led to complications of any kind. In any case, it is usually possible to cut down on to the umbilical vein above the umbilicus and, failing this, the saphenous vein can be used (Arnold and Alford, 1948). Before carrying out repeat transfusions it is wise to estimate the level of unconjugated bilirubin (not just total bilirubin) because the level of conjugated bilirubin also tends to rise in severe cases with poor liver function, and conjugated bilirubin is not toxic to brain cells. The reserve binding capacity should also be estimated because a repeat exchange is not necessary if this is adequate.

It is possible that an exchange transfusion may still be of some use even after early signs of kernicterus have appeared if the serum bilirubin level is still high.

Other forms of treatment are now in the experimental stage. One is phototherapy. Cremer *et al.* (1958) first suggested that exposure to ultraviolet light could reduce the serum bilirubin level but Franklin (1958) thought the photochemical products of bilirubin might themselves be toxic. It is now known that photodecomposed bilirubin is water-soluble, does not cross the blood-brain barrier and is rapidly excreted in the bile and urine, so does not accumulate (Diamond, 1969); it also does not bind with albumin (Porto *et al.*, 1969). Considerable evidence is accumulating to show that the photochemical products are not toxic (Hsia, 1970; Lucey, 1970; Gorodischer *et al.*, 1970). In fact, it is likely that photodecomposition is a normal route of excretion for bilirubin which can be increased by the use of extra light.

Phototherapy has produced the best results when a phototherapy unit (broad spectrum light) is fixed over the incubator or cot (Lucey *et al.*, 1968); but a significant, though smaller, reduction in physiological jaundice has been achieved by increasing the general lighting of the nursery, especially at night (Giunta and Rath, 1969). The infant's eyes must be covered to prevent the light from injuring the retina; and the body temperature must be monitored. So far, no-one knows the

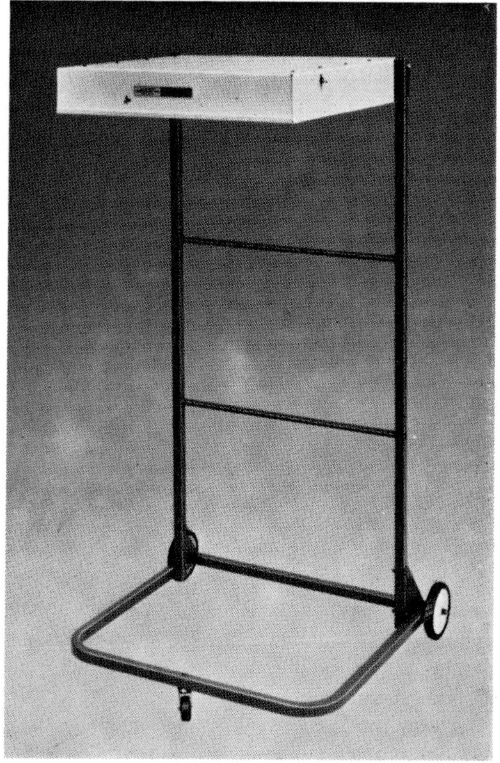

(Photograph by courtesy of Air-Shields (U K.) Ltd.)

FIG. 46. *Air-Shields* ® *Phototherapy Unit*. This can be placed over any incubator or cot.

minimum dose required to achieve the maximum effect on the bilirubin level and more research is needed into the correct use of light in suitable cases. Fig. 46 shows a phototherapy unit which can be placed over an incubator or cot.

At a symposium of phototherapy for hyperbilirubinaemia in Chicago (Behrman and Hsia, 1969) all participants agreed that phototherapy should not be employed as a routine measure but that it could be used to treat jaundiced pre-term infants when the risks of phototherapy are less than the risks of jaundice or of treating jaundice by some other method. The main risk of phototherapy is injury to the cornea from the eye-covering. Even if phototherapy is used there is the same necessity to monitor the serum bilirubin level and the reserve albumin binding capacity so that an exchange transfusion can be performed if this should become necessary.

Another form of treatment in the experimental stage is the use of phenobarbitone which is believed to reduce the bilirubin level by activating the transferase enzyme and so increasing conjugation and excretion of bilirubin (Yaffe *et al.*, 1966; Trolle, 1968; McMullin *et al.*, 1970); but Walker *et al.* (1969) and Cunningham *et al.* (1969) could not confirm this. Further investigations are required, with a long term follow-up, before this treatment can be recommended for routine use.

The development of kernicterus should always be regarded as a failure of treatment.

Prognosis. This should be guarded in all cases in which marked jaundice has occurred, whether obvious signs of kernicterus have developed or not.

In tissue cultures, damage to nerve cells begins at bilirubin levels of 20 mg.%, while at 40 mg.% most of the cells are killed (Küster and Dortmann, 1958) so it is probable that infants will suffer some brain damage even before they develop clinical signs of kernicterus.

Shiller and Silverman (1961) followed up 100 low-weight babies who had high bilirubin levels after birth, and found 22 with neurological anomalies at the age of 3 years. Koch (1964) took serial bilirubin levels in 100 low-weight babies: eight died (two with kernicterus at levels of 24·8 and 30·7 mg./100 ml.). At the age of 7 years, 68 were examined. He found no neurological abnormalities except mental retardation among those with levels less than 20 mg./100 ml., but there were 22% with major neurological abnormalities among those with levels over 20 mg./100 ml. McDonald (1967) examined 1,066 children, with a birth weight of 1,800 g. or less, at the age of 6–8 years. Among those who had been jaundiced, spastic diplegia and deafness were significantly more common, especially among those with a gestational age less than 31 weeks at birth; but there was no depression of the IQ in the jaundiced children who were neurologically normal. Culley *et al.* (1970) found no reduction in intelligence in non-haemolytic jaundiced babies with serum bilirubin levels below 20 mg./100 ml. These investigations all emphasize the importance of keeping the serum bilirubin level below 20 mg./100 ml.

Haemolytic Disease of the Newborn (Erythroblastosis)

The incidence of haemolytic disease, as given by different investigators, shows a variation from 1 in 150 births to 1 in 300 births among Caucasians. It is less frequent among Asiatics and Negroes. Rh incompatibility (anti-D) causes most of the severe cases of haemolytic disease of the newborn. Many relatively mild cases (and a few severe) are caused by anti-A or anti-B immunization (anti-A being more common than anti-B) and occasionally the disease is caused by other Rh antigens or by incompatibilities within other blood groups, e.g. Kell, Duffy etc.

Rh incompatibility. An Rh negative woman is usually immunized as the result of a pregnancy with an Rh positive baby but immunization can also occur after a transfusion or intramuscular injection with Rh positive blood. If sufficient Rh positive foetal erythrocytes enter the mother's circulation, she will develop antibodies; but a small transplacental haemorrhage may only lead to sensitization, a situation in which a further Rh positive pregnancy is needed to produce detectable antibodies. There is a direct relationship between the size of the transplacental haemorrhage and the risk of developing antibodies (Woodrow and Donohoe, 1968). If the Rh positive foetal erythrocytes are ABO incompatible with the mother's blood they are usually rapidly destroyed and the mother may be protected. There are two kinds of Rh antibodies, saline agglutinating antibodies (in 19 S fraction of the gamma globulin) and blocking antibodies (in 7 S fraction). The blocking antibodies can pass through the placenta to the foetus where they attach themselves to the Rh positive red blood cells, which are then destroyed by macrophages. Large transplacental haemorrhages of foetal blood (more than 1 ml.) may occasionally occur during pregnancy, but normally occur during delivery (Woodrow *et al.*, 1965); and operative trauma at this time has been shown to increase their incidence (Wimhofer *et al.*, 1962).

Among white skinned people (Caucasians) approximately 15% are Rh negative, 38% are Rh positive homozygous and 47% are Rh positive heterozygous. It has been estimated that 11–13% of marriages are between Rh negative women and Rh positive men, but only 1 in 20 of these marriages will at some time produce an affected infant. The first Rh positive child is rarely affected unless the mother has had a previous Rh positive miscarriage, blood transfusion, or intramuscular blood injection or there has been a considerable "foetal bleed" during pregnancy. The second or subsequent children may be affected, but some

Rh negative mothers may never produce antibodies even after many pregnancies with Rh positive children. However, once a mother has produced antibodies, all her subsequent Rh positive children will be affected although some may be mildly affected. If the husband is homozygous Rh positive, all their children will be Rh positive, but if he is heterozygous approximately half of their children will be Rh negative and unaffected.

All the findings in haemolytic disease of the newborn are the result of an excessive destruction of red blood cells, to which the infant responds with an increased red cell production. The excessive destruction of the red blood cells causes (a) anaemia which may lead to heart failure and hydrops and (b) an excessive production of bilirubin which causes jaundice after birth (when the mother's liver is no longer available for its metabolism) and this can lead to kernicterus if untreated, especially in a pre-term infant with poor liver function. The foetus attempts to compensate for the anaemia by the production of new red blood cells, many of which are immature and nucleated (erythroblasts). The foetus may therefore die *in utero* with erythroblastosis; or develop hydrops, jaundice and anaemia. The severity of the disease can vary considerably.

Death in utero. This may be with or without hydrops, but even in the absence of hydrops the face usually shows slight oedema. The spleen is enlarged, and the placenta is disproportionately heavy. On histological examination, generalized erythroblastosis is found if the foetus has been dead for a short time only. If maceration is advanced, erythroblasts may often still be seen in the pulmonary capillaries.

Hydrops foetalis. The degree of oedema varies; at times it is so slight that it may be mistaken for subcutaneous fat by a casual observer, while at other times it is very severe and associated with fluid in all the serous cavities. Jaundice is rare but subcutaneous haemorrhages occur. The liver and spleen are enlarged from an abnormal degree of haemopoiesis. The serum proteins are low, usually being less than 2 g./100 ml. A severe degree of anaemia is present and many immature red blood cells are seen. The placenta is oedematous and may weigh as much as one-third of the infant's weight. Recovery may occur in infants showing subcutaneous oedema only but severe cases are either stillborn or die shortly after birth.

About half the mothers who are carrying a hydropic foetus develop symptoms resembling toxaemia. At the 7th or 8th month of pregnancy the mother's weight increases rapidly and she develops oedema, albuminuria (John and Duncan, 1964) and sometimes hypertension and hydramnios (Goodlin, 1957). The foetus usually dies soon after the onset of these symptoms in the mother.

Jaundice and anaemia. The degree of anaemia depends solely on the amount of blood destruction while the degree of jaundice depends also on the ability of the liver to conjugate and excrete the extra bilirubin. Due to the immaturity of the liver in pre-term infants, marked anaemia is rarely seen without jaundice.

The infant may look normal or pale at birth and the cord may be yellow. Jaundice develops early (within 24 hours) and may deepen rapidly. The infant becomes lethargic and feeds badly. The liver and spleen are usually enlarged. A blood count within 48 hours of birth shows anaemia and an increased number of nucleated red blood cells (10,000–100,000 per c.mm.), while later counts show an increasing degree of anaemia with a decreasing number of immature red cells. The number of platelets is reduced and in many cases there is a decrease in Factor V (de Brunijne and van Creveld, 1955) and the infants may suffer from subcutaneous, pulmonary and other haemorrhages. The serum bilirubin level in the cord blood is generally above the mean normal values of 1·5–1·8 mg./100 ml. (Valquist, 1941; Mollison and Cutbush, 1951), and the concentration of bilirubin in the serum rises as the jaundice increases, this bilirubin being mainly unconjugated.

The most serious complication is the development of kernicterus (see p. 184). This may occur in any baby with a high level of unbound bilirubin and an inadequate serum binding capacity (see section on hyperbilirubinaemia).

Diagnosis. Haemolytic disease must be differentiated from oedema and jaundice due to other causes (see pp. 228 and 230); also from anaemia present at or shortly after birth due to such causes as haemorrhagic disease and the rare condition of intrauterine loss of foetal blood due to various causes (see p. 203).

Preventive treatment. Prevention is now possible in the majority of mothers not already immunized.

No Rh negative woman, from birth until the end of child-bearing age, should be transfused with Rh positive blood or given such blood by intramuscular injection.

To reduce the risk of sensitization by an Rh positive foetus, any procedures which might cause trauma to the placental site during late pregnancy and labour (e.g. induction by Drew Smythe catheter, external version, manual removal of the placenta) should be avoided if possible in non-immunized Rh negative women. Surgical termination of pregnancy at 2–3 months can lead to sensitization if the foetus is Rh positive (Gallén *et al.*, 1965); but Voight and Britt (1969) found the risk before 12 weeks gestation was very small.

Research at the Nuffield Unit of Medical Genetics (Liverpool) suggested that immunization might be prevented if transplacental haemorrhages occurring at delivery could be neutralized by the administration of anti-Rh (anti-D) antibodies after delivery (Finn, 1960).

Clinical trials have now shown that 1 ml. anti-D gammaglobulin (containing 200 μg. anti-D) given to an Rh negative mother after her first Rh positive ABO compatible infant can suppress immunization if given within 48–72 hours after birth (Combined Study, 1966; Freda *et al.*, 1967; Clarke, 1968). Occasional failures occur and these may be due to transplacental haemorrhages during pregnancy causing an antibody titre too low to detect, so that the mother appears to be unimmunized when the Rh immunoglobulin is given after birth (Finn, 1970); or they may be due to a particularly large transplacental haemorrhage which is not completely neutralized by the Rh immunoglobulin (Hugh-Jones and Mollison, 1968; de Wit and Borst-Eilers, 1968).

The present practice is to give 1 ml. (200 μg.) anti-D antibody to all non-immunized Rh negative women, regardless of parity, who have just delivered an Rh positive baby whether the baby is ABO compatible or not because the protection from an ABO incompatible baby is not complete. The same dose should be given to any Rh negative woman who has had an abortion induced after 12 weeks gestation, if supplies are available. When a large transplacental haemorrhage is believed to have occurred during delivery, the foetal red cells in the maternal blood should be counted (foetal score), e.g. by the Kleihauer technique (Kleihauer and Betke, 1960) and the dose of immunoglobulin can be increased up to 1,000 μg. or more if the foetal score is high. Terry (1970) suggests that the foeto-maternal transplacental haemorrhage might be reduced if only one clamp is placed on the cord (near the baby) and the placental end is allowed to bleed during the third stage of delivery.

Protection given by Rh immunoglobulin only covers one following Rh positive pregnancy, and a further dose is required after each delivery of an Rh positive child.

The incidence of Rh haemolytic disease will gradually be reduced but not for some time. Women already immunized cannot be treated with Rh immunoglobulin; immunization due to other blood factors (e.g. ABO, other Rh antigens, etc.) cannot be neutralized by anti-D gammaglobulin; transplacental haemorrhages during pregnancy are not covered by this treatment, and sometimes the transplacental haemorrhage at birth is too large to be completely neutralized

Curative treatment. Careful management of pregnancy is still necessary in some cases to detect a severely affected child *in utero* so as to be able to prevent still-birth and hydrops; and careful management of the affected child is necessary to prevent kernicterus.

The previous obstetric history is extremely important. If there has been a previous stillbirth or severely affected infant, there is a 60% risk of intrauterine death before 35 weeks gestation. With a history of a less severely affected infant requiring treatment, the risk is 33%; and if a previous child was mildly affected and did not require treatment, this risk falls to 20% (Walker, 1968).

All expectant mothers must have their blood investigated for ABO grouping and Rh typing as part of their routine prenatal care. Rh negative mothers must have the blood examined at regular intervals for the presence of antibodies; and if antibodies develop, the husband's blood must also be examined. If the husband is heterozygous some of the children will be Rh negative and unaffected; and if the baby is likely to be ABO compatible, the mother is more likely to be affected than if it is ABO incompatible.

Any mother who is already immunized, or who develops antibodies for the first time, must be booked for delivery in a hospital with full facilities for intensive care of mother and baby.

The selection of mothers likely to have a stillbirth or severely affected infant is not easy. The maternal antibody titre is of some value in the first affected pregnancy but after this the previous history is of more value. The best assessment of the condition of any particular foetus is obtained by estimating the bilirubin content of the liquor amnii, obtained by amniocentesis. In 1956 Bevis reported that spectrophotometric examination of the liquor amnii revealed an increase in blood pigments in cases of haemolytic disease. Walker (1957) used the shape of the curve (relative to bilirubin) to predict whether a foetus was affected or not and, since then, this method has been used successfully by many investigators. The bilirubin level in the liquor can be estimated chemically (Gambino and Freda, 1966) as well as spectrophotometrically (Walker, 1957 and 1970) but the latter method is usually preferred.

If a previous pregnancy has resulted in a stillbirth or very severe disease, the risk of death *in utero* is so great that the initial amniocentesis is usually performed at 20 weeks gestation; but if previous babies were only moderately affected, or if it is the first affected pregnancy, the initial amniocentesis (if indicated) is usually done at 30 weeks gestation.

The mean liquor bilirubin levels at different stages of normal pregnancy have been assessed by Walker (1970). The level rises to a maximum at 18–20 weeks, and this level is maintained until about 26 weeks, then there is a continuous fall until term. No decision should be taken on a single estimation unless the level is extremely high. With two consecutive estimations a falling level gives reassurance while a high and rising level suggests a bad prognosis and labour should be induced if the foetus has reached a gestational age of 35 weeks.

If intrauterine death is expected before there is a reasonable chance of survival after birth, an intrauterine transfusion should be attempted. Liley first used this technique in 1963 to keep the foetus alive until it had a chance of survival. The various techniques are well described by Walker and Ellis (1970). The procedure is not without risk and should only be undertaken by a skilled staff and only to prevent death *in utero*. The risks include trauma to the foetus and placenta (and this may release more foetal erythrocytes into the maternal circulation); infection of mother and foetus; onset of premature labour; runt disease (Cohen *et al.*, 1965) and abnormalities in the immunoglobulin pattern (Hobbs *et al.*, 1968) if viable lymphocytes are injected.

Because an exchange transfusion is more beneficial than a simple transfusion this has been tried *in utero* by Freda and Adamson (1964) using a leg delivered through an incision in the uterus; and by Seelen *et al.* (1966) who incised the uterus along the placental margin and used a large placental vein; and also by Asensio *et al.* (1968) who actually delivered the foetus by Caesarean section, carried out an exchange transfusion and returned the foetus to the uterus. These procedures have not met with much success; serious maternal infection has occurred and foetal death and onset of premature labour have been common.

The proper place of intrauterine transfusion in the management of Rh immunization is not yet known but it is certain that cases must be very carefully selected. More controlled studies are required.

Opinions vary as to whether mildly affected infants should be delivered before term or not. However, labour should never be induced before 37–38 weeks gestation unless there are special indications because pre-term infants are more liable to develop hyperbilirubinaemia and kernicterus than term infants and, in addition, a low gestation age itself carries an increased risk of neonatal death.

During labour the use of sedatives and anaesthetics should be restricted to a minimum if the mother has antibodies. Sulphonamides and salicylates must be avoided. The condition of the infant must be carefully monitored (see p. 18). In severe cases a foetal blood sample can be obtained during labour (see p. 19) for the haemoglobin level, Coombs' test and the blood group, and this will allow an early assessment of the severity of the disease and cross-matching of the blood before birth. All facilities for resuscitation must be available (see p. 20). The umbilical cord must be clamped immediately after birth to prevent more blood containing antibodies from entering the infants circulation. Terry (1970) recommends using one clamp only (on the baby) and leaving the placental end of the cord to bleed in order to reduce foeto-maternal transplacental haemorrhage during the third stage. In any case, some of this cord blood is required for examination.

In every case where the mother is Rh negative (even if no antibodies have been found during pregnancy) cord blood must be sent for (1) Rh typing (2) Coombs' test and (3) ABO group. If the infant is pale, oedematous or jaundiced, or if the Coombs' test is positive, the cord blood must also be examined for (4) haemoglobin level and (5) unbound bilirubin level; and it should also be cross-matched.

Meanwhile the infant must be kept warm, drugs which compete with bilirubin for albumin binding and glucuronyl conjugation must be avoided, and feeding should be started as soon as possible. If the infant is severely affected it may require oxygen (see p. 134 for administration of oxygen) and even assisted ventilation (see p. 142). In such cases the umbilical artery may have to be catheterized for the purpose of monitoring the Pa_{O_2}, pH and blood sugar; and any acidosis and hypoglycaemia should be corrected before an exchange transfusion is given (see p. 136).

If a pre-term infant is found to be Rh positive and Coombs positive, the author believes that an exchange transfusion should be undertaken as soon as possible, regardless of the haemoglobin and bilirubin levels, because a pre-term infant is one of the chief indications for an exchange. The purpose of the first exchange is to reduce any increased venous pressure, correct any anaemia and remove sensitized red blood cells. Because of the pre-term baby's poor ability to convert and excrete indirect-acting bilirubin, it is essential to reduce the degree of haemolysis by removing the infant's own blood cells as soon as possible. The best route for an exchange transfusion is the umbilical vein (Diamond *et al.*, 1951). The blood should be as fresh as possible (never more than 3 days old for fear of dangerous levels of potassium): it must be Rh negative and compatible in regard to the infant's ABO grouping and with the mother's serum, and warmed. At least 80 ml./lb. (180 ml./kg.) should be exchanged in order to obtain replacement of approximately 90% of the Rh positive red cells and 25% of the antibodies. The infant's anaemia will be corrected during the process of replacement if the P C V of the blood is kept up (40%) by reducing the volume of the citrate-dextrose used as an anticoagulant. If the infant's venous pressure is raised, which is common in severe cases, it is advisable to remove 20–25 ml. of the infant's blood (according to the condition of the infant) during the early stages of the exchange, and to give the transfusion slowly. The technique of an exchange transfusion has been discussed on p. 190. In a severe case, acidosis may develop during an exchange transfusion with citrated blood. This can be prevented by adding sodium bicarbonate, i.e. 1·8 mEq/100 ml. to the blood given in the first half of the exchange and 0·9 mEq/100 ml. to that given during the second half of the exchange transfusion (Gandy *et al.*, 1968). If severe acidosis is present before the exchange it is wise to correct it before starting the exchange.

After the exchange, the infant's blood must be examined regularly for the haemoglobin and serum bilirubin levels, and reserve serum binding capacity (12-hourly at first, then daily and finally at longer intervals) until it is certain that the bilirubin level is falling. One, or possibly more, repeat exchanges may be necessary to prevent kernicterus. The purpose of these repeat exchanges is solely for the removal of bilirubin in order to prevent kernicterus. For details as to how this is best done, and for the possible use of phototherapy, see curative treatment in the section on hyperbilirubinaemia (p. 191).

No affected infant should be given its own mother's milk unboiled during the first week of life, because the antibody titre in the milk can be high during this period and absorption of traces of unaltered antibodies cannot be precluded (Boorman *et al.*, 1958). Hirszfeldowa *et al.* (1960) have reported several cases of anaemia and one case of jaundice due to absorption of antibodies from the milk.

After the first 7–10 days, the danger of kernicterus should be over, but the level of haemoglobin will continue to fall for 10–12 weeks, the normal fall being increased by the continued action of antibodies, traces of which may still be found up to 6–8 weeks after birth. Until the danger of kernicterus is over (10 days in a pre-term infant) the haemoglobin should be maintained above 12·0 g.% to avoid stimulation of the bone marrow which would produce more sensitized red blood cells susceptible to the antibodies present (Gairdner *et al.*, 1952). This is usually achieved by giving blood with a suitable P C V for the first exchange. Occasionally the blood used for a repeat exchange during the 1st week of life may have to be slightly "packed", but this is rare. After this period, a "top-up" transfusion is only required if the haemoglobin falls below 7·0 g.% before the 8th–10th weeks of life, or if there is any complicating infection, or failure to gain weight. For these "topping-up" transfusions the quantity of blood required may be calculated from the fact that an infant has approximately 40 ml. of blood per lb. (90 ml./kg.). If the haemoglobin has fallen to 6·0 g./100 ml. (40%) then 16 ml./lb. (36 ml./kg.) of blood will be required to bring the haemoglobin level back to 12·0 g./100 ml. (80%): citrated blood is usually equivalent to 80% whole blood, therefore 20 ml./lb. (44 ml./kg.) of citrated blood will be required. No more than 10 ml./lb. (20 ml./kg.) should be given in one operation, so either "packed" cells (prepared by removing half the supernatant plasma citrate) must be used or the transfusion should be given as a slow drip over 12 hours. The most useful route for such a transfusion is a scalp vein, but any superficial vein may be used.

Prognosis. This depends on the gestational age of the infant (the lower the gestational age the worse the prognosis), the severity of the disease, and the facilities available for prenatal, natal, and postnatal care. The best results are obtained if mothers known to be immunized are cared for in hospitals with full facilities for assessing gestational age and well-being of the foetus, for performing intrauterine transfusion if necessary, and for exchange transfusion in the infant after birth.

Many of the cases which develop kernicterus die, and those that survive suffer from varying degrees of cerebral palsy, mental deficiency and deafness; *but kernicterus should now be regarded as a preventable complication.*

Green staining of the deciduous teeth, and a persistent obstructive jaundice due to liver damage ("inspissated bile syndrome") which sometimes used to follow haemolytic disease are rarely seen nowadays due to the use of exchange transfusions, repeated if necessary.

It is wise to follow up all infants who have suffered from haemolytic disease to at least the age of 3 years to exclude minor degrees of cerebral palsy, mental retardation and high tone deafness.

ABO incompatibility. In 20% of all pregnancies, the mother's serum contains antibodies (anti-A or anti-B) which are incompatible with the red blood cells of her baby but most of these are naturally occurring saline agglutinating antibodies in the 19 S fraction of the gamma globulin which do not cross the placenta. It is these naturally occurring anti-A, or occasionally anti-B, antibodies which are protective against Rh immunization.

Occasionally, however, the mother's serum contains strongly haemolytic "immune" antibodies (blocking antibodies in the 7 S fraction of the gamma globulin) which can cross the placenta. "Immune" antibodies are found as the result of a transfusion with blood of an incompatible ABO group, or from a pregnancy with a foetus with an incompatible ABO group. Luckily few pre-term Caucasian babies are seriously affected (Schellong, 1964). However, this condition is seen quite commonly in Negro and Asian babies, and may easily be missed because of the difficulty of diagnosing jaundice in coloured babies. The condition is most likely to occur if the mother is group O and the baby group A, but it occurs with a group B baby of a group O mother; also rarely when the mother is B and the infant A, and very rarely, vice versa.

Weiner *et al.* (1960) said there were two patterns of anti-A haemolytic disease (1) a mild condition in which the first-born incompatible baby is affected as well as all subsequent incompatible ones and (2) a more severe condition in which the mother is sensitized by the birth of one or more incompatible unaffected babies before the birth of a severely affected incompatible one.

The importance of the condition is that kernicterus can occur if the bilirubin level rises unduly high.

It is now possible to predict ABO haemolytic disease. Sera from group O mothers are screened for haemolysis of group A pig cells: if positive, they are further tested by an antibody absorption test for 7 S antibodies, to predict the severity of the disease in the baby. At birth the cord blood is tested by a direct Bromelin test (Tovey and Lockyer, 1965).

In the absence of prenatal tests, haemolytic disease due to ABO incompatibility should be suspected if:

(1) Jaundice develops within 24 hours of birth.

(2) The blood groups of the mother and baby show potential incompatibility (the mother usually being group O).

(3) The infant is Coombs negative (it may occasionally be weakly positive).

(4) The fragility of the infant's red blood cells is increased and spherocytosis is present.

The diagnosis can be confirmed by finding a positive direct Bromelin test.

Blood used for exchange transfusion must be group O, and the same Rh group as the infant; and it must be free from immune anti-A or there will be a further rise in the bilirubin level necessitating another exchange transfusion (Morris and King, 1961).

Affected infants should not be given their own mother's milk as antibodies may be present in high concentrations and cause an increase in jaundice (Hirszfeldowa *et al.*, 1960).

Anaemia

Although the pre-term baby with a maturity more than 30 weeks starts life with just as high a haemoglobin level and red cell count as a baby born at term (see p. 5) the postnatal fall in both is greater, more rapid and more prolonged; and the final rise is slower especially in regard to the level of haemoglobin (Mackay, 1933).

More immature red cells (normoblasts and reticulocytes) are present in the blood at birth and throughout the first week of life, and the greater fragility of these cells accounts for part of the greater initial falls in the haemoglobin level and red cell count (see p. 5). These immature cells disappear rapidly after the first week of life. Reticulocytes reappear in the blood at the age of 5–6 weeks (van Creveld and Heybrock, 1932), but as the cell count and haemoglobin level both continue to fall until 8–10 weeks of age the cell production does not exceed the cell destruction until then. After this age, any low-weight baby may develop a late anaemia which is due to iron deficiency.

Anaemia can also be due to, or aggravated by, such conditions as:

(1) Haemolytic disease.

(2) Infections.

(3) Haemorrhages from various causes, e.g. haemorrhagic disease, bleeding of foetus into maternal circulation (Chown, 1955) or into twin (Klingberg *et al.*, 1955), bleeding from a separated or damaged placenta or from abnormal umbilical vessel (Michaels, 1955), or bleeding from the cord after delivery.

(4) Chemical agents such as naphthalene from moth balls (Cock, 1957), resorcin in medicaments (Cunningham, 1956), and vitamin K.

(5) Hereditary spherocytosis.

(6) Nutritional disturbances, including folic acid deficiency (a megaloblastic anaemia), and vitamin E deficiency with characteristic vitamin E deficient erythrocytes and low tocopherol levels (Chadd, 1970).

(7) Blood taken for investigations.

When taking blood samples it should be remembered that, during the first week of life, samples taken by skin prick have a higher level of haemoglobin and a higher red cell count than venous samples, and that it is desirable to use venous samples whenever an accurate haemoglobin estimation is required.

Early anaemia. The "physiological" anaemia is exaggerated by the relatively faster growth of low-weight babies, and the smallest babies show the most marked degrees of anaemia. In the pre-term baby it may be partly haemolytic in origin, the greater fragility of the immature red cells present at birth accounting for the greater cell destruction (Foconi and Sjölin, 1959). According to Schulman *et al.* (1954) the main cause is a marked decrease in red cell production during the early neonatal period; and this is coupled with a slight decrease in the life of the red cells. This decrease in cell production is believed to be due to a poor response of erythropoiesis to the stimulus of anaemia (Gairdner *et al.*, 1955). This type of anaemia shows no response to the administration of iron or liver (Josephs, 1934). It can be exaggerated by a folic acid deficiency, other nutritional disturbances and infections.

Preventive treatment. Attention should be given to the mother's diet during pregnancy because it is likely that infants of mothers whose diets are low in iron, or who suffer from an iron deficiency anaemia, may show a greater degree of anaemia than usual (Parsons *et al.*, 1937; Smith, 1959; McFarlane, 1964). If a mother has a folic acid deficiency during pregnancy, this must also be treated; and the infant should be given oral tocopherol acetate (10 mg. t.d.s.) daily after birth until it can be put to the breast (untreated breast milk has a high level of vitamin E but heat treated breast milk and cow's milk have not).

Although it is generally believed that the cord should not be clamped in the healthy term baby until it has ceased to pulsate, clamping of the cord should probably not be delayed in a pre-term baby (see p. 20). As blood is the major source of iron to be used later for the maintenance of the haemoglobin level (Josephs, 1953) any early haemorrhage should be treated with a blood transfusion. The dosage of vitamin K should be kept within safe limits. Attention must be paid to the feeding, and to the correct administration of vitamins (including vitamin E). General hygiene must be good and the infant protected from infection. Sunlight and fresh air are of great importance and when the infant is strong enough it should be put out in the open air for a short period daily.

This type of anaemia cannot be prevented by administration of iron before the age of 4 weeks unless the infant has lost blood by haemorrhage. This is understandable since the iron derived from destruction of the red cells is retained in the body and there is already more iron available than can be utilized. As the amount of iron in the body depends on the weight at birth (Widdowson and Spray, 1951) and as babies with a low birth weight grow relatively more rapidly than heavier ones, the smallest babies will require an earlier administration of iron to prevent a later iron deficiency anaemia but even the smallest ones should not require extra iron before the age of 4 weeks.

Curative treatment. If the haemoglobin falls below 7·0 g./100 ml. before the age of 8–10 weeks, in spite of the administration of iron and the treatment of any folic acid deficiency, a blood transfusion should be given. The amount of blood required to raise the level of haemoglobin is calculated as on p. 201. As it is not safe to give more than 10 ml./lb. (20 ml./kg.) in one short operation, "packed" cells may be used and the transfusion given as a slow scalp vein drip. Such a transfusion is usually only necessary for the smallest pre-term infants unless there has been an infection or a haemorrhage.

Late anaemia (Iron deficiency anaemia). The late anaemia, or anaemia occurring after the first 3 months of life, is characterized by a low colour index, due to the level of haemoglobin rising more slowly than the red cell count. Any low-weight infant is liable to suffer from this hypochromic microcytic iron deficiency anaemia for the following reasons:

(1) A relatively poor iron store (the store is proportional to the body weight, i.e. is small).

(2) A relatively greater growth after birth with a correspondingly greater increase in blood volume.

(3) A great susceptibility to infection.

(4) A greater chance of being a twin, with a reduced iron reserve.

This type of anaemia responds well to the administration of iron except in the presence of infection; and it can also be prevented to some extent by the administration of iron after the age of 4 weeks.

Preventive treatment. Good feeding, good hygiene and protection from infection are all necessary. Babies fed on human milk are less likely to develop severe anaemia than those fed on cow's milk (Crosse *et al.*, 1954). The iron content is higher in human milk and the lower phosphate content causes less inhibition of iron absorption. In addition, infants fed on human milk suffer less from infections (see p. 104).

The administration of iron can be commenced at the age of 4–6 weeks, for although it is known that this will not prevent the development of the early type of anaemia it accelerates the expected rise in the haemoglobin after the initial drop (Mackay, 1933) and thus prevents the development of the late anaemia.

Curative treatment. This condition is cured by the administration of iron. Iron can be given as ferric ammonium citrate, 140 mg./kg./day (Mist. ferric ammonium 80 mg. per ml.); as ferrous sulphate (20% elemental iron) 20–30 mg./kg./day or as ferrous gluconate (12% elemental iron) 30–50 mg./kg./day.

Because iron may not be well tolerated by small infants, small doses must be given at first. Ferric salts should be given in the feeds, so that the iron is well diluted; but ferrous salts should be given between feeds because the phosphorus in the milk reduces absorption of the iron. Iron supplements are required until the end of the first year of life, and sometimes longer.

For infants resistant to or intolerant of oral iron, or for a rapid response to iron, Jectofer (iron-sorbitol-citric-acid complex) can be used intramuscularly. A single dose (1·5 mg./kg.) is given daily, or on alternate days, until the haemoglobin reaches the desired level.

Transfusions are usually only necessary when anaemia is associated with infection, which reduces the efficiency of iron.

Retrolental Fibroplasia

What is now known to be the final stage of this disease was first described in pre-term babies by Terry in 1942. Earlier signs were described 7 years later (Owens and Owens, 1949) but it was only in 1953 that exposure to oxygen was finally proved to be the cause of the condition. Animal experiments by Ashton *et al.* (1953) and Patz *et al.* (1953) showed that exposure of suitable animals to oxygen resulted in spasm, then obliteration, of the developing retinal vessels (proportional to the duration of exposure and concentration of the oxygen) which was followed later by neovascularization, haemorrhage and retinal detachment; as in retrolental fibroplasia.

In the pre-term infant the disease has three stages. The first occurs during the administration of oxygen and is directly related to the concentration of oxygen in the arterial blood and the maturity of the retina. Vasoconstriction of the retinal vessels is the first sign, and this is followed by vaso-obliteration if excessive administration of oxygen continues. The second, or active, stage usually begins between the ages of 3 weeks and 3 months; the smaller the birth weight, the later the onset. The first sign is dilatation and tortuosity of the retinal blood vessels; the fundus then becomes pale and haemorrhages appear alongside the blood vessels; these haemorrhages spread into the vitreous either in the periphery or near the optic disc; this is followed by separation of the retina which usually commences at the periphery and is most marked at the sites of the haemorrhages. New vessel formation and vitreous opacities may be seen at the junction of the attached with the separated retina (Figs. 47 and 48).

After several weeks, the active stage passes gradually into the third or cicatrical stage, this being characterized by organization of the vitreous and formation of a retrolental membrane. The "foetal blue" of the iris may be retained for a longer period than usual, the anterior chamber becomes shallow and impairment of vision may be accompanied by squint, nystagmus and photophobia. Microphthalmia is a common sequel to a severe case and secondary glaucoma is a possible complication. Both eyes are affected, although different stages may be present in the two eyes, and spontaneous arrest may occur at any stage.

The damage done during the cicatricial stage depends on the severity of the acute stage and the time at which the disease is arrested. Mild or abortive cases may be followed by little or no abnormality. Owens (1951) stated that 60% of his cases showing early manifestations underwent spontaneous regression with no residual damage. The exact stage at which the condition becomes irreversible is not known.

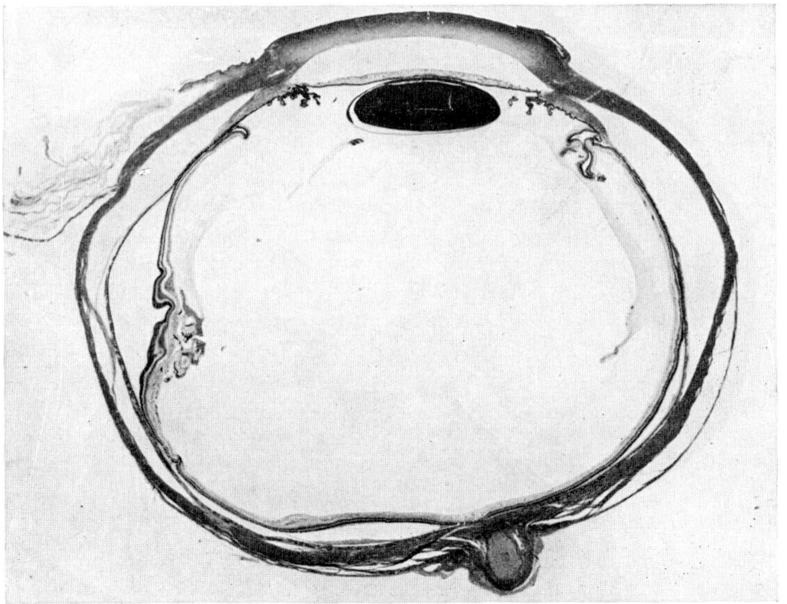

(Photograph by courtesy of Norman Ashton)

Fig. 47. Whole eye showing retrolental fibroplasia (Active stage). At the equator on one side there is a localized proliferation of vasoformative tissue which extends out of the nerve fibre layer into the vitreous.

It is well established (Reece *et al.*, 1952; Ashton *et al.*, 1953) that the active stage of retrolental fibroplasia (R L F) consists of an irregular localized proliferation of capillary endothelial cells associated with a more diffuse proliferation of "glial" cells, confined initially to the nerve fibre layer of the retina. If this vaso-formative tissue becomes too exuberant, it bursts through the limiting membrane into the vitreous. Protein transudate then seeps through the new vessels growing into the vitreous and this becomes organized into fibrous strands which distort or detach the retina. Detachment of the retina is followed by absorption of the vitreous and pulling together of the retina behind the lens, leaving only a stalk of rolled-up retinal tissue connected posteriorly with the optic disc. New vessels may appear on the iris and glaucoma may develop as a sequel to shallowing of the anterior chamber and angle block, and late atrophic changes cause a shrunken eye.

Cause. The occurrence of R L F coincided with the increase in the use of oxygen, and cases occurred in the U.S.A. some years before they occurred elsewhere.

The incidence of the condition is known to depend on:

(1) The level of arterial oxygen tension.

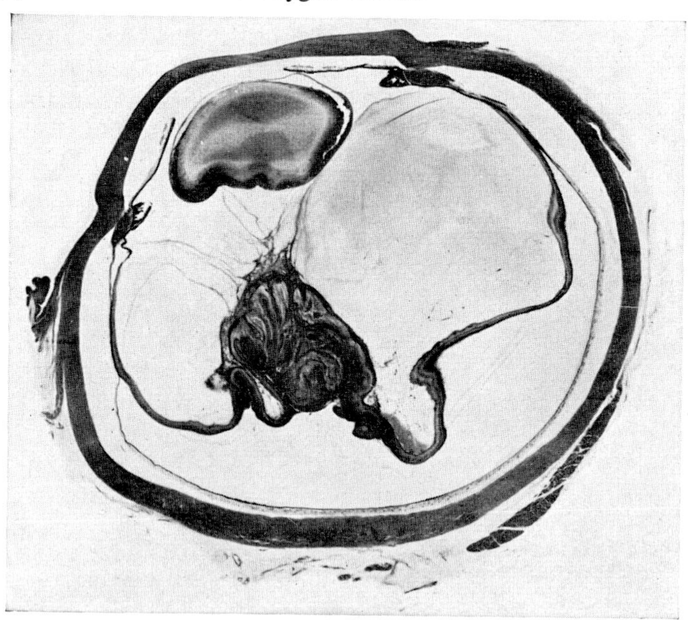

(Photograph by courtesy of Norman Ashton)

FIG. 48. Whole eye showing retrolental fibroplasia (Cicatricial stage). Protein transudate seeps through the new vessels growing into the vitreous and becomes organized into fibrous strands which distort and detach the retina.

(2) The length of time of administration of oxygen.

(3) The degree of immaturity of the eyes at the time when oxygen is given (see p. 8 for development of eye).

Distribution of cases of R L F relative to the number of days in high concentrations of oxygen shows an increase in incidence with duration of exposure. The curve rises rapidly during the first few days after birth and then flattens out, showing that the critical period is immediately after birth (Report of M. and R. Pediatric Research Conference, 1955).

The risk of developing R L F from exposure to oxygen diminishes as the birth weight increases, i.e. as the retina becomes more mature; R L F rarely occurs in infants weighing more than 2,000 g. at birth.

R L F must be differentiated from other forms of pseudoglioma, congenital cataract, glioma of retina (retinoblastoma), remains of posterior vascular sheath, and retinitis due to congenital toxoplasmosis, rubella and cytomegalic inclusion disease.

Preventive treatment. The use of oxygen must be restricted to babies who become cyanosed without it, and this is particularly important for babies weighing less than 2,000 g. (4 lb. 6 oz) at birth, or having a gestational age less than 34 weeks. If oxygen is necessary, the minimum amount should be used for the minimum period of time.

Now that oxygen is being used more freely more cases of R L F will occur unless oxygen is used carefully. Many believe that the administration of 40% oxygen is safe without being monitored but the safe concentration is not yet known. It is certainly below 40% (Report of 16th M. & R. Pediatric Research Conference, 1955; de Leon *et al.*, 1970); and cases have been reported from units using concentrations between 30% and 40% (Zacharias, 1964). In the author's experience 30% is the highest level which should be given without monitoring the level of Pao_2.

It is now known that monitoring the level of arterial oxygen tension (Pao_2) is much more important than monitoring the concentration of inspired oxygen because the Pao_2 level (in the same concentration of oxygen) will vary according to the amount of $R \rightarrow L$ shunt present. But the safe Pao_2 level is also unknown. Some believe it should be kept below 160 mm. Hg. which is the level found in normal infants breathing 40% oxygen, but others (including the author) think it should be kept between 90 and 100 mm. Hg. (Roberton and Dahlenburg, 1969; de Leon *et al.*, 1970) which is the level reached by normal babies by the age of 48 hours breathing air (Gupta, 1965).

The minimum concentration must be given to maintain the Pao_2 at the required level. This entails monitoring the Pao_2 during the administration of oxygen in concentrations over 30% (de Leon does not believe this can be omitted up to 40%). The necessary frequency of testing is not yet known because the Pao_2 level can change quickly in the same oxygen concentration without any noticeable change in the condition of the infant, e.g. during alveolar expansion of primary atelectasis in very small infants, or after the administration of alkalis in idiopathic respiratory distress, or during recovery from respiratory distress. In the light of present knowledge the frequency must be dependent on the possibility of changes occurring in the Pao_2 at the time in question.

Garner and Ashton (1971) have established the principle that intermittent (as opposed to continuous) oxygen can prevent damage to the growing retinal vessels by allowing reversal of vasoconstriction before vaso-obliteration can occur. Oxygen should never be given continuously when intermittent use will suffice, e.g. for cyanosis following apnoeic attacks. Where high concentrations are used for long periods (especially after the first few days when frequent blood sampling becomes extremely difficult) it may be possible and safer to replace oxygen by air for short periods at definite intervals. This should be a profitable area for research.

It has been suggested that careful observation of the retinal vessels for spasm might be an alternative to Pao_2 monitoring (Patz, 1967). Baum (1971) does not agree because the retina is difficult to see in infants of less than 30 weeks gestation (due to persistent vasculosa lentis); a 24 hour service of expert opthalmologists would be required; and the signs they would be looking for are probably due to established retinal damage. In addition, the absence of vasospasm is not an indication that the Pao_2 is within safe limits (Robertson *et al.*, 1968). If facilities are not available for monitoring the Pao_2, any infant weighing less than 2,000 g., or with a gestational age less than 34 weeks, which requires the administration of oxygen for more than a very short period should be transferred to an intensive care unit.

The eyes of all infants weighing less than 2,000 g., or with a gestational age less than 34 weeks, who have been given oxygen during the first 2 weeks of life should be examined with an ophthalmoscope before being discharged and again at the age of 3 months. R L F has never developed after this age, so only doubtful cases need to be seen after this.

Curative treatment. There is no cure for a fully developed case. In the early stages of the disease many forms of treatment have been tried but the only one believed to have any effect is A C T H (Houlton, 1956; Brown, 1960). A C T H may be tried if spontaneous regression does not occur but new vessels are growing into the vitreous and the vitreous is becoming hazy. Brown uses 5 mg. 6-hourly intramuscularly. Once A C T H has been started, it should be given without interruption until the disease has burnt itself out (normally from the 5th–7th week until the 12th–13th week (Brown and Corner, 1952). If stopped before this (even for 24 hours), the condition deteriorates and the final result may be worse than if no treatment had been given. Brown thinks this is the reason why some observers reported A C T H as ineffective.

Rickets

Rickets is a preventable disease but, in the absence of preventive treatment, rickets not only occurs more frequently in low-weight (especially pre-term) infants but it also occurs at an earlier age and tends to be more severe.

Pre-term infants are more prone to develop rickets for the following reasons:

(1) They have a deficient store of calcium and phosphorus, and possibly also of vitamin D, at birth.

(2) A relatively small part of the skeleton is calcified at birth.

(3) Their growth after birth is relatively more rapid, creating extra needs.

(4) Their absorption of fat and vitamin D tends to be deficient, although their absorption of calcium and phosphorus is normal.

(5) Renal function tends to be poor, and vitamin D may not promote tubular reabsorption of phosphate.

(6) Because of their small size and general frailty, low-weight babies are less exposed to natural sunlight.

(7) The increased incidence of infections and digestive disturbances may reduce still further the absorption of fat and mineral salts.

Term infants which are light-for-dates are also more prone to rickets for reasons (1), (3) and (6).

The earliest clinical signs are craniotabes, beading of the ribs and chest deformities. Evidence of tetany may be the first sign of rickets. Craniotabes may be seen as early as 6–8 weeks of age and is usually in the posterior half of the skull (but this may also be found in very small infants without rickets). Radiological examination may show the presence of rickets when there are no clinical signs. Rarefaction and splaying of the distal end of the ulna may be seen at the age of 3 months, or even earlier. Chemical changes in the blood develop several weeks before the radiological changes in the bones. The serum phosphatase is usually increased when active rickets is present; in low-weight babies high levels of serum phosphatase are suggestive of rickets if liver disease and obstructive jaundice can be excluded. The levels of serum calcium and serum phosphorus vary considerably (Sydow, 1946).

Preventive treatment. During the prenatal period the mother should take an adequate diet containing mineral salts and vitamins, and after birth the child should be treated with vitamin D and later with fresh air and sunlight.

In earlier literature large daily prophylactic doses of vitamin D were considered necessary for pre-term babies (Davidson and Merritt, 1934; Eliot and Park, 1942) but later work showed that there was no need for the large doses which had been recommended in the past: indeed there is even a danger of hypercalcaemia from overdosage in infants who are hypersensitive to vitamin D (Creery and Neill, 1954; de Luca and Cozzi, 1964) especially as vitamin D is added to many of the proprietary infant foods. Glaser *et al.* (1949) stated that although 100 i.u. of vitamin D was a satisfactory prophylactic dose for the majority of pre-term babies, 400–800 i.u. allowed a greater margin of safety; while Harrison *et al.* (1955) showed that relatively small doses of vitamin D (250–400 i.u.) were effective for prophylaxis. The administration of vitamin D should be started at the age of 1 week (see p. 119).

The older and stronger babies should be put out in the open air as soon as possible, provided chilling is avoided.

Curative treatment. Vitamin D is used for cure as well as prevention, but treatment must be more intensive for cure. Ultraviolet light may also be used.

Hypocalcaemia and Hypomagnesaemia

Low-weight infants occasionally develop tetany during the first week of life, due to a decrease in the serum calcium associated with an increase in the serum phosphorus. This may be caused by a transient hypoparathyroidism, an inadequate excretion of phosphorus due to poor kidney function, or to an excessive intake of phosphorus, e.g. the early administration of a concentrated cow's milk formula.

Gittleman *et al.* (1956) demonstrated a significant correlation between the level of blood calcium on the first day of life and birth weight; the lower the birth weight, the lower the level of calcium. Brück and Weintraub (1955) found that the calcium level fell during the initial fasting period; the longer the fast, the lower the level. These investigators also found that the calcium level rose in all babies to whom human milk was given, but it fell at first in 40% of babies to whom cow's milk was given. Tetany rarely occurs in infants fed on human milk because of its low phosphate content (Oppé and Redstone, 1968).

Babies of diabetic mothers, light-for-dates babies, and babies of mothers with a deficient calcium intake (Watney *et al.*, 1971) are particularly liable to develop low blood calcium levels.

Neonatal tetany is characterized by irritability, twitching and convulsions, and often vomiting, and must be differentiated from intracranial birth injury and infections. Laryngeal and carpopedal spasms are uncommon; and in a pre-term infant, Chvostek's sign is not significant before the age of 2–3 months. The serum calcium is below 7·0 mg./100 ml., the serum phosphorus level is low in early tetany, but high when associated with high phosphate feeding, while the phosphatase level is normal.

Hypocalcaemic tetany must be differentiated from tetany due to other causes, e.g. alkalosis (from vomiting or hyperventilation), vitamin D deficiency (which usually occurs at a later age), iatrogenic tetany from large amounts of citrate given during an exchange transfusion, and hypomagnesaemia.

Attention has been drawn recently to the association of *hypomagnesaemia* with tetany of the newborn (Mizrahi *et al.*, 1968; Wong and Teh, 1968). Although hypomagnesaemia is usually associated with hypocalcaemia Wong and Teh reported cases with normal calcium levels. Hypomagnesaemia should be suspected if tetany occurs without a low serum calcium level or if the condition fails to respond to calcium salts. It is recommended that the serum magnesium level should be determined as well as the serum calcium level in all babies with tremors or convulsions.

Prevention. During pregnancy the mother should have an adequate calcium intake; and vitamin D supplements should be given (Watney *et al.*, 1971). The infant should be fed on human milk if possible. If cow's milk is used, it should be diluted during the first week of life.

Treatment. In mild cases, calcium gluconate (0·5 g./kg./day) solution may be given by mouth, *in feeds*. In severe cases, 3–5 ml. of 10% solution of calcium gluconate should be given intravenously (never intramuscularly) at the rate of 1 ml. per minute and sedatives administered to control the convulsions, e.g. chloral grain 1 (60 mg.) orally; or soluble phenobarbitone grains $\frac{1}{8}$–$\frac{1}{4}$ (7$\frac{1}{2}$–15 mg.) intramuscularly if oral feeding has not been started. These sedatives can be repeated as required. Infants fed on cow's milk should either be given human milk, or have their feeds diluted. An adequate dose of vitamin D should be ensured.

If hypomagnesaemia is present, this may be corrected by an intramuscular injection of 50% magnesium sulphate (2 ml./kg./4 hours) or an oral dose of 30 mEq. daily.

Hypoglycaemia

Hypoglycaemia may be associated with many conditions which occur in the low-weight baby, e.g. severe birth asphyxia, idiopathic respiratory distress, intracranial haemorrhage, infections, severe haemolytic disease, "cold injury", etc.; it also occurs in babies of diabetic mothers but in many cases it is idiopathic.

Idiopathic hypoglycaemia most frequently occurs among infants who are light-for-dates (Cornblath *et al.*, 1961; Brown and Wallis, 1963;

Pildes *et al.*, 1967; Raivio, 1968; Gentz *et al.*, 1969; Sparrevohn, 1969); and male infants are more often affected than females. Clinical signs may result when the blood sugar level has fallen below 20 mg./100 ml. but many low-weight babies still appear quite normal with a blood sugar below this level.

The aetiology of idiopathic hypoglycaemia is unknown but there are many theories, e.g.:

(1) The relatively large brain of the light-for-dates baby may require more glucose than the relatively small liver can supply (Cornblath *et al.*, 1963).

(2) Some abnormality in blood glucose regulation (Raivo, 1969b).

(3) Prenatal brain damage or congenital abnormality of the brain which is responsible for both hypoglycaemia and subsequent abnormal neurological development (Cornblath *et al.*, 1964; Knobloch *et al.*, 1967).

(4) Lack of free fatty acids to counteract a sensitive insulin release (Randle *et al.*, 1963; Creery *et al.*, 1964) but Raivo (1969a) does not support this theory.

Signs usually develop on the 2nd or 3rd day of life and vary from slight tremors, hypertonicity and feeding difficulties to apnoea and cyanosis, convulsions and coma. Hypoglycaemia should always be remembered when a previously healthy infant (especially if light-for-dates) suddenly develops any of these signs, and the blood glucose should be investigated immediately. The Dextrostix enzyme test strip is a useful preliminary test. When the colour change is present (brown to grey) hypoglycaemia can be eliminated because the lowest reading is 30 mg./100 ml. If the colour change is absent or doubtful, blood must be sent for laboratory examination. A true blood glucose level (measured by the glucose oxidase method) should be requested rather than the total reducing substances present.

The condition must be differentiated from all other causes of apnoea (see p. 220) and convulsions (see p. 232), etc.

Preventive treatment. Every effort should be made to reduce the incidence of light-for-dates babies and pre-term babies. All low-weight babies (especially those light-for-dates) must be kept warm and fed as soon as possible after birth, if necessary by intragastric drip. It is probably better to use milk rather than glucose (Haas, 1966). There is ample evidence that early milk feeding can prevent hypoglycaemia (Smallpeice and Davies, 1964; Wharton and Bower, 1965; Cornblath *et al.*, 1966; Rabor *et al.*, 1968). Milk supplies fat which spares glucose for its essential cerebral function, and fat stores are low in low-weight infants.

Infants at risk, i.e. babies which are light-for-dates, very small pre-term babies and babies of diabetic mothers should be screened at 6-hourly intervals for the first few days of life (by Dextrostix, followed by laboratory tests if necessary). If two consecutive blood glucose estimations are less than 20 mg./100 ml. the infant should be treated at once, even if there are no abnormal signs.

Curative treatment. As an immediate rise in blood glucose is required in order to reduce the risk of brain damage an immediate injection of 50% glucose (1 ml./kg.) should be given, followed by a glucose drip. Usually the scalp vein is used and 10% glucose given (100 ml./kg./day). Intravenous hydrocortisone (10 mg. four times daily) may be given in addition. Oral or intragastric milk feeds should be continued and the feed can be made up with 5% glucose instead of water. Cyanotic attacks and convulsions must be suitably treated (see pp. 220 and 232).

The blood glucose level must be carefully monitored and if it does not rise above 20 mg./100 ml. fairly rapidly, the glucose drip can be supplemented with 1 ml./kg. of 50% glucose, injected into the drip tubing every 1–2 hours until normal blood glucose levels are sustained (Beare and Gould-Hurst, 1968). If this fails, intramuscular injections of glucagon (1 mg. 2-hourly) can be given. The effectiveness of glucagon should be checked by estimating the blood glucose levels immediately before and half-an-hour after its administration. In affected infants of diabetic mothers glucagon is often used routinely since these babies are known to have excessive glycogen stores; but it also seems to be efficient in babies who are light-for-dates (Blum *et al.*, 1969).

The use of diazoxide to raise the blood glucose level (Ehrlich and Martin, 1969) is still in the experimental stage, especially as there are side effects.

As prolonged intravenous administration of hypertonic glucose can result in electrolyte imbalance, this must be corrected if it occurs.

Prognosis. The prognosis for light-for-dates babies with symptomatic hypoglycaemia is poor, even with treatment. Many of the survivors have permanent brain damage, i.e. mental retardation, cerebral palsy or epilepsy (Brown & Wallis, 1963; Chance and Bower, 1966; Creery, 1966; Cox and Dunn, 1967; Eeg-Olofsson *et al.*, 1967; Beare and Gould-Hurst, 1968). Anderson *et al.* (1966) found very severe brain damage in two cases which died.

The tendency to hypoglycaemia may sometimes persist into childhood (Broberger & Zetterström, 1961; Neligan *et al.*, 1963; Raivio, 1969b).

It is not yet known if neurological damage can be prevented by early diagnosis and treatment, as this condition occurs in infants already prone to neurological damage. Nor is it yet clear whether pre-term infants which are not light-for-dates can suffer permanent brain damage from symptomatic hypoglycaemia which is promptly treated. The prognosis for babies of diabetic mothers seems to be good with prompt treatment.

Babies of Diabetic Mothers

Although babies of diabetic mothers form only a small fraction of all births, they are important because of their high mortality rate. In the majority of cases labour is induced at 36–38 weeks gestation and although the infants usually weigh more than 2,500 g. they are often pre-term babies requiring special care.

The weight and length of the baby are in proportion to each other but often greatly in excess of those proportional to the gestation age; and the umbilical cord and placenta are correspondingly large. The baby looks fat and plethoric. In severe maternal diabetes (with placental infarction and insufficiency) the infant may be light-for-dates with a thin cord, little vernix and a dry skin; and such a baby has a particularly high mortality.

Babies of diabetic mothers tend to be lethargic and hypotonic. They are particularly liable to develop respiratory distress and acidosis, even when the maturity is greater than 36 weeks. They are also liable to sudden attacks of apnoea and cyanosis. They may develop hypoglycaemia, especially if the mother was hypoglycaemic during labour or if her diabetes was poorly controlled during pregnancy. Tetany may occasionally occur, due to hypocalcaemia, and they are liable to develop hyperbilirubinaemia. Renal thrombosis may develop (Takeuchi and Benirschke, 1961), and it is generally believed that these babies are more liable to have congenital malformations (Joslin, 1943; Gellis and Hsia, 1959; Tiisala *et al.*, 1967) although some investigators do not believe this (Cardell, 1953; Farquhar, 1965). Watson (1968) found no increase in the incidence of malformation but a tendency for malformations to be more severe.

Treatment. Some of the complications can be avoided by meticulous control of the mother's diabetes during pregnancy, expert obstetric care during delivery, skilled resuscitation at birth and expert paediatric care during the neonatal period.

On the whole, mortality is lowest when the infant is delivered at 37–38 weeks: earlier delivery increases the risk of respiratory distress and later delivery increases the risk of intrauterine death.

If possible, a member of the paediatric staff should be present at birth to receive the baby and resuscitate it if necessary. The stomach should be aspirated to prevent later regurgitation and inhalation which might lead to respiratory distress, and the baby should be examined for abnormalities.

Later care must be based on the gestational age of the infant and not on its weight. It must be kept warm, and feeding should be commenced as soon as possible to reduce the risk of hypoglycaemia and acidosis. The blood glucose level should be monitored 6-hourly. The umbilical cord should be carefully watched for haemorrhage (due to shrinking of a thick cord). Any complications arising must be suitably treated (see sections on hypoglycaemia, idiopathic respiration distress, cyanotic attacks, hypocalcaemia and hyperbilirubinaemia). Because of the possibility of renal thrombosis, intravenous infusions should be given into veins other than the umbilical vein, if possible.

Temporary Idiopathic Neonatal Diabetes

Low weight babies who are light-for-dates may develop a diabetic state in the neonatal period (Hutchison *et al.*, 1962; Lewis and Mortimer, 1964; Osborne, 1965). The infant rapidly loses weight and becomes dehydrated in spite of adequate calories and fluid (calculated on maturity and age, and not on weight). The infant is thirsty and has polyuria; and glycosuria and hyperglycaemia are found. The condition sometimes follows hypoglycaemia (Chance and Bower, 1966). It must be distinguished from hyperglycaemia associated with infections and cerebral abnormalities. The aetiology is unknown but defective insulin production or the presence of insulin antagonism have been suggested (Lewis and Mortimer, 1964; Chance and Bower, 1966).

Treatment. Insulin should be given, the dose being decided by the results of urine testing. The condition usually disappears after some weeks or perhaps months.

Babies of Mothers addicted to Narcotics

As drug addiction is becoming increasingly frequent, the drug withdrawal syndrome will become more common among the newborn. The taking of drugs by the mothers can cause retardation of intrauterine growth and also curtailment of pregnancy.

The first signs in the infant appear any time during the first 3 days of life, the time being dependent on the interval between the last narcotic dose taken by the mother and her delivery.

The infant becomes irritable; it may have a high-pitched shrill cry, tremors (perhaps convulsions), rigidity of the limbs, vomiting and loose stools, and it may even collapse into a coma. This condition may easily be confused with intracranial haemorrhage or meningitis.

Treatment. Sedation must be given and any necessary supportive measures taken. Sedatives which may be used include: chloral hydrate (given orally up to 60 mg. hourly if necessary), soluble phenobarbitone (6 mg./kg./day divided into four doses and given orally or intramuscularly) or Chlorpromazine (2 mg./kg./day divided into four doses given orally or intramuscularly).

Neonatal Necrotizing Enterocolitis

This condition is reported as becoming more frequent in neonatal units (Leading Article, *Brit. med. J.*, 1970). It usually occurs in preterm infants during the first week of life, especially among those who have had exchange transfusions (Brennan, 1967; Wilson and Woolley, 1969). Affected infants have often suffered from birth asphyxia, idiopathic respiratory distress, apnoeic attacks or jaundice. The early signs are those of intestinal obstruction but a small blood-stained stool may be passed. A straight X-ray of the abdomen shows dilated loops of bowel and usually streaks or bubbles of gas beneath the intestinal mucous membrane. If perforation has occurred free gas is seen in the peritoneal cavity.

The cause is unknown but suggestions include:

(1) Infection.

(2) Stasis of intestinal contents, e.g. delay in passing meconium or obstruction by inspissated milk curds (Cook and Rickham, 1969).

(3) Intestinal ischaemia, possibly caused by umbilical catheters (Orme and Eades, 1968).

Doubts have been expressed about the safety of polyvinyl chloride (PVC) tubing in exchange transfusion sets, and PVC umbilical catheters (Rogers and Dunn, 1969).

Treatment. Oral feeding must be stopped; and intravenous fluids and gastric suction started. Umbilical catheters must not be used as they may compromise the splanchnic circulation; and any umbilical catheter already in use must be removed at once. Antibiotics should be given.

Surgery is necessary if the bowel perforates and, in any case, a surgical opinion will help to eliminate other conditions which may require surgery.

SYMPTOMS

Hyperpyrexia

Hyperpyrexia is very liable to occur during the early life of a low-weight baby and may be due to:

(1) Overheating.

(2) Lack of sufficient fluid (inanition fever).

(3) Infection.

(4) Administration of certain drugs, e.g. sulphonamides.

(5) Massive haemorrhage into the ventricles of the brain, or into the suprarenals (rare).

The infant becomes restless, the respiration becomes rapid and shallow, and the skin feels hot and dry. Infants who can suck take fluids avidly.

Overheating is the commonest cause unless the body temperature is controlled by a "Servo" unit. Pre-term infants have a poor heat regulating centre and an inadequate production of sweat; and overheating can easily occur if, for example, the sun shines directly onto the incubator or cot. Inanition fever rarely occurs in pre-term babies. Infective conditions can occur within a few days after birth and this cause should be eliminated before the fever is attributed to overheating or lack of fluid (serious infections however can occur without any febrile response). Intraventricular haemorrhage can be diagnosed by the presence of signs of intracranial and/or respiratory difficulty (apnoea and cyanosis); and haemorrhage into the suprarenals by cyanosis, pallor, shock and perhaps a palpable abdominal mass.

Treatment. For preventive treatment see control of body temperature p. 61. If hyperpyrexia occurs, sufficient fluids must be ensured and the temperature inside the incubator or cot suitably reduced. Any drug suspected of causing a febrile reaction should be discontinued and any other cause of the condition suitably treated.

Hypothermia

This is much more common among low-weight babies than hyperpyrexia. Both pre-term and light-for-dates babies have little subcutaneous fat, and pre-term babies also have little brown fat and a poor heat-regulating centre. The commonest cause is under-heating but hypothermia can also occur with intracranial birth injury and infections.

The infant is lethargic and takes feeds badly. It may feel cold to the touch and there may be slight oedema and cyanosis of the hands and feet. In severe cases the "cold injury" syndrome may develop.

Low weight babies being nursed in their own homes during cold weather are particularly liable to suffer from the "cold injury" syndrome (Mann and Elliott, 1957; Bower *et al.*, 1960), especially if they are wrapped up too tightly. In addition to lethargy, refusal to feed and a falling temperature, a generalized oedema develops with hardness and rigidity of the limbs. The face and extremities are surprisingly red while the rest of the body is pale. Hypoglycaemia develops and, unless treated, death may occur from infection, renal failure or pulmonary haemorrhage. Babies dying from "cold injury" have little or no brown fat (Aherne and Hull, 1964).

Treatment. Preventive treatment consists of proper control of body temperature (see p. 61). If hypothermia should develop the cause must be treated, e.g. intracranial birth injury, infection, etc.; and the temperature inside the incubator or cot suitably raised. Babies suffering from "cold injury" should be warmed up gradually, hypoglycaemia must be treated if present, and oxygen given if necessary. ACTH or cortisone are sometimes used.

Cyanosis and Apnoeic Attacks

Low-weight infants, especially those weighing less than 3 lb. (1,360 g.) at birth are liable to cyanosis during the first few weeks of life.

The following are possible causes of cyanosis:

(1) The poorly developed respiratory system, i.e. primary atelectasis.
(2) Idiopathic respiratory distress.
(3) Intracranial birth injury, with pressure on, or damage to, the respiratory centre.
(4) Infections, e.g. pneumonia, meningitis or septicaemia.
(5) Congenital malformations of the respiratory tract, oesophagus, diaphragm, heart or brain.
(6) Obstruction of the air passages by aspiration during birth or at a later date.
(7) Errors in feeding and general management.
(8) Drugs or poisons which produce sulphaemoglobinaemia or methaemoglobinaemia.
(9) Kernicterus.
(10) Biochemical disturbances, e.g. hypoglycaemia and hypocalcaemia.

The cyanosis may be continuous as in extreme degrees of atelectasis, severe intracranial birth injury, severe infections, congenital heart disease, sulphaemoglobinaemia or methaemoglobinaemia; but, more commonly, it occurs in attacks and these must be differentiated from convulsions (see p. 232). The attacks may come on insidiously: the respiration becomes feeble, irregular and finally ceases and cyanosis develops during the period of apnoea. When cyanosis is due to obstruction of the air passages by inhalation of vomit or mucus, the onset is usually sudden.

In order to discover the cause of the cyanosis a full history is required in addition to a thorough physical examination of the infant. The differential diagnosis is extremely important, as the treatment depends on the cause.

Atelectasis, intracranial birth injury, infections of the lung, meningitis, septicaemia, kernicterus, hypoglycaemia and hypocalcaemia are described in this chapter.

Congenital malformation of the oesophagus (most commonly with a tracheo-oesophageal fistula) should be suspected in any infant with a persistent excess of mucus or saliva after adequate mucus extraction. The condition is confirmed by the inability to pass a feeding catheter into the stomach. Choanal atresia (rare) is suspected if the infant cannot breathe with the mouth shut, and this is confirmed by finding that a catheter cannot be passed through either side of the nose.

Diaphragmatic hernia is another rare cause of cyanosis from birth; severe cases do not survive for long and are characterized by the sunken abdomen and over-distended thorax in association with cyanosis and rapid respiration. Dyspnoea is the most prominent symptom in infants who survive more than a few hours. The physical signs depend on the amount of intestine in the thoracic cavity; the heart may be displaced (diaphragmatic hernia is one of the commonest causes of a right sided heart), and radiography will show some part of the alimentary tract in the thorax. Early diagnosis and treatment are necessary if the infant is to survive.

The diagnosis of congenital malformation of the heart is often difficult as a murmur may or may not be present. A radiological examination and an electrocardiogram may provide supporting evidence. The cyanosis in these cases shows little response to the administration of oxygen and increases with crying. The commonest cause of cyanotic heart disease with an unobtrusive or absent murmur is transposition of the great arteries. As surgery can now save some of these babies, diagnosis is a matter of urgency.

Obstruction of air passages due to inhalation of food, vomit or mucus is sudden in onset, and in many cases it is associated with a faulty feeding technique or with errors in the general management of the infant. Errors leading to vomiting are discussed in the section on regurgitation and vomiting. Inhalation and cyanosis may occur if a bottle or pipette is offered to an infant unable to swallow, or if catheter feeds are badly given.

The possibility of any infant suffering from sulphaemoglobinaemia or methaemoglobinaemia must always be considered if the cyanosis is continuous and does not respond to the administration of oxygen, especially if the infant seems well in all other respects. The commonest cause of such a condition is the administration of sulphonamides, but the presence of other poisons must be eliminated, one possibility being aniline from napkins and other garments marked with marking ink, and used before being sent to the laundry (Howarth, 1951).

Treatment. This entails preventive and curative treatment of all causes of cyanosis and cyanotic attacks.

In regard to cyanosis due to congenital malformations, appropriate surgical treatment is indicated and, until this can be done, supportive treatment must be given, e.g. a baby with a tracheo-oesophageal fistula will require suction of the air passages; and in the case of a severe diaphragmatic hernia it may be necessary to pass an endotracheal tube and ventilate the lungs by intermittent positive pressure.

Obstruction due to inhalation is treated by clearing the air passages, re-establishing respiration with the minimum of handling and exposure (see p. 142) and the administration of oxygen and prophylactic antibiotics.

Errors in feeding technique and general management must be corrected and drugs causing cyanosis eliminated.

Treatment of methaemoglobinaemia is intravenous administration of either methylene blue (1–2 mg./kg.) or ascorbic acid (500 mg.).

Anorexia

One of the chief difficulties in the feeding of a small baby is its lack of desire for food. Occasionally, however, infants show a surprising desire to feed during the first few days of life, when their requirements are relatively small. If over-feeding is allowed at this time it may lead to digestive disturbances and be followed by severe anorexia.

Anorexia may accompany many conditions, e.g. infections, intracranial birth injury, jaundice, hypothermia, metabolic disorders, etc., but it is a common condition even in the absence of these complications and it is often difficult to get a pre-term infant to take sufficient food.

Treatment. Any complication should be treated. Small frequent feeds may be tried but if there is any real difficulty in getting a small infant to take sufficient food for its needs, catheter feeds should be given without hesitation.

It has been of interest to find that the appetite is improved if the older infants are transferred to a cooler ward when a weight of $4\frac{1}{2}$ lb. (2,040 g.) is reached.

Regurgitation and Vomiting

Owing to the poor development of the mechanism for the closure of the cardiac end of the stomach, and the relatively strong pyloric sphincter, regurgitation frequently occurs in the pre-term baby.

Regurgitation or vomiting is a dangerous complication, because the vomitus may be inhaled causing asphyxia, atelectasis from a blocked bronchus, or inhalation pneumonia. In addition, vomiting causes a loss of calories, fluid and electrolytes which can be ill afforded by the low-weight baby.

The more common causes of vomiting or regurgitation in the low-weight baby are:

(1) Obstruction due to congenital malformations of the digestive tract.
(2) Infection.

(3) Intracranial birth injury.
(4) Excessive handling, especially after a feed.
(5) Incorrect feeding.

Atresia of the oesophagus should be suspected if hydramnios was present; and can be recognized soon after birth by the flow of frothy saliva from the mouth and the impossibility of passing a feeding catheter into the stomach. Radiography may show air in the stomach and intestines (if the lower segment of the oesophagus communicates with the trachea), but no fluid levels will be seen. A radio-opaque tube or a water soluble contrast medium (such as Dionosil or Hypaque) will show the level of the atresia: barium must not be used because it might spill over into the air passages. The infant must not be given any fluid by mouth before operation. The head should be lowered and the pharynx kept clear by aspiration until the operation can be performed.

Partial thoracic stomach or hiatus hernia should be suspected when vomiting occurs early, is blood-stained, and is controlled by small frequent feeds and keeping the infant in the sitting position, day and night. The diagnosis can be finally confirmed by radiological examination after a small barium or gastrograffin meal.

Atresia of the duodenum causes early vomiting, with bile in the vomitus if the obstruction is below the ampulla of Vater.

Malformation of the lower gut. Vomiting starts later and is generally preceded by abdominal distension. Meconium may be passed even if the obstruction is complete (without cornified epithelial cells from swallowed amniotic fluid), but the subsequent passage of a changing stool depends on whether the obstruction is partial or complete. The site of obstruction can be confirmed by radiological examination, films being made in the upright position in order to distinguish the air- and fluid-filled gut above the obstruction from the empty gut below. Barium should be avoided because it tends to clog the intestinal tract: also it may be aspirated during vomiting.

Obstructions due to anal abnormalities should be recognized by direct inspection or by the inability to put a thermometer into the rectum.

Less common causes of vomiting should be excluded, such as Hirschsprung's disease, volvulus from malrotation and malfixation of the gut, abnormal mesenteric bands, intestinal duplication, strangulated hernia or neonatal necrotizing enterocolitis (see p. 218). Meconium ileus is also a cause of obstructive vomiting and should be suspected if there is a family history of fibrocystic disease of the pancreas, and confirmed by X-ray.

Vomiting due to pyloric stenosis is not often met in the pre-term baby while in the special care unit. When it occurs, symptoms start later than in a term child. The vomit is projectile and the characteristic signs of visible peristalsis and a pyloric tumour can be found.

Vomiting due to infection or intracranial birth injury should be diagnosed by the presence of other signs of these conditions. When vomiting is due to handling, it usually occurs during or immediately after the handling, and the cause is thus easily recognized.

If all these conditions are absent, the vomiting must be due to errors of feeding, the commonest being:

(1) General overfeeding or underfeeding.
(2) Too large an individual feed, causing distension.
(3) Unsuitable formula: vomiting is usually caused by an excess of fat.
(4) Incorrect administration of feed; the child in the wrong position; the feed given too rapidly or too slowly; or failure to bring up wind after feeding.

In bottle fed infants, the hole in the teat may be too large or too small: too small a hole leads to excessive air swallowing and too large a hole allows excessively rapid feeding and both lead to distension of the stomach and may result in vomiting.

Treatment. Prevention of vomiting entails careful feeding and handling of the infant and prevention of infection.

Handling should be reduced to a minimum, and any procedure such as cleaning, weighing and dressing should take place *before* a feed and *not after*.

Immediate treatment consists of lowering the head of the cot or incubator mattress, clearing the mouth and pharynx, and administering oxygen if cyanosed. Antibiotics should be given if aspiration has occurred.

The treatment of vomiting due to congenital malformations, infection or intracranial birth injury is that of the cause.

The feeding should be thoroughly investigated, as regards the digestibility of the formula, the quantity given, frequency of feeds, and method of giving them, and any error found must be corrected. The head of the cot or incubator mattress should be well raised during the administration of feeds and can be left in this position for 15–20 minutes after the feed has been completed.

In mild cases the condition can be cured by giving small, frequent dilute feeds. In severe cases it may be necessary to wash out the stomach and omit all feeding by the mouth for 6–12 hours. During this period sufficient water, electrolytes and glucose must be given parenterally to prevent and correct dehydration and acidosis (see p. 159). When the vomiting has been controlled, small frequent feeds can be commenced; a suitable feed for a mild case being the child's usual formula diluted to half strength. If the vomiting has been severe, the stomach will be intolerant of food for some time and modified feeds should be given, i.e. with high protein, low fat and moderate sugar content. As the child's digestion improves, the strength of the feeds can be increased and the modified feeds replaced gradually by a suitable normal feed.

When vomiting is due to gastric distension, the child should be sat up, in order to get up the wind, during and after feeds. If the infant is too feeble to allow of this and simple raising of the head of the cot fails, the distension may be relieved by placing the infant in the head-up prone position. The oesophagus enters the stomach posteriorly and this makes it difficult to bring up wind in the supine position (Hughes-Davis, 1967). If this also fails, the distension must be relieved by passing a catheter into the stomach.

Diarrhoea

Diarrhoea may be infective, parenteral or dietetic in origin: it can also be the result of giving broad spectrum antibiotics. Owing to a low resistance to infection and poor digestive powers the low-weight baby is particularly prone to all these types of diarrhoea. Dehydration occurs very rapidly and is a serious complication. Luckily diarrhoea is rarely seen nowadays in a well run unit.

Infective diarrhoea is considered in the section on infections (p. 156). Parenteral diarrhoea must be excluded by careful examination of the infant for signs of infection in the urine, ears, nasopharynx or lungs. The dietetic variety usually occurs in artificially fed infants and is due to some error of feeding, such as general overfeeding or an excess of one particular food element. General overfeeding may give rise to vomiting as well as diarrhoea and it is likely that the infant gained unduly before the onset of diarrhoea; the stools are large, loose and sometimes even watery. An excess of fat is a common cause of fermentative diarrhoea, but excess of sugar rarely causes diarrhoea in a healthy low-weight infant because the tolerance for sugar is good if non-fermentative sugars are used (see p. 111).

Preventive treatment. Includes protection from infection, careful feeding and care with the administration of broad spectrum antibiotics (see p. 180). The slightest degree of diarrhoea must be recognized and treated at the earliest possible opportunity. Nurses must realize the importance of a careful examination of each stool and the necessity of reporting the slightest abnormality without delay. To do this the nurses must know what the stool looks like at each stage, i.e. meconium; "changing" stool (often green, curded and watery); and "normal" stool.

Curative treatment. The treatment *of infective diarrhoea* has been dealt with already. In cases of *parenteral diarrhoea* the infection must be located and treated, for unless this is done the treatment of the diarrhoea is unlikely to be effective. All milk feeds should be stopped until the stools improve but sufficient fluid, electrolytes and glucose must be given to combat dehydration and acidosis (see p. 159). If vomiting is present, fluids must be given by the intravenous route. As the condition improves, dilute milk feeds may be introduced and these gradually strengthened until the infant is back on normal feeds.

In the *dietetic variety* errors in the feeding must be corrected. The size and frequency of feeds must be reduced in the overfed infants, and in cases due to excess of fat or sugar these elements must be suitably reduced. If the condition is due to an excess of fat or inability to digest fat, human milk must be partially skimmed and half-skimmed dried milk substituted for full-cream evaporated or dried milks: in addition to the reduction of fat, an adequate quantity of sugar should be ensured. In the rare cases of sugar intolerance, the fats must be reduced as well as the sugar and a high-protein feed will have to be given to ensure sufficient calories. In all these cases a preliminary "starve" is advisable, but sufficient water and electrolytes must be given to combat dehydration. In all cases of diarrhoea the child must be kept warm: undue handling must be avoided and oxygen should be administered if required. If dehydration occurs the treatment of this complication must have prior consideration (see p. 227).

Sore Buttocks

Low-weight babies are particularly liable to this condition, owing to the delicacy of their skin and their susceptibility to digestive disturbances, thrush, urinary infections and seborrhoeic dermatitis.

Preventive treatment. This consists of care in the washing and rinsing of napkins or the use of disposable ones, frequent and careful changing of napkins, attention to the feeding, and early diagnosis and treatment of thrush and urinary infections. The tendency to develop perianal excoriation during the administration of broad spectrum antibiotics may be reduced by the administration of vitamin B, and the local use of a barrier cream.

Curative treatment. In addition to the local treatment of the buttocks it is necessary to find and remove the cause of the condition.

Fat indigestion should be treated by reduction of the fat in the feeds, and sugar intolerance by reduction of both fat and sugar. Oral thrush, urinary infections, and infections causing diarrhoea must be treated. If the excoriation is due to the administration of a broad spectrum antibiotic, this drug should be stopped as soon as possible.

Exposure of the buttocks to light and air promotes healing. The napkin should be placed under the infant instead of being pinned on. Various local applications are advocated, such as tannafax jelly, zinc and castor oil, calamine lotion, or a barrier cream. Boric acid should not be used as a rinse for the napkins or in a local application because of the risk of poisoning. In severe cases, exposure of the buttocks to ultra violet light is helpful. Cases due to thrush may be treated locally with a saturated aqueous solution of gentian violet; and those due to seborrhoeic dermatitis with a mild tar paste.

Dehydration

This subject is of extreme importance in the low-weight baby, not only because of its greater possibility, but also because of the great care required in its treatment.

Dehydration is usually due to a deficiency of both electrolytes and water, and can only be cured if both are replaced. It may be caused by:

(1) Deficient intake.
(2) Excessive loss: Vomiting.
Diarrhoea.
Perspiration (slight in low-weight babies).
Increase in respiration rate.

Any infant becomes dehydrated more easily than an adult because its body water content is relatively greater (75–80% as compared with 60–65%). In addition, the kidneys in infancy have poor powers of concentration (Young, 1943), and in order to maintain the electrolytic and water balance of the body sufficient fluid is required to ensure a free flow of dilute urine. For this reason an infant requires more fluid per pound of body weight than an adult, i.e. 2½ oz. as compared with less than 1 oz./lb. (160 ml. as compared with less than 64 ml./kg.).

Dehydration is liable to occur in a pre-term baby because:

(1) Feeding difficulties may lead to an insufficient intake.

(2) The body water content is even greater than that of a baby born at term.

(3) The kidneys have an even lower mineral clearance than those of a baby born at term, and a still greater amount of fluid is required per pound body weight, i.e. 3 oz./lb. (192 ml./kg.).

(4) There is an increased liability to infection which may cause vomiting, diarrhoea and increase in respiratory rate.

(5) There is an increased liability to diarrhoea and vomiting from digestive disorders.

(6) The risk of over-heating is greater.

In a light-for-dates baby, dehydration is liable to occur if insufficient food is given, i.e. if it is not fed for its "expected" weight. A light-for-dates baby is also prone to infection.

Preventive treatment. As dehydration is such a serious condition in the low-weight baby preventive treatment is most important.

Special precautions must be taken to protect low-weight infants from infection; digestive disturbances must be avoided by careful feeding; and each infant must be given its full daily fluid requirement (see p. 112). The relative humidity of the incubator or nursery must be carefully controlled, because a small infant becomes dehydrated if the humidity falls below 30% and this may easily occur, in a badly ventilated nursery heated by electricity and with no added moisture.

If fluid is lost by a vomit or a loose stool, or by an increased respiration rate, it should be replaced at once (by the mouth if possible, or intravenously). For practical purposes, fluid lost by an increased respiration rate can be counted as water and the nurse should give extra water if an infant is feverish and the respiration is rapid; but fluid lost in a vomit or in a loose stool contains electrolytes and the nurse should replace this with one-fifth strength physiological saline. For this temporary use (until the doctor has seen the infant), salts other than sodium chloride need not be considered.

Curative treatment. This has already been dealt with in the section on infective diarrhoea earlier in this chapter (see p. 158).

Oedema

Generalized oedema in the low-weight baby may be associated with:

(1) Haemolytic disease (hydrops).
(2) Congenital heart disease.
(3) Urinary infection.
(4) Excessive administration of electrolytes (salt retention).
(5) "Cold injury" syndrome.
(6) Idiopathic respiratory distress.
(7) Syphilis.

In pre-term infants generalized oedema may occur in the absence of any of the causes mentioned; and the lower the gestational age, the more frequently is this type of oedema seen. The oedema develops within 2–3 days of birth and usually affects the lower limbs, face, hands and genitalia. It is a soft pitting oedema which shifts when the position of the infant is changed. As a rule, it subsides in a few days but occasionally it spreads to involve the whole body. The general condition of the child tends to be poor and the temperature to be subnormal; feeds may be taken badly. Oedema is particularly liable to occur in pre-term babies because of the increased permeability of their blood capillaries, the relatively poor function of their immature kidneys (associated with salt and water retention) and their greater degree of hypoproteinaemia.

Preventive treatment. Includes prevention of hydrops (haemolytic disease), infection and hypothermia, and the avoidance of excessive administration of electrolytes. A concentrated cow's milk formula should be avoided during the first few weeks of life and care must be taken to avoid any sudden increase in administration of electrolytes when changing from human milk to cow's milk formula, even after the first few weeks. The administration of parenteral electrolytes must also be carefully controlled in small babies.

Curative treatment. Curative treatment is that of the cause, i.e. idiopathic respiratory distress, congenital heart disease, urinary infection, "cold injury" syndrome, etc. Oedema due to a low serum protein level subsides rapidly after a blood transfusion; and oedema due to immaturity of the kidneys usually disappears without any special treatment.

Constipation

This condition can occur relatively frequently in the low-weight baby unless the management is good, and may be due to:

(1) Immaturity of the intestinal musculature.
(2) Insufficient intake of foods.
(3) Insufficient intake of fluids, or too concentrated milk feeds.
(4) Loss of food and fluid by vomiting.

Congenital atresia or stenosis of the digestive tract, neonatal necrotizing enterocolitis, congenital aganglionic megacolon, meconium ileus or meconium plug are all possible causes; and the condition may be aggravated in the artificially fed child by an incorrect balance between the various food elements. Constipation may be associated with abdominal distension.

Treatment. If meconium has not been passed by the age of 36 hours, a doctor should examine the infant in order to discover the cause.

The treatment depends on the cause. Cases due to congenital atresia and meconium ileus can only be dealt with surgically, but a partial anal stenosis is relatively common and this is easily dilated by inserting a well lubricated catheter into the anus. A meconium plug will also be dislodged by this procedure.

The passage of infrequent normal stools in an infant who is healthy and gaining weight satisfactorily needs no treatment.

Constipation due to underfeeding is characterized by the infrequent passage of small stools associated with a poor gain in weight, and this type is treated by an increase in the size or frequency of the feeds.

When the condition is due to insufficient fluids the stools are larger, but hard and dry. It is easily cured by the administration of extra fluids.

In artificially fed infants an excess of protein causes a constipated, alkaline and offensive stool. In these cases the sugar should be increased.

Drugs are not required as a rule and should be avoided if possible.

In older and larger infants, Milk of Magnesia can be used if attention to diet and habit fails. Liquid paraffin should be avoided because of its effect on the absorption of vitamin D (Smith and Spector, 1940). The administration of vitamin B is sometimes helpful.

Sudden development of constipation may be due to acquired intestinal obstruction and the infant must be examined carefully to exclude such causes as strangulated hernia or volvulus. Radiological examination should be undertaken if there is any doubt as to the cause of the obstruction.

Abdominal Distension

Abdominal distension occurs readily in the low-weight infant, and its prevention is important because the distension causes embarrassment to both heart and lungs and may precipitate cyanotic attacks. The usual cause is an error in the feeding but it may also result from constipation, infections, intracranial birth injury or idiopathic respiratory distress. Over-heating occasionally gives rise to distension, by causing impairment of digestion. Atresia of the lower bowel must be considered among the possible causes of abdominal distension; and of course enlargement of the liver, spleen, kidneys, bladder, etc., must be excluded.

Preventive treatment. This entails a good feeding routine and avoidance of constipation, infection and over-heating.

Curative treatment. If the distension is gastric in origin, infants should be propped up in order to get up the wind, then placed in the prone position with the head end of the cot or incubator mattress raised. If the distension persists, a feeding catheter should be passed into the stomach and the air expressed by gentle pressure on the upper abdomen.

If the distension is intestinal the treatment depends on the cause. Constipation, atresias, intracranal injury, idiopathic respiratory disorders, infections and over-heating must be suitably treated, and errors in feeding corrected. In severe cases, oral feeding should be discontinued until the distension subsides, suitable fluids being given parenterally instead. In mild cases, it is sufficient to give small frequent weak feeds for a short period.

Jaundice

In addition to hyperbilirubinaemia associated with low birth weight, the commonest types of jaundice in low-weight infants are:

(1) "Physiological" jaundice.
(2) Jaundice due to haemolytic disease.
(3) Jaundice due to septicaemia.
(4) Obstructive jaundice.

Rare causes include:

(1) Transplacental infections such as cytomegalic inclusion disease, generalized toxoplasmosis, neonatal listeriosis, virus hepatitis, rubella and congenital syphilis.

(2) Haemolysis resulting from congenital defects in erythrocytes or haemoglobin, e.g. hereditary spherocytosis, deficient glucose-6-phosphate dehydrogenase (Doxiadis *et al.*, 1964), thalassaemia, sickle-cell disease, etc.

(3) Haemolysis due to toxic agents, e.g. naphthaline (vapour from shawls kept with moth balls. Valaes *et al.*, 1963), resorcin ointment (Cunningham, 1956), vitamin K analogues (especially if associated with deficiency of G-6-PD. Doxiadis and Valaes, 1964).

(4) Metabolic conditions, e.g. galactosaemia and hypothyroidism (Åkerrén, 1954).

Jaundice has sometimes developed from an absorption of bilirubin from extensive haemorrhages into the tissues (Rausen and Diamond, 1961; Davis and Shiff, 1966); or from large haematomata (Zuelzer and Brown, 1961). Administration of drugs which compete with bilirubin for albumin binding and glucuronyl conjugation increase the chances of jaundice developing.

Kernicterus is a possible complication of any haemolytic jaundice in which the serum level of unconjugated bilirubin rises to dangerous levels in the absence of an adequate reserve albumin binding capacity.

"Physiological" Jaundice

This occurs more frequently in the pre-term infant than in the term infant and is usually more severe and prolonged. It is partly accounted for by an exaggeration of the normal red cell destruction which takes place immediately after birth due to the relatively greater number of fragile immature cells, but the chief factor is the poor ability of the immature liver to excrete bilirubin. The light-for-dates infant also has a high incidence of jaundice, due to poor liver function.

Diagnosis. "Physiological" jaundice usually develops after the second day of life, reaches its peak on about the fifth or sixth day in a low-weight baby, then diminishes rapidly. The stool and urine are normal, the liver and spleen are not enlarged and there is no undue degree of anaemia. The general condition of the infant is good unless hyperbilirubinaemia develops.

Treatment. The serum bilirubin level must be watched. No treatment is required unless hyperbilirubinaemia develops (see p. 184).

Obstructive Jaundice

In addition to the various congenital abnormalities of the biliary tract which result in obstruction to the flow of bile into the intestine, this heading includes cases of obstruction due to mucus, inspissated bile, hepatitis, and also the rare cases due to pressure on the common bile duct by tumour masses.

Diagnosis. Jaundice due to atresia usually appears at or shortly after birth but may be delayed. It is slight at first and gradually deepens. The urine becomes deeply bile-stained and contains bile salts but not urobilinogen. The meconium is normal but the stool is persistently pale. The serum bilirubin (conjugated) level is high. The liver is much enlarged and the spleen may be slightly enlarged. There is a tendency to haemorrhage. In a pre-term baby the level of unconjugated bilirubin may also be raised and this tends to complicate the picture.

Jaundice due to obstruction by mucus or inspissated bile or following hepatitis appears rather later; it varies in intensity and bile may appear intermittently in the stool. This type of jaundice may respond to medical treatment.

The differential diagnosis between these two conditions is not easy, and liver function tests are not very helpful.

Treatment. Medical treatment should be tried, based on a low fat formula with full fluid and caloric requirements. The administration of cortisone may be useful in hepatitis (Miller, 1957). Surgical treatment should be attempted before the age of 6–8 weeks if obstruction has been confirmed by careful observation, repeated stool examinations, cholangiography and liver biopsy. Undue delay leads to liver damage.

Convulsions

Severe convulsions are rare in low-weight babies, but cerebral irritability (twitchings, tremors, etc.) occurs relatively frequently because these babies are more liable to suffer from certain conditions which are associated with convulsions or twitching, such as:

(1) Intracranial birth injury.
(2) Intracranial infections, e.g. meningitis.
(3) Extracranial infections.
(4) Congenital defects of the brain.
(5) Kernicterus.
(6) Anoxia.
(7) Hypocalcaemia and hypomagnesaemia.
(8) Hypoglycaemia.

The use of certain stimulants, e.g. Lethidrone (N-allylnormorphine), Vandid (vanillic acid di-ethylamide) and Coramine (nikethamide) can cause convulsions; and babies of mothers addicted to narcotics may have convulsions.

Treatment. The cause of the convulsion must be treated. During the convulsion, or twitching, the airway must be kept clear and oxygen should be given if required. The infant should be disturbed as little as possible and sedatives should be given (see p. 217 for sedatives with dosage).

REFERENCES

ABALLI, A. J. and DE LAMERENS, S. (1962). *Ped. Clin. N. Amer.*, **9**, 785.

ADAMS, F. H., FUJIWARA, T., EMMANOUILIDES, G. and SCUDDER, A. (1965). *J. Pediat.*, **66**, 357.

ADAMSON, T. M., COLLINS, L. M., DEHAN, M., HAWKER, J. M., REYNOLDS, E. O. R. and STRANG, L. B. (1968). *Lancet*, **3**, 227.

AGERS, T. E. (1964). *A.M.A. Arch. Ophthal.*, **71**, 58.

AHERNE, W. and HULL, D. (1964). *Proc. roy. Soc. Med.*, **57**, 1172.

AHVENAINEN, E. K. (1965). *Ann. Paediat. Fenn.*, **11**, 1.

AIDIN, R., CORNER, B. and TOVEY, G. H. (1950). *Lancet*, **1**, 1153.

AINSWORTH, P. and DAVIES, P. A. (1969). *Develop. Med. Child. Neurol.*, **11**, 297.

ÅKERRÉN, Y. (1954). *Acta Paediat.* (Uppsala), **43**, 411.

ALFORD, C. A., NEVA, F. and WELLER, T. H. (1964). *New Engl. J. Med.*, **271**, 1275.

ALLISON, A. C. (1955). *Lancet*, **1**, 669.

AMBRUS, C. M., WEINTRAUB, D. H., NISWANDER, K. R. and AMBRUS, J. L. (1965). *Pediatrics*, **35**, 91.

ANDERSON, K.E., COULTER, J. R. and KEYNES, D. R. (1961). *J. Hyg. Camb.*, **59**, 15.

ANDERSON, J. M., MILNER, R. D. G. and STRICH, S. J. (1966). *Lancet*, **1**, 1278.

APGAR, V. (1953). *Anesth. and Analg.*, **32**, 260.

APT, L. and DOWNEY, W. S. Jr. (1953). *Amer. J. Dis. Child.*, **86**, 639.

ARNOLD, D. P. and ALFORD, K. M. (1948). *J. Pediat.*, **32**, 113.

ASENSIO, S. H., FIGUEROA-LONGO, J. G. and PELEGRINA, I. A. (1968). *Obstet. and Gynec.*, **32**, 350.

ASHTON, N., WARD, B. and SERPELL, G. (1953). *Brit. J. Ophthal.*, **37**, 513.

ASHWORTH, A. M., NELIGAN, G. A. and ROGERS, J. E. (1959). *Lancet*, **1**, 801.

ASTERIADOU-SAMARTZIS, E. and LEIKIN, S. (1958). *Pediatrics*, **21**, 397.

ASTRUP, P., JORGENSEN, K., ANDERSEN, O. S. and ENGEL, K. (1960). *Lancet*, **1**, 1035.

AVERY, M. E. and DROLETTE, M. (1958). *Lancet*, **2**, 960.

AVERY, M. E. and MEAD, J. (1959). *Amer. J. Dis. Child.*, **97**, 517.

BABER, K. G., CORNER, B., DUNCAN, E. H. L., EADES, S. M., GILLESPIE, W. A. and WALKER, S. C. B. (1967). *J. Hyg. (Lond.)*, **65**, 381.

BANNISTER, P. and LOCKE, J. C. (1957). *Canad. med. Ass. J.*, **76**, 81.

BARBER, M. and WATERWORTH, P. M. (1962). *Brit. med. J.*, **1**, 1159.

BARBER, M., HAYHOE, F. G. J. and WHITEHEAD, J. E. M. (1949). *Lancet*, **2**, 1120.

BARBER, M. and OKUBADEJO, O. A. (1965). *Brit. med. J.*, **2**, 735.

BARBER, M., WILSON, B. D. R., RIPPON, J. E. and WILLIAMS, R. E. O. (1953). *J. Obstet. Gynaec. Brit. Emp.*, **60**, 476.

BARRIE, D. (1966). *Brit. med. J.*, **2**, 1574.

BAUM, J. D. (1971). *Proc. roy. Soc. Med.*, **64**, 777.

BEARD, A. G., PANOS, T. C., MARASIGAN, B. V., EMINIANS, J., KENNEDY, H. F. and LAMB, J. (1966). *J. Pediat.*, **68**, 329.

BEARE, T. H. and GOULD-HURST, P. R. S. (1968). *S. Aust. Clin.*, **3**, 125.

BEHRMAN, R. E. (1970). *J. Pediat.*, **76**, 169.

BEHRMAN, R. E. and HSIA, D. Y. Y. (1969). *J. Pediat.*, **75**, 718.

BERDINOFF, G. (1958). *Ann. Anat. Path. Paris*, **3**, 369.

BEVIS, D. C. A. (1956). *J. Obstet. Gynaec. Brit. Emp.*, **63**, 68.

BIEMOND, A. and VAN CREVELD, S. (1937). *Arch. Dis. Childh.*, **12**, 173.

BILLING, B. H., COLE, P. G. and LATHE, G. H. (1954). *Brit. med. J.*, **2**, 1263.

BLACK, J. A. (1962). *Practitioner*, **189**, 99.

BLUM, D., DODION, J., LOEB, H., WILKIN, P. and HUBINONT, P. O. (1969). *Arch. Dis. Childh.*, **44**, 304.

BLYSTAD, W. (1956). *Acta paediat.*, **45**, 103.

BOORMAN, K. E., DODD, B. E. and GUNTHER, M. (1958). *Arch. Dis. Childh.*, **33**, 24.

BOUND, J. P. and TELFER, T. P. (1956). *Lancet*, **1**, 720.

BOWER, B. D., JONES, L. F. and WEEKS, M. M. (1960). *Brit. med. J.*, **1**, 303.

BRAY, J. (1945). *J. Path. Bact.*, **60**, 395.

BRENNAN, M. F. (1967). *N. Z. med. J.*, **66**, 385.

BROBERGER, O. and ZETTERSTRÖM, R. (1961). *J. Pediat.*, **59**, 215.

BROWN, C. A. (1960). p. 464 in "Prematurity" by B. D. Corner. Cassell, London.

BROWN, C. A. and CORNER, B. D. (1952). *Brit. J. Ophthal.*, **36**, 281.

BROWN, R. J. K. and WALLIS, P. G. (1963). *Lancet*, **1**, 1278.

BROWN, A. K. and ZUELZER, W. W. (1957). *Amer. J. Dis. Child.*, **93**, 263.

BRÜCK, E. and WEINTRAUB, D. H. (1955). *Amer. J. Dis. Child.*, **90**, 653.

BRUNS, W. T., LOKEN, K. O. and SIEBENS, A. A. (1961). *Pediatrics*, **28**, 388.

BURKE, B. S., BEALE, V. A., KIRKWOOD, S. B. and STUART, H. C. (1943). *J. Nutrit.*, **26**, 569.

BURNARD, E. D. (1959). *Brit. med. J.*, **1**, 1495.

BUTLER, N. R. and ALBERMAN, E. D. (1969). "Perinatal Problems". E. & S. Livingstone Ltd., Edinburgh and London.

BUTLER, R. N. and BONHAM, D. G. (1963). "Perinatal Mortality". E. & S. Livingstone Ltd., Edinburgh and London.

CADE, J. F., HIRSH, J. and MARTIN, M. (1969). *Brit. med. J.*, **2**, 281.

CARDELL, B. S. (1953). *J. Obstet. Gynaec. Brit. Emp.*, **60**, 834.

CEDERGREN, B., LAGERCRANTZ, R. and NOREN, L. (1962). *Acta Paediat.*, **51**, 45.

CHADD, M. A. (1970). Paper presented by title only at Second European Congress of Perinatal Medicine, London. April 8–10.

CHANCE, G. W. and BOWER, B. D. (1966). *Arch. Dis. Childh.* **41**, 279.

CHOWN, B. (1955). *Amer. J. Obstet. Gynec.*, **70**, 1298.

CHU, J., CLEMENTS, J. A., COTTON, E., KLAUS, M. H., SWEET, A. Y., THOMAS, M. A. and TOOLEY, W. H. (1965). *Pediatrics*, **35**, 733.

CHU, J., CLEMENTS, J. A., COTTON, E., KLAUS, M. H., SWEET, A. Y. and TOOLEY, W. H. (1967). *Pediatrics*, **40**, 709.

CLARKE, C. A. (1968). *Lancet*, **2**, 1.

CLEMENTS, J. A., BROWN, E. S. and JOHNSON, R. F. (1958). *J. appl. Physiol.*, **12**, 262.

COCK, T. C. (1957). *Amer. Dis. J. Child.*, **94**, 77.

COHEN, M. M., WEINTRAUB, D. H. and LILIENFELD, A. M. (1960). *Pediatrics*, **26**, 42.

COHEN, F., ZUELZER, W. W., KADOWAKI, J., THOMPSON, R. and KENNEDY, D. (1965). *J. Pediat.*, **67**, 937.

COHLAN, S. Q., BEVELANDER, T. and TRIAMSIE, T. (1959). *New Engl. J. Med.*, **261**, 1318.

COLMAN, H. I. and RIENZO, J. (1962). *Obstet. and Gynec.*, **19**, 87.

COMBINED STUDIES (1966). *Brit. med. J.*, **2**, 907.

COMLEY, A. and WOOD, B. (1968). *Arch. Dis. Childh.*, **43**, 151.

CONN, N. K. (1969). *Scott. med. J.*, **14**, 23.

COOK, J., PARRISH, J. A. and SHOOTER, R. A. (1958). *Brit. med. J.*, **1**, 74.

COOK, R. C. M. and RICKHAM, P. P. (1969). *J. Ped. Surg.*, **4**, 599.

CORNBLATH, M., BAENS, G. S. and LUNDEEN, E. (1961). *Amer. J. Dis. Child.*, **102,** 729.

CORNBLATH, M., FORBES, E. A., PILDES, R. S., LUEBBEN, G. and GREENGARD, J. (1966). *Pediatrics*, **38,** 547.

CORNBLATH, M., WYBREGT, S. H. and BAENS, G. S. (1963). *Pediatrics*, **32,** 1007.

CORNBLATH, M., WYBREGT, S. H., BAENS, G. S. and KLEIN, R. I. (1964). *Pediatrics*, **33,** 388.

CORNER, B. (1955). Paper given at combined meeting of American, British and Canadian paediatricians at Quebec, June, 1955.

COX, M. and DUNN, H. G. (1967). *Devel. Med. Child. Neurol.*, **9,** 430.

CREERY, R. D. G. (1966). *Devel. Med. Child. Neurol.*, **8,** 746.

CREERY, R. D. G. and NEILL, D. W. (1954). *Lancet*, **2,** 110.

CREERY, R. D. G., WYBREGT, S. H., BAENS, G. S. and KLEIN, R. I. (1964). *Pediatrics*, **33,** 388.

CREMER, J. R., PERRYMAN, P. W. and RICHARDS, D. H. (1958). *Lancet*, **1,** 1094.

CROSSE, V. M. (1957). *Ann. Paediat. Fenn.*, **3,** 153.

CROSSE, V. M. (1959a). *Pediatria Internazionale*, **9,** 115.

CROSSE, V. M. (1959b). Report of IX International Congress of Paediatrics, Montreal.

CROSSE, V. M. (1959c). Panel discussion "Kernicterus" IX International Congress of Paediatrics, Montreal.

CROSSE, V. M., HICKMANS, E. M., HOWARTH, B. E. and AUBREY, J. (1954). *Arch. Dis. Childh.*, **29,** 178.

CROSSE, V. M. and MACKINTOSH, J. M. (1953). *Brit. med. J.*, **1,** 1374.

CROSSE, V. M., MEYER, T. C. and GERRARD, J. W. (1955). *Arch. Dis. Childh.*, **30,** 501.

CROSSE, V. M., WALLIS, P. G., LOW, A. and HENLY, A. A. (1960). *Nutrition*, **14,** 65.

CULLEY, P., POWELL, J., WATERHOUSE, J. and WOOD, B. (1970). *Brit. med. J.*, **3,** 383.

CUNNINGHAM, A. A. (1956). *Arch. Dis. Childh.*, **31,** 173.

CUNNINGHAM, M. D., MACE, J. W. and PETERS, E. R. (1969). *Lancet*, **1,** 550.

DARROW, D. C. and GOVAN, C. D. Jr. (1946). *J. Pediat.*, **28,** 515 and 541.

DAVIS, J. A. and SHIFF, D. (1966). *Lancet*, **1,** 636.

DAVIDSON, L. T. and MERRITT, K. K. (1934). *Amer. J. Dis. Child.*, **48,** 281.

DAY, R. L. (1954). *Amer. J. Dis. Child.*, **88,** 504.

DE BRUNIJNE, J. I. and VAN CREVELD, S. (1955). *Neonatal Studies*, **3,** 149.

DE LEON, A. S., ELLIOTT, J. H. and JONES, D. B. (1970). *Ped. Clin. N. Amer.*, **17,** 309.

DE LUCA, G. and COZZI, M. (1964). *Minerva Pediat.*, **16,** 210.

DESA, D. J. (1967). *D. Phil. Thesis*, Univ. of Oxford.

DESA, D. J. (1969). *J. Obstet. Gynaec. Brit. Cwlth.*, **76,** 148.

DE WIT, C. D. and BORST-EILERS, E. (1968). *Brit. med. J.*, **1,** 152.

DIAMOND, I. (1969). *Advances in Pediatrics*, **16,** 99.

DIAMOND, L. K., ALLEN, F. H. and THOMAS, W. O. (1951). *New Engl. J. Med.*, **224,** 39.

DONALD, I. (1964). "Practical Obstetric Problems", 3rd ed. Lloyd-Luke, London.

DOWLING, H. F. (1957). *J. Amer. med. Ass.*, **164,** 44.

DOXIADIS, S. A. and VALAES, T. (1964). *Arch. Dis. Childh.*, **39,** 545.

DOXIADIS, S. A., VALAES, T., KARAKLIS, A. and STAVRAKAKIS, D. (1964). *Lancet*, **2,** 1210.

DRAGE, J. S. and BERENDES, H. (1966). *Pediat. Clin. N. Amer.*, **13,** 625.

DRILLIEN, C. M. (1970). *Pediat. Clin. N. Amer.*, **17**, 9.
DUDGEON, J. A. (1963). p. 157, "Infection in Hospitals". Blackwell Scientific Publications, Oxford.
DUNCAN, J. T. and WALKER, J. (1942). *J. Hyg. (Camb.)*, **42**, 474.
DUNHAM, E. C. (1955). "Premature Infants", 2nd ed. Hoeber-Harper, N.Y.
DUNN, P. M. (1965). *Arch. Dis. Childh.*, **40**, 62.
DURAN-JORDA, F., HOLZEL, A. and PATTERSON, W. H. (1956). *Arch. Dis. Childh.*, **31**, 113.
DUTTON, G. J. (1959). Panel discussion "Kernicterus" IX International Congress of Paediatrics, Montreal.
EEG-OLOFSSON, O., GENTZ, J., JODAL, V., NILSSON, L. R. and ZETTERSTRÖM, R. (1967). *Acta paediat. Scand., Suppl.* 177, p. 85.
EHRLICH, R. M. and MARTIN, J. M. (1969). *Amer. J. Dis. Child.*, **117**, 411.
ELIOT, M. M. and PARK, E. A. (1942). "Practice of Pediatrics", Maryland, p. 97.
ELLIOTT, G. B. and ELLIOTT, K. A. (1962). *Arch. Dis. Childh.*, **37**, 34.
ERNSTER, L., HERLIN, L. and ZETTERSTRÖM, R. (1957). *Pediatrics*, **20**, 647.
EVANS, P. R. and POLANI, P. E. (1950). *Quart. J. Med.*, **19**, 129.
FARQUHAR, J. W. (1962). *Arch. Dis. Childh.*, **37**, 321.
FARQUHAR, J. W. (1965). "Recent Advances in Paediatrics". 3rd ed., p. 121. Edited by D. Gairdner. C. & A. Churchill, London.
FEDRICK, J. and BUTLER, N. R. (1970). *Biol. Neonat. (Basel)*, **15**, 229.
FELDMAN, H. A. (1959). "Textbook of Pediatrics", 7th ed., p. 616. Nelson, W. B. Saunders Co., Philadelphia and London.
FICHTER, E. G. and CURTIS, J. A. (1955). Paper given at combined meeting of American, British and Canadian paediatricians at Quebec, June, 1955.
FINN, R. (1960). *Lancet*, **1**, 526.
FINN, R. (1970). *Brit. med. J.*, **2**, 219.
FOCONI, S. and SJÖLIN, S. (1959). *Acta Paediat. Uppsala*, **48**, 18.
FORFAR, J. O., BALF, C. L., ELIAS-JONES, T. F. and EDMONDS, P. N. (1953). *Brit. med. J.*, **2**, 170.
FORFAR, J. O., GOULD, J. C. and MACCABE, A. F. (1968). *Lancet*, **2**, 177.
FORKNER, C. E., FREI, E., EDGCOMB, J. H. and UTZ, J. P. (1958). *Amer. J. Med.*, **25**, 877.
FRANKLIN, A. W. (1958). *Lancet*, **1**, 1227.
FREDA, V. J. and ADAMSONS, K. (1964). *Amer. J. Obstet. Gynec.*, **89**, 817.
FREDA, V. J., GORMAN, J. G., POLLACK, W., ROBERTSON, J. G., JENNINGS, E. R. and SULLIVAN, J. F. (1967). *J. Amer. med. Assoc.*, **199**, 390.
FREYRE, E. A. and KENNEDY, E. R. (1963). *Med. Ann. D.C.*, **32**, 175.
FROEHLICH, L. A. and FUJIKURA, T. (1966). *Amer. J. Obstet. Gynec.*, **94**, 274.
GAIRDNER, D. (1965). "Recent Advances in Paediatrics". 3rd ed. J. & A. Churchill, London.
GAIRDNER, D., MARKS, J. and ROSCOE, J. D. (1952). *Arch. Dis. Childh.*, **27**, 214.
GAIRDNER, D., MARKS, J. and ROSCOE, J. D. (1955). *Arch. Dis. Childh.*, **30**, 203.
GAIRDNER, D., MARKS, J., ROSCOE, J. D. and BRETTELL, R. O. (1958). *Arch. Dis. Childh.*, **33**, 489.
GAISFORD, N. and JENNISON, R. F. (1955). *Brit. med. J.*, **2**, 700.
GAJL-PECZALSKA, K. (1964). *Arch. Dis. Childh.*, **39**, 226.
GALLÉN, J., KOVÁCS, Z., SZONTÁGH, F. E. and BODA, D. (1965). *Brit. med. J.*, **2**, 1471.
GAMBINO, S. R. and FREDA, V. J. (1966). *Amer. J. clin. Pathol.*, **46**, 198.
GANDY, G., PARTRIDGE, J. W. and GAIRDNER, D. (1968). *Arch. Dis. Childh.*, **43**, 147.
GANDY, G., JACOBSON, W. and GAIRDNER, D. (1970). *Arch. Dis. Childh.*, **45**, 289.
GARNER, A. and ASHTON, N. (1971). *Proc. roy. Soc. Med.*, **64**, 774.

GELLIS, S. G. (1952). *Amer. J. Dis. Child.*, **83,** 402.
GELLIS, S. S. and HSIA, D. Y. (1959). *Amer. J. Dis. Child.*, **97,** 1.
GENTZ, J., PERSSON, B. and ZETTERSTRÖM, R. (1969). *Acta Paediat. Scand.*, **58,** 449.
GERRARD, J. W. (1952). *Brain,* **75,** 526.
GEZON, H. M. (1960). Conference on environmental aspects of institutional infections. Atlanta Georgia. U.S.A. November.
GEZON, H. M., THOMPSON, D. J., ROGERS, K. D., HATCH, T. E. and TAYLOR, P. M. (1964). *New Engl. J. Med.*, **270,** 379.
GILLESPIE, W. A., SIMPSON, K. and TOZER, R. C. (1958). *Lancet,* **2,** 1075.
GILLESPIE, W. A. and WALKER, S. C. B. (1967). *J. Hyg.* (*Lond.*), **65,** 381.
GITLIN, D. and CRAIG, J. M. (1956). *Pediatrics,* **17,** 64.
GITTLEMAN, I. F., PINCUS, J. B., SCHMERZLER, E. and SAITO, M. (1956). *Pediatrics,* **18,** 721.
GIUNTA, F. and RATH, J. (1969). *Pediatrics,* **44,** 162.
GLASER, K., PARMELEE, A. H. and HOFFMAN, W. S. (1949). *Amer. J. Dis. Child.*, **77,** 1.
GLUCK, L. and WOOD, H. F. (1961). *New Engl. J. Med.*, **265,** 1177.
GOODLIN, R. C. (1957). *Obstet. and Gynec.*, **10,** 299.
GORDON, H. H. and NITOWKI, H. M. (1956). *Amer. J. Clin. Nutrit.*, **4,** 391.
GORODISCHER, R., LEVY, G., KRASNER, J. and YAFFE, S. J. (1970). *New Engl. J. Med.*, **282,** 375.
GOSSETT, I. H. (1960). *Lancet,* **1,** 87.
GOVAN, A. D. T. and SCOTT, J. M. (1953). *Lancet,* **1,** 611.
GRAY, O. P., ACKERMAN, A. and FRAZER, A. J. (1968). *Lancet,* **1,** 545.
GREGG, N. M. (1941). *Trans. Opthal. Soc. Australia,* **3,** 35.
GROSSMAN, H., BERDON, W. E., MIZRAHI, A. and BAKER, D. H. (1965). *Radiology,* **85,** 409.
GRUBER, H. S. and KLAUS, M. H. (1970). *J. Pediat.*, **76,** 194.
GRUENWALD, P. (1964). *Acta Paediat. Scand.*, **53,** 470.
GUPTA, J. M. (1965). M. D. Thesis. Singapore.
GUPTA, J. M., DAHLENBURG, G. W. and DAVIS, J. A. (1967). *Arch. Dis. Childh.*, **42,** 416.
HAAS, L. (1966). *Develop. Med. Child. Neurol.*, **8,** 773.
HARDISTY, R. M. and INGRAM, G. I. C. (1965). "Bleeding Disorders". Blackwell, Oxford.
HARE, R. and RIDLEY, M. (1958). *Brit. med. J.*, **1,** 69.
HARGREAVES, T. and HOLTON, J. B. (1962). *Lancet,* **1,** 7234.
HARRIS, R. C., LUCEY, J. F. and MACLEAN, R. J. (1958). *Pediatrics,* **21,** 875.
HARRISON, H. C., HARDY, J., PARK, E. A. and HARRISON, H. E., quoted in "Premature Infants", by E. C. Dunham, 2nd ed., 1955. Hoeber-Harper, New York.
HELMRATH, T. A., HODSON, W. A. and OLIVER, T. K. Jr. (1970). *J. Pediat.*, **76,** 202.
HEY, E. N., KOHLINSKY, S. and O'CONNELL, B. (1969). *Lancet,* **1,** 335.
HIRSZFELDOWA, H., DRAKOWA, D. and PODOLAK, O. (1960). *Arch. Franç de Péd,* **17,** 215.
HOBBS, J. R., HUGHS, M. I. and WALKER, W. (1968). *Lancet,* **1,** 1400.
HOEPRICH, P. D. (1958). *Medicine,* **37,** 143.
HOULTON, A. C. L. (1956). *Trans. Ophthal. Soc. U.K.*, **76,** 519.
HOWARTH, B. E. (1951). *Lancet,* **1,** 934.
HSAI, Y. H., ALLEN, F. H., DIAMOND, L. K. and GELLIS, S. S. (1953). *J. Pediat.*, **42,** 277.

HSAI, D. Y.-Y., DRISCOLL, S. G., DOWBEN, R. M., GRANA, L. and WILKINSON, A. (1959). Panel Discussion "Kernicterus" IX International Congress of Paediatrics, Montreal.

HSIA, D. Y. (1970). Symposium on Bilirubin Metabolism. Original Article Series, National Foundation, New York City.

HUGHES-DAVIS, T. H. (1967). *Brit. med. J.*, **4,** 172.

HUGH JONES, K., SLACK, J., SIMPSON, K., GROSSMAN, A. and HSIA, D. Y. (1960). *New Engl. J. Med.*, **263,** 1223.

HUGH-JONES, N. C. and MOLLISON, P. L. (1968). *Brit. med. J.*, **1,** 150.

HUTCHISON, J. H., KEAY, A. J. and KERR, M. M. (1962). *Brit. med. J.*, **2,** 426.

HUTCHISON, J. H., KERR, M. M., DOUGLAS, T. A., INALL, J. A. and CROSBIE, J. C. (1964). *Pediatrics*, **33,** 956.

HUTCHISON, W. M., DUNACHIE, J. F., SIIM, J. C. and WORK, K. (1970). *Brit. med. J.*, **1,** 142.

HYMAN, C. B., KLASTER, J., HANSON, V., HARRIS, I., SEDGWICK, R., WURSTEN, H. and WRIGHT, A. R. (1969). *Amer. J. Dis. Child.*, **117,** 395.

JELLARD, J. (1957). *Brit. med. J.*, **1,** 925.

JOHN, A. H. and DUNCAN, A. S. (1964). *J. Obstet. Gynaec. Brit. Cwlth.*, **71,** 61.

JOHNSON, L., FIGUEROA, E., GARCIA, M. L. and NEWMARK, H. (1959). *Abstract. Amer. J. Dis. Child.*, **98,** 602.

JOHNSON, W. C. and MEYER, J. R. (1925). *Amer. J. Obstet. Gynec.*, **9,** 151.

JOSEPHS, H. (1934). *Amer. J. Dis. Child.*, **48,** 1237.

JOSEPHS, H. W. (1953). *Medicine*, **32,** 125.

JONES, P. F. and REID, D. H. S. (1966). *Lancet*, **2,** 573.

JOSLIN, E. P. (1943). *New Engl. J. Med.*, **228,** 645.

KALBERG, P., COOK, C. D., O'BRIEN, D., CHERRY, R. B. and SMITH, C. A. (1954). *Acta paediat.*, **43,** (Suppl. 100), 397.

KEITH, J. D., ROSE, V., BRANDO, M. and ROWE, R. D. (1961). *J. Pediat.*, **59,** 167.

KEMPE, C. H. (1958). *J. Pediat.*, **53,** 19.

KIRBY, W. M. M. and AHERN, J. J. (1953). *Antibiot. Chemother.*, **3,** 831.

KITCHEN, W. H., KRIEGER, V. I. and SMITH, M. A. (1960). *J. Pediat.*, **57,** 876.

KLEIHAUER, E. and BETKE, K. (1960). *Internist*, **1,** 292.

KLEINSCHMIDT, H. (1930). *Klin. Wschr.* Part II, 1951.

KLINGBERG, W. G., JONES, B., ALLEN, W. M. and DEMPSEY, E. (1955). *Amer. J. Dis. Child.*, **90,** 519.

KNOBLOCK, H., SOTOS, J. F., SHERARD, F. S. Jr., HODSON, W. A. and WEHE, R. A. (1967). *J. Pediat.*, **70,** 876.

KNUTSEN, C. A. and BREWER, G. J. (1966). *Amer. J. Clin. Path.*, **45,** 82.

KOCH, C. A. (1964). *J. Pediat.*, **65,** 1.

KOCH, C. A., JONES, D. V., DINE, M. S. and WAGNER, E. A. (1959). *J. Pediat.*, **55,** 23.

KRAVITZ, H., ELEGANT, L., BLOCK, B., BABAKITIS, M. and LUNDEEN, E. (1958). *Pediatrics*, **22,** 432.

KÜSTER, F. and DORTMANN, A. (1958). *Dtsch. med. Wschr.*, **83,** 1193.

KÜSTER, F. and KRINGS, H. (1950). *Z. Kinderheilk*, **67,** 503.

LABORATORY REPORTS (1969). *Brit. med. J.*, **4,** 375.

LAMBDIN, M. A., WADDELL, W. N. Jr. and BIRDSONG, M. McL. (1960). *Pediatrics* **25,** 935.

LANZKOWSKY, P. (1960). *Brit. med. J.*, **2,** 1777.

LAPATSANIS, P. D. and IRVING, I. M. (1963). *Acta Paediat.*, **52,** 436.

LAURANCE, B. M. (1955). *Lancet*, **1,** 819.

LAURANCE, B. M. and SMITH, B. H. (1962). *Lancet*, **1,** 589.

LEADING ARTICLE (1970). *Brit. med. J.*, **3,** 121.

LEPPER, M. H., MOULLIN, B., DOWLING, H. F., JACKSON, G. G. and KOFMAN S. (1954). *Antibiot. ann.*, 1953–54, p. 308.

LEWIN, J. E. (1969). *Lancet*, **2,** 667.

LEWIS, S. R. and MORTIMER, P. E. (1964). *Arch. Dis. Childh.*, **39,** 618.

LEWIS, T. L. T. (1964). "Progress in Clinical Obstetrics and Gynaecology", 2nd ed. J. & A. Churchill, London.

LIEBERMAN, J. (1959). *New Engl. J. Med.*, **260,** 619.

LIGHT, I. J., WALTON, R. L., SUTHERLAND, J. M., SHINEFIELD, H. R. and BRACKVOGEL, V. (1967). *Amer. J. Dis. Child.*, **113,** 291.

LIGHT, I. J., SUTHERLAND, J. M., COCHRAN, M. L. and SUTORIUS, J. (1968). *New Engl. J. Med.*, **278,** 1243.

LILEY, A. W. (1963). *Brit. med. J.*, **2,** 1107.

LINHARTOVA, A. and CHUNG, W. (1963). *J. Clin. Path.*, **16,** 56.

LLOYD-STILL, J. (1969). *Acta Paediat. Scand.*, **58,** 147.

LOWBURY, E. J. L. (1955). *Lancet*, **1,** 985.

LUCEY, J. F. (1960). *Pediatrics*, **25,** 690.

LUCEY, J. F. (1970). Symposium on Bilirubin Metabolism. Original Article Series. National Foundation, New York City.

LUCEY, J. F. and DOLAN, R. G. (1959). *Pediatrics*, **23,** 553.

LUCEY, J. F., FERREIRO, M. and HEWITT, J. (1968). *Pediatrics*, **41,** 1047.

LUDLAM, G. B. and HENDERSON, J. L. (1942). *Lancet*, **1,** 64.

MANN, T. P. and ELLIOTT, R. I. K. (1957). *Lancet*, **1,** 229.

MACKAY, H. M. M. (1933). *Arch. Dis. Childh.*, **8,** 251.

MARTONI, L., BABINI, B. and SCORZA, P. (1965). *Minerva Med.*, **56,** 2409.

MCCORD, J. R. (1935). *J. Amer. med. Assoc.*, **105,** 89.

MCDONALD, A. (1967). "Children of very low Birthweight". Spastic Society (in association with W. Heinemann, London).

MCFARLANE, J. (1964). *Med. J. Aust.*, **2,** 364.

MCKAY, E. and RICHARDSON, J. (1959). *Lancet*, **2,** 713.

MCMULLIN, G. P., HAYES, M. F. and ARORA, S. C. (1970). *Lancet*, **2,** 949.

MEDEARIS, D. N. Jr. (1957). *Pediatrics*, **19,** 467.

MEYER, T. C. (1956). *Arch. Dis. Childh.*, **31,** 75.

MEYER, T. C. and ANGUS, J. (1956). *Arch. Dis. Childh.*, **31,** 212.

MICHAELS, J. P. (1955). *Amer. J. Obstet. Gynec.*, **70,** 1251.

MIKHAILOV, G. (1959). *Arkl. Patol. Moska.*, **21,** 46.

MILLER, B. (1957). *Amer. J. Dis. Child.*, **94,** 318.

MILLER, C. A. and REED, H. R. (1958). *Pediatrics*, **21,** 362.

MILLER, H. C. (1962). *J. Pediat.*, **61,** 2.

MILLER, H. C., BEHRLE, F. C., SMULL, N. W. and BLIM, R. D. (1957). *Pediatrics*, **19,** 387.

MILLER, H. C. and FUTRAKUL, P. (1968). *J. Pediat.*, **72,** 62.

MIZRAHI, A., LONDON, R. D. and GRIBETZ, D. (1968). *New Engl. J. Med.*, **278,** 1163.

MINKOWSKI, A. (1965). *Proc. roy. Soc. Med.*, **58,** 1.

MOLLISON, P. L. and CUTBUSH, M. (1951). *Blood*, **6,** 777.

MORRIS, M. B. and KING, J. (1961). *Arch. Dis. Childh.*, **36,** 610.

MOSS, P. D. (1962). *Arch. Dis. Childh.*, **37,** 452.

M.R.C. REPORT, "Retrolental Fibroplasia in the United Kingdom" (1955). *Brit. med. J.*, **2,** 78.

MURDOCH, A. I., KIDD, B. S. L., LLEWELLYN, M. A., REID, M. MC. C. and SWYER, P. R. (1970). *Biol. Neonat. (Basel)*, **15,** 1.

MUTO, E. (1969). *Acta Paed. Jap. Overseas ed.*, **11,** 105.

MURRAY, J. O. and WALKER, J. H. C. (1958). *Med. Offr.*, **100,** 221.

NASRALLA, M., GAWRONSKA, E. and HSIA, D. Y. (1958). *J. Clin. Invest.*, **37,** 1403.

NELIGAN, G., ROBSON, E. and WATSON, J. (1963). *Lancet*, **1,** 1282.

NOONE, P., GRIFFITHS, R. J. and TAYLOR, C. E. D. (1970). *Lancet*, **1,** 1202.

NORTHWAY, W. H., ROSAN, R. C. and PORTER, D. Y. (1967). *New Engl. J. Med.*, **276,** 357.

NOVAK, M., POLACEK, K. and MELICHAR, V. (1962). *Biol. Neonat. (Basel)*, **4,** 310.

ODELL, G. B. (1959). Panel discussion "Kernicterus" IX International Congress of Paediatrics, Montreal.

ODELL, G. B. (1964). *J. Pediat.*, **35,** 1108.

ODELL, G. B., COHEN, S. N. and GORDES, E. H. (1962). *Pediatrics*, **30,** 613.

ODELL, G. B., COHEN, S. N. and KELLY, P. C. (1969). *J. Pediat.*, **74,** 214.

OPPÉ, T. E. and REDSTONE, D. (1968). *Lancet*, **1,** 1045.

ORME, R. L'E. and EADES, S. M. (1968). *Brit. med. J.*, **4,** 349.

OSBORNE, G. R. (1965). *Arch. Dis. Childh.*, **40,** 332.

OSKI, F. A. and NAIMAN, J. L. (1966). "Hematologic Problems in the Newborn". Saunders, Philadelphia.

OWENS, W. C. (1951). M. and R. Pediatric Research Conference Report, 28th April, 1951.

OWENS, W. C. and OWENS, E. U. (1949). *Amer. J. Ophthal.*, **32,** 1.

OWREN, P. A. (1959). *Lancet*, **2,** 754.

PARKER, M. T. and HEWITT, J. H. (1970). *Lancet*, **1,** 800.

PARSONS, L. G. (1944). *Lancet*, **1,** 267.

PARSONS, L. G., HICKMANS, E. M. and FINCH, E. (1937). *Arch. Dis. Childh.*, **12,** 369.

PATZ, A. (1967). *Arch. Ophthal.*, **78,** 565.

PATZ, A., EASTHAM, A., HIGGINBOTHAM, D. K. and KLEH, T. (1953). *Amer. J. Ophthal.*, **36,** 1511.

PILDES, R. S., FORBES, A. E., O'CONNOR, S. M. and CORNBLATH, M. (1967). *J. Pediat.*, **70,** 76.

PLUM, P. (1965). *Amer. J. Dis. Child.*, **40,** 376.

POLLARD, B. R. and PERRY, S. E. (1959). *Mon. Bull. Minist. Hlth. Lab. Serv.*, **18,** 46.

PORTO, S. O., PILDES, R. S. and GOODMAN, H. (1969). *J. Pediat.*, **75,** 1048.

POTTER, E. L. (1961). "Pathology of the Foetus", 2nd ed., Year Book, Medical Publishers, Chicago.

PUBLIC HEALTH LABORATORY SERVICE (1970). *Brit. med. J.*, **2,** 497.

PUSEY, V. A., MACPHERSON, R. I. and CHERNICK, V. (1969). *Canad. med. Ass. J.*, **100,** 451.

RABOR, I. F., OH, W., WU, P. Y. K., METCOFF, J., VAUGHAN, M. A. and GABLER, M. (1968). *Pediatrics*, **42,** 261.

RAIVIO, K. O. (1968). *Acta Paediat. Scand.*, **57,** 540.

RAIVIO, K. O. (1969). *Ann. Paediat. Fenn.*, **14,** 105(a) and 110(b).

RAMMELKAMP, C. H., MORTIMER, E. A. and WOLMSKY, E. (1964). *Ann. Intern. Med.*, **60,** 753.

RANDLE, P. J., GARLAND, P. B., HALES, C. N. and NEWSHOLME, E. A. (1963). *Lancet*, **1,** 785.

RAUSEN, A. R. and DIAMOND, L. K. (1961). *Amer. J. Dis. Child.*, **101,** 164.

RAY, C. G. and WEDGWOOD, R. J. (1964). *Pediatrics*, **34,** 378.

REECE, A. B., BLODI, F. C. and LOCKE, J. C. (1952). *Amer. J. Ophthal.*, **35,** 1407.

REISNER, S. H., WYBREGT, S. H., BAENS, G. S. and CORNBLATH, M. (1964). *J. Pediat.*, **65,** 107.

REPORT OF SIXTEENTH M. and R. PEDIATRIC RESEARCH CONFERENCE (1955). M. and R. Laboratories, Columbus, 16, Ohio.

REYNOLDS, O. (1968). *Brit. med. J.*, **4**, 320.
REYNOLDS, E. O. R., ORZALESI, M. M., MOTOYAMA, E. K., CRAIG, J. M. and COOK, C. D. (1965). *Acta Paediat. Scand.*, **54**, 51.
REYNOLDS, E. O. R., ROBERTSON, N. R. C. and WIGGLESWORTH, J. S. (1968). *Pediatrics*, **42**, 758.
ROBERTSON, B. (1963). *Acta Paediat.*, **52**, 569.
ROBERTON, N. R. C. (1967). *Proc. roy. Soc. Med.*, **60**, 1106.
ROBERTON, N. R. C. and DAHLENBURG, G. W. (1969). *Pediat. Res.*, **3**, 149.
ROBERTON, N. R. C., GUPTA, J. M., DAHLENBURG, G. W. and TIZARD, J. P. M. (1968). *Lancet*, **1**, 1323.
RODRIGUEZ, S. U., LEIKIN, S. L. and HILLER, M. C. (1964). *New Engl. J. Med.*, **270**, 881.
ROGERS, A. F. and DUNN, P. (1969). *Lancet*, **2**, 1246.
ROGERS, K. B. (1951a). *Proc. roy. Soc. Med.*, **44**, 519.
ROGERS, K. B. (1951b). *J. Hyg. Camb.*, **49**, 140.
ROGERS, K. B. (1963). p. 131, "Infection in Hospitals". Blackwell Scientific Publications, Oxford.
ROGERS, K. B., KOEGLER, S. J. and GERRARD, J. W. (1949). *Brit. med. J.*, **2**, 1501.
ROOTH, G. and SJÖSTEDT, S. (1958). *Neonatal Studies*, **7**, 121.
ROSEN, L., KERN, J. and BELL, J. A. (1964). *Amer. J. Hyg.*, **79**, 1.
ROSSIER, A. (1953). p. 42, "Anoxia of the Newborn Infant". Blackwell Scientific Publications, Oxford.
ROZDILSKY, B. (1959). Panel Discussion "Kernicterus" IX International Congress of Paediatrics, Montreal.
RUBELLA SYMPOSIUM (1965). *Amer. J. Dis. Child.*, **110**, 345.
RUSSELL, G. and COTTON, E. K. (1968). *Pediatrics*, **41**, 1063.
RUYS, J. H. and GELDEREN, H. H. (1962). *J. Pediat.*, **61**, 413.
SAINTE-ANNE DARGASSIES, S. (1962). *Biol. Neonat. (Basel)*, **4**, 174.
SANZ, M. C. (1957). *Clin. Chem.*, **3**, 406.
SCARPELLI, E. M. (1969). *Advances in Pediatrics*, **16**, 177.
SCHELLONG, G. (1964). *Z. Kinderheilk.*, **90**, 134.
SCHIFF, D. (1967). *Proc. roy. Soc. Med.*, **60**, 1108.
SCHULMAN, I., SMITH, C. H. and STERN, G. S. (1954). *Amer. J. Dis. Child.*, **88**, 567.
SCOPES, J. W. (1970). *Brit. J. hosp. Med.*, **3**, 579.
SELBIE, F. R. (1953). *Arch. Middlx. Hosp.*, **3**, 1.
SEELEN, J. and 9 colleagues (1966). *Amer. J. Obstet. Gynec.*, **95**, 872.
SERGOVICH, F. R. and LEONG, E. K. (1970). Personal Communication to Chen *et al.*, *J. Pediat.*, **76**, 393.
SEVER, J. L. (1968). Personal Communication to Dudgeon. *Proc. roy. Soc. Med.*, **61**, 1236.
SHAFFER, T. E., SYLVESTER, R. F., BALDWIN, J. N. and RHEIMS, M. S. (1957). *Amer. J. Pub. Hlth.*, **47**, 990.
SHILLER, J. G. and SILVERMAN, W. A. (1961). *Amer. J. Dis. Child.*, **101**, 587.
SHNIER, M. H. and LEVIN, S. E. (1959). *Brit. med. J.*, **1**, 1004.
SILVERMAN, W. A. and ANDERSEN, D. H. (1956). *Pediatrics*, **17**, 1.
SILVERMAN, W. A. and SILVERMAN, R. H. (1958). *Lancet*, **2**, 588.
SILVERMAN, W. A., SINCLAIR, J. C., GANDY, G. M., FINSTER, M., BAUMAN, W. A. and AGATE, F. J. (1967). *Pediatrics*, **39**, 740.
SILVERMAN, W. A., ANDERSON, D. H., BLANC, W. A. and CROZIER, D. N. (1956). *Pediatrics*, **18**, 614.
SIMON, H. J., ALLWOOD-PAREDES, J. and TREJOS, A. (1965). *Pediatrics*, **35**, 254.
SIMPSON, K., TOZER, R. C. and GILLESPIE, W. A. (1960). *Brit. med. J.*, **1**, 315.

SINCLAIR, J. C., ENGEL, K. and SILVERMAN, W. A. (1968). *Pediatrics*, **42**, 565.
SMALLPEICE, V. and DAVIES, P. A. (1964). *Proc. roy. Soc. Med.*, **57**, 1173.
SMANGOEN, I. (1957). *J. Trop. Med. Lond.*, **3**, 13.
SMITH, N. J. (1959). *J. Pediat.*, **54**, 654.
SMITH, M. C. and SPECTOR, H. (1940). *J. Nutrit.*, **20**, 19.
SPARR, R. A. and PRITCHARD, J. A. (1958). *Obstet. and Gynec.*, **12**, 131.
SPARREVOHN, S. (1969). *Acta Paediat. Scand.*, **58**, 651.
STAHLMAN, M. (1964). *Pediat. Clin. N. Amer.*, **11**, 364.
STENBÄCK, F., DUMMERT, K. and RÄSÄNEN, O. (1968). *Ann. Paediat. Fenn.*, **14**, 61.
STERN, L. and DENTON, R. L. (1965). *Pediatrics*, **35**, 483.
STEWART, G. T. and HOLT, R. J. (1963). *Brit. med. J.*, **1**, 308.
STONEMAN, M. E. R. and ORME, R. L'E. (1969). *Proc. roy. Soc. Med.*, **63**, 485.
STRONG, S. J. and CORNEY, G. (1967). "The Placenta in Twin Pregnancy". Pergamon, Oxford.
STUHLFAUTH, K. (1958). *Med. Klin. (Munich)*, **53**, 1554.
STULBERG, C. S. and ZUELZER, W. W. (1956). *Ann. N.Y. Acad. Sci.*, **66**, 90.
STULBERG, C. S., ZUELZER, W. W., NOLKE, A. C. and THOMPSON, A. L. (1955). *Amer. J. Dis. Child.*, **90**, 125.
SURGERY FOR THE NEWBORN (1968). H.M. Stationery Office, London.
SVIRSKY-GROSS, S. (1958). *Ann. Paediat. (Basel)*, **190**, 109.
SYDOW, G. (1946). *Acta Paediat. Stockh.*, **33**, 101, Suppl. 2.
TAKEUCHI, A. and BENIRSCHKE, K. (1961). *Biol. Neonat. (Basel)*, **2**, 237.
TAYLOR, P. M., BRIGHT, N. H., BIRCHARD, E. L., DERINOZ, M. N. and WATSON, D. W. (1963). *Biol. Neonat. (Basel)*, **5**, 299.
TAYLOR, J., POWELL, B. W. and WRIGHT, J. (1949). *Brit. med. J.*, **2**, 117.
TERRY, M. F. (1970). *J. Obstet. Gynaec. Brit. Cwlth.*, **77**, 129.
TERRY, T. L. (1942). *Amer. J. Ophthal.*, **25**, 1409.
THALER, M. M. and STOBRE, H. C. (1963). *New Engl. J. Med.*, **269**, 606.
THOMAS, D. V., FLETCHER, G., SUNSHINE, P., SCHAFER, I. A. and KLAUS, M. H. (1965). *J. Amer. med. Assoc.*, **193**, 183.
TIBBLES, J. A. R. and PRITCHARD, J. S. (1965). *Pediatrics*, **35**, 778.
TIISALA, R., MICHELSSON, K. and WIST, A. (1967). *Ann. Paediat. Fenn.*, **13**, 9.
TIZARD, J. P. M. (1971). *Proc. roy. Soc. Med.*, **64**, 771.
TOVEY, G. H. and LOCKYER, J. W. (1965). Proceedings of Xth Congress International Soc. of Blood Transfusion, Karger, Basle.
TROLLE, D. (1968). *Lancet*, **2**, 705.
TUNSTALL, M. E., CATER, J. I., THOMSON, J. S. and MITCHELL, R. G. (1968). *Arch. Dis. Childh.*, **43**, 486.
USHER, R. H. (1959). *Pediatrics*, **24**, 562.
USHER, R. H. (1961a). p. 92. Ciba Foundation Symposium on Somatic Stability in the newly-born. Ed. Wolstenholme, G. E. N. and O'Connor, M. J. and A. Churchill Ltd., London.
USHER, R. H. (1961b). *Pediat. Clin.* N. Amer., **8**, 525.
USHER, R. H. (1963). *Pediatrics*, **32**, 966.
USHER, R. H. and CARRIER, C. (1961). *Amer. J. Dis. Child.*, **102**, 775.
USHER, R. H., MCLEAN, F. and MAUGHAN, G. B. (1964). *Amer. J. Obstet. Gynec.*, **88**, 806.
USHER, R. H., SHEPHERD, M. and LIND, J. (1963). *Acta Paediat.*, **52**, 497.
VALAES, T. (1963). *Acta Paediat.*, **52**, 149. Suppl.
VALAES, T., DOXIADIS, S. A. and FESSAS, P. (1963). *J. Pediat.*, **63**, 904.
VAHLQUIST, B. (1960). *Amer. J. Dis. Child.*, **99**, 729.
VALQUIST, B. (1941). *Acta Paediat. Stockh.*, **28**, Suppl. 5.
VAN BREEMEN, V. L., NEUSTEIN, H. B. and BRUNS, P. D. (1957). *Amer. J. Path.*, **33**, 769.

VAN CREVELD, S. (1959). *J. Pediat.*, **54**, 633.
VAN CREVELD, S. and HEYBROCK, N. (1932). *Rev. franç. péd. Paris*, **8**, 158.
VANÉK, J., JÉROVIC, O. and LUKÉS, J. (1953). *Ann. Paediat.*, **180**, 1.
VERGER, P., MARTIN, C., KERMAREC, Y., BATTIN, J. J., TRICOTTET, J. C., MOSS, A. J., DUFFIE, E. R. and FAGAN, L. M. (1963). *J. Amer. med. Assoc.*, **184**, 48.
VEST, M. (1958). *Schweiz. Med. Wschr. Basel*, **88**, 969.
VIVELL, O. and MAAS, R. (1962). *Mschr. Kinderheilk.*, **110**, 387.
VOIGHT, J. C. and BRITT, R. P. (1969). *Brit. med. J.*, **4**, 395.
WADE-EVANS, T. (1962). *Arch. Dis. Childh.*, **37**, 470.
WALKER, A. H. C. (1957). *Brit. med. J.*, **2**, 376.
WALKER, W. (1968). *Brit. med. J.*, **3**, 368.
WALKER, W. (1970). *Brit. med. J.*, **2**, 220.
WALKER, W., HUGHES, M. I. and BARTON, M. (1969). *Lancet*, **1**, 548.
WALKER, W. and ELLIS, M. I. (1970). *Brit. med. J.*, **2**, 223.
WATNEY, P. J. M., CHANCE, G. W., SCOTT, P. and THOMPSON, J. M. (1971). *Brit. med. J.*, **2**, 432.
WHARTON, B. A. and BOWER, B. D. (1965). *Lancet*, **2**, 969.
WATERS, W. J. (1967). *J. Pediat.*, **70**, 185.
WATERS, W. J., DUNHAM, R. and BOWEN, W. R. (1958). *Proc. Soc. Exper. Biol. and Med.*, **99**, 175.
WATERS, W. J. and PORTER, E. (1964). *Pediatrics*, **33**, 749.
WATSON, C. (1968). *Arch. Dis. Childh.*, **43**, 746.
WELLER, T. H. and HANSHAW, J. B. (1962). *New Engl. J. Med.*, **266**, 1233.
WESTPHAL, N. W., VIERGIVER, E. and ROTH, R. (1962). *Pediatrics*, **30**, 12.
WEINER, A. S., FREDA, V. J., WEXLER, I. B. and BRANCATO, G. J. (1960). *Amer. J. Obstet. Gynec.*, **79**, 567.
WIDDOWSON, E. M. and SPRAY, C. M. (1951). *Arch. Dis. Childh.*, **26**, 205.
WILLIAMS, R. E. O. (1961). *Lancet*, **2**, 173.
WILLIAMS, R., WILLIAMS, E. D. and HYAMS, D. E. (1960). *Lancet*, **1**, 376.
WILSON, M. G. and MIKITY, V. G. (1960). *Amer. J. Dis. Child.*, **99**, 489.
WILSON, S. E. and WOOLLEY, M. M. (1969). *Archs. Surg.*, **99**, 563.
WIMHOFER, H., SCHNEIDER, J. and LEIDENBERGER, F. (1962). *Geburtsh. u Frauenheilk.*, **22**, 589.
WITKOP, C. J. and WOLF, R. O. (1963). *J. Amer. med. Assoc.*, **185**, 1008.
WOLFF, O. H., PETTY, B. W., ASTLEY, R. and SMELLIE, J. M. (1955). *Lancet*, **1**, 991.
WOLINSKY, E., LIPSITZ, P. J., MORTIMER, E. A. and RAMMELKAMP, C. H. (1960). *Lancet*, **2**, 620.
WONG, H. B. and TEH, Y. F. (1968). *Lancet*, **2**, 18.
WOODROW, J. C., CLARKE, C. A., DONOHOE, W. T., FINN, R., MCCONNELL, R. B., SHEPPARD, P. M., LEHANE, D., RUSSELL, S. H., KULKE, W. and DURKIN, C. (1965). *Brit. med. J.*, **1**, 279.
WOODROW, J. C. and DONOHOE, W. T. A. (1968). *Brit. med. J.*, **4**, 139.
YAFFE, S. J., CRIGLER, J. F. and GOLD, N. (1966). *New Engl. J. Med.*, **275**, 1461.
YOUNG, W. F. (1943). *Proc. roy. Soc. Med.*, **36**, 219.
ZACHARIAS, L. (1964). *J. Pediat.*, **64**, 156.
ZIMMERMAN, H. M. and YANNET, H. (1933). *Amer. J. Dis. Child.*, **45**, 740.
ZINKHAM, W. H. (1959). Panel Discussion "Kernicterus". IX International Congress of Paediatrics, Montreal.
ZINKHAM, W. H. and CHILDS, B. (1957). *J. Clin. Invest.*, **36**, 938.
ZNELZER, W. W. (1960). *A.M.A. Arch. Gen. Psychiat.*, **3**, 127.
ZUELZER, W. W. and BROWN, A. K. (1961). *Amer. J. Dis. Child.*, **101**, 87.
ZUELZER, W. W. and MUDGETT, R. T. (1950). *Pediatrics*, **6**, 452.

CHAPTER 8

REDUCTION OF MORTALITY AND MORBIDITY DUE TO LOW BIRTH WEIGHT

To achieve this it is necessary to know the causes of low birth weight, and the causes of mortality and morbidity (long term prognosis) in low weight babies.

Causes of Low Birth Weight

Low birth weight may be due to a curtailed pregnancy (pre-term infant), retarded growth *in utero* (light-for-dates infant), or a combination of both factors.

Conditions which are associated with both curtailed pregnancy and retarded intrauterine growth include:

(1) Maternal complications during pregnancy.
(2) Multiple pregnancy.
(3) Congenital malformation.
(4) Sex of the infant.
(5) Biological factors.
(6) Socio-economic conditions.
(7) Smoking by mother.

Curtailed pregnancy may result from blood incompatibility, incompetent cervix, premature separation of the placenta, premature rupture of membranes and, occasionally, physical or emotional trauma. Spontaneous premature rupture of membranes plays a relatively important part in causing a curtailed pregnancy. Early rupture may be due to such causes as abnormal presentation, placenta praevia, multiple pregnancy or hydramnios; but in many cases the cause is unknown and there may be some abnormality of the membranes.

Growth retardation *in utero* usually occurs if the mother lives at a high altitude (see later).

Maternal complications during pregnancy. In a special survey undertaken in the City of Birmingham, the incidence of maternal complications during pregnancy was 35·7% among 1,139 single-born infants weighing 2,500 g. or less at birth, and free from malformation, while among 2,821 controls (every seventh single-born baby weighing more than 5½ lb. or 2,500 g. at birth and free from malformation) the incidence was 12·4%. On analysis of the complications it appeared that the majority of diseases or abnormal conditions of the mother during pregnancy exerted some influence on the incidence of low-weight babies.

Donnelly *et al.* (1964) and Abramowicz and Kass (1966) have also reported an increased incidence of low birth weight associated with complications of pregnancy.

In the British Perinatal Mortality Survey (Butler and Bonham, 1963), it was found that the incidence of curtailed pregnancies was increased among mothers with severe toxaemia and essential hypertension-toxaemia but not with essential hypertension only. Women with accidental antepartum haemorrhage and placenta praevia also had an increased incidence of curtailed pregnancy. The following table, compiled from figures in the Survey (Butler and Alberman, 1969) shows that the incidence of both curtailed pregnancy and low birth weight increase as the severity of pre-eclamptic toxaemia increases; but the effect on intrauterine growth is greater than the effect on the length of gestation.

Pre-eclamptic toxaemia	Single-born infants	
	2,500 g. and less at birth (% of births in each group)	Less than 37 weeks gestation (% of births in each group)
None or mild ..	5·4	4·2
Moderate ..	5·8	3·5
Severe	18·0	8·9
All cases	6·7	4·9

Multiple birth. It is well known that multiple birth is associated with low birth weight. McKeown and Record (1952) found the mean birth weights for twins, triplets and quadruplets were: 5¼ lb. (2,390 g.), 4 lb. (1,820 g.) and 3 lb. (1,360 g.) respectively.

Butler and Alberman (1969) found that 54·1% of multiple births weighed 2,500 g. and less at birth, compared with 6·7% of single births; and Dunn (1965) reported 55% of multiple births as weighing 2,500 g. or less.

In the survey (Butler and Alberman, 1969), 26·2% of all the multiple births occurred before 37 completed weeks gestation (29·4% of the like sex pairs and 17·6% of the unlike sex pairs). The figure for single births was 4·7%. Mutliple birth has a greater effect on intrauterine growth than on the length of gestation.

Naeye *et al.* (1966) stated that the birth weights were similar for multiple-born and single-born infants delivered at 29 weeks gestation; but after 33 weeks the birth weight of the multiple-born infant was definitely less than that of the single-born infant of the same gestational age.

Congenital malformation. Babies with congenital malformations tend to have a curtailed pregnancy (Murphy, 1947) and also a lower birth weight (Donnelly *et al.*, 1964). Butler and Alberman (1969) found a lower mean birthweight and a lower gestational age for nearly all types of malformation.

Light-for-dates babies have more malformations than pre-term babies, who in their turn have more malformations than normal term babies (van den Bergh and Yerushalmy, 1966) and the incidence of malformation increases as the weight for gestational age decreases (Drillien, 1964).

Ahvenainen (1959) found that the incidence of malformation among low-weight babies was ten times that found among babies weighing more than 2,500 g. at birth; and Butler and Bonham (1963) found the incidence among babies weighing less than 1,000 g. was twenty times that of babies weighing more than 2,500 g.

Congenital malformation is a cause of both curtailed pregnancy and low birthweight.

Sex. Butler and Bonham (1963) found (among single-born infants) 6·0% of the males and 7·4% of the females weighed 2,500 g. or less at birth; and Bonham and Alberman (1969) found that 5·34% of the males and 4·48% of the females were born before 37 completed weeks gestation.

The increased incidence of low birth weight among the females is due to their lower average birth weight, which is exhibited as early as 29–30 weeks gestation (Tyson, 1946; Drillien, 1947; Gibson and McKeown, 1952a). The reason for slightly more males than females being born before 37 weeks is not known.

Other factors. Certain biological and socio-economic factors influence the incidence of low birth weight, and these factors are closely interrelated.

Drillien and Richmond (1956) have shown the interrelationship between social class, parity, maternal height and physical condition, prenatal care, living conditions, etc., and how all these factors together resulted in a proportion of babies with birth weights of 2,500 g. or less in Classes IV and V (Classification of Registrar General) which was twice as high as that in Classes I and II.

Low birth weight which is not explained by an obvious cause, such as a prenatal complication, multiple pregnancy, etc., has a very complex social etiology.

Social class. Many investigators have shown that the average birth weight is lower (and therefore the incidence of low birth weight is higher) among the poorer sections of any community (Douglas, 1950; Bundersen *et al.*, 1951; McKeown and Gibson, 1951; Baird, 1952; Nørregaard, 1953; del Mundo and Cruz-Adiao, 1953; Knobloch and Pasamanick,

1959; W H O Technical Report Series No. 217, 1961; Udani, 1963; Butler and Bonham, 1963; Donnelly *et al.*, 1964; Drillien, 1964; Rantakallio, 1969).

Mothers in the upper social classes tend to be taller and heavier than those in the lower classes and the former have fewer low-weight babies than the latter (Baird, 1945).

Illesley (1955) has suggested that tall, healthy, intelligent women tend to migrate upward into a higher social class by marriage, while less well-endowed women move downward to replenish the stock of small mothers in the lower socio-economic levels.

The following table has been compiled from Butler and Alberman's figures and shows the incidence of

(1) infants with birth weights of 2,500 g. or less,
(2) infants born before 37 weeks gestation,

in each of the Registrar General's social classes.

Social class of father	Single-born infants	
	2,500 g. or less at birth (% of births in each social class)	Less than 37 weeks gestation (% of births in each social class)
I and II	4·9	4·0
III	6·6	4·8
IV	7·2	4·9
V	8·2	5·5
No husband ..	10·8	5·9
All classes ..	6·7	4·9

Social class has a greater effect on weight than on gestational age: there are more babies who are light-for-dates among social classes IV and V than among I and II (Ounstead, 1965), and still more among illegitimate babies.

There is a definite association between social class and the incidence of congenital malformations. Butler and Bonham (1963) found that malformations occurred less frequently among the Registrar General's Social Classes I and II than among Classes IV and V; and most frequently among illegitimate infants.

Age of mother. The highest incidence of low birth weight has been found among mothers under the age of 20 years; the incidence then falls as the mother's age increases but it rises again after the age of 30–35 (Woodbury, 1925; Anderson *et al.*, 1941; Blegen, 1952; Nørregaard, 1953; Drillien and Richmond, 1956; Heady and Morris, 1959; Butler and Bonham, 1963; Drillien, 1964; Donnelly *et al.*, 1964; Butler and Alberman, 1969).

The following table (from figures by Butler and Alberman, 1969) shows the incidence of

(1) infants with a birth weight of 2,500 g. or less,
(2) infants born before 37 weeks gestation,

in various maternal age groups.

Age of mother (years)	Single-born infants	
	2,500 g. and less at birth (% of births in each age group)	Less than 37 weeks gestation (% of births in each age group)
Less than 20 ..	8·0	7·3
20–29	6·3	4·4
30–34	7·1	4·8
35 and over ..	7·3	5·9
All ages	6·7	4·9

From this table it can be seen that both birth weight and gestational age are associated with maternal age.

The age of marriage is lower and large families are more common in the lower social classes. The numbers of both very young mothers and much older mothers tend therefore to be higher at the lower socio-economic levels and more pre-term and low-weight babies are produced.

Von der Ahe and Bach (1951) believed that the high incidence of low birth weight among young mothers was due to factors other than age because they found that 136 girls between 12 and 16 years of age only had 5·9% low-weight babies (compared with 7·2% for all births in the area) when they received excellent prenatal care.

Maternal height. The association between maternal height and low birth weight has also been recognized (Baird, 1945; Thompson, 1951; Douglas and Mogford, 1953b; Drillien, 1957; W H O, 1961; Butler and Bonham, 1963; Donnelly *et al.*, 1964; Ounstead, 1965; Walker, 1967; Rantakallio, 1969; Butler and Alberman, 1969).

The following table (compiled from figures of Butler and Alberman) shows the incidence of

(1) babies weighing 2,500 g. or less at birth,
(2) babies born before 37 weeks gestation,

among mothers of different heights.

Maternal height (in.)	Single-born infants	
	2,500 g. or less at birth (% of births in each maternal height group)	Less than 37 weeks gestation (% of births in each maternal height group)
65+	4·7	4·1
62–64	6·1	4·5
<62	9·2	5·5
All heights ..	6·7	4·9

From this table it can be seen that maternal height has more effect on weight than on gestational age.

Maternal height has a definite association with social class. In the British Perinatal Mortality Survey there were 40·9% tall women (65 in. and over) among social class I, but only 26·0% among social classes IV and V.

Baird (1945) suggested that small stature might be associated with socio-economic factors operative since early childhood. Poor social conditions rarely occur in isolation: poor education, housing, nutrition and income may have existed for years and led to deficient growth.

Birth order. The incidence of low birth weight is high among first born infants, and lowest among second babies (Woodbury, 1925; Anderson *et al.*, 1941; Douglas, 1950; Blegen, 1952; Heady and Morris, 1959; Butler and Bonham, 1963; Donnelly *et al.*, 1964; Butler and Alberman, 1969); it then rises with subsequent births except in social classes I and II (Drillien and Richmond, 1956).

The following table (compiled from figures of Butler and Alberman) shows the incidence of

(1) infants with a birth weight of 2,500 g. or less,

(2) infants born before 37 weeks gestation,

in each birth order.

Birth Order	Single-born infants	
	2,500 g. or less at birth (% of births in each birth order)	Less than 37 weeks gestation (% of births in each birth order)
1	7·6	4·8
2	5·4	4·0
3 and 4	6·8	5·4
5+	7·4	5·5
All births ..	6·7	4·9

Previous obstetric history. A low-weight baby is more likely if the mother has had a previous miscarriage, stillbirth or low-weight baby (Anderson *et al.*, 1941; Alm, 1953; Drillien, 1964; Donnelly *et al.*, 1964; Terris and Gold, 1969). Ounsted (1965) has shown that this family incidence of low birth weight is due to a tendency to have light-for-dates babies, not pre-term babies. Walker (1967) found that 10% of mothers of light-for-dates babies were true "repeaters" and had several light-for-dates babies, while 25% had at least one other baby weighing less than 2,500 g. with a gestational age over 37 weeks.

Nutrition. Diet is closely associated with socio-economic conditions, and the relationship between malnutrition and low birth weight has been shown by many investigators (Toverud, 1939; Ebbs *et al.*, 1941; Burke *et al.*, 1943a and b; People's League of Health, 1942; Tyson, 1946; Smith, 1947; Blegen, 1952; Nørregaard, 1953; del Mundo and Cruz-Adiao, 1953; Thomson, 1962; Udani, 1963).

Living conditions. Blegen (1952) reported an association between overcrowding and the incidence of low birth weight.

The following table shows the incidence of low birth weight in different housing conditions for the City of Birmingham during 1963.

Living conditions are closely associated with social class.

Persons per room	Infants weighing 2,500 g. or less at birth (% of births in each housing group)
Less than 1	6·7
1 and less than 1½ ..	6·7
1½ and less than 2 ..	7·3
2 or more	9·5
All groups	8·0

Altitude. The birthweight is likely to be smaller than usual at all periods of gestation if the mother lives at a high altitude (Boder, 1952; Lichty *et al.*, 1957; Howard *et al.*, 1957); and the birthweight decreases as the altitude increases (Grahn and Kratchman, 1963; Abramowicz and Kass, 1966).

Smoking during pregnancy. A number of studies have now shown that women who smoke during pregnancy have, on average, smaller babies than women who do not smoke (Simpson, 1957; Lowe, 1959; Frazier *et al.*, 1961; Simpson, 1964; Yerushalmy, 1964; Russell *et al.*, 1968; Terris and Gold, 1969). The small weight cannot be explained by differences in parity or length of gestation (Lowe, 1959); nor by maternal height or social class (Herriot *et al.*, 1962). Russell *et al.* (1968) have confirmed these findings and also show that maternal age, education and work done during pregnancy do not account for the differences in birthweight.

The following table has been compiled from figures in the British Survey (Butler and Alberman, 1969) and shows that smoking has more effect on weight than on gestational age.

Groups	Single-born infants	
	2,500 g. and less (% of births in each group)	Less than 37 weeks gestation (% of births in each group)
Smokers	8·6	6·0
Non-smokers ..	4·9	4·2
Total	6·2	4·9

The extent to which intrauterine growth is impaired depends on the amount of smoking (Ravenholt and Levinski, 1965). If the mother stops smoking early in pregnancy, normal foetal growth can be expected (MacMahon *et al.*, 1965).

Lowe (1959) suggests that smoking reduces the blood flow to the placenta, so reducing the quantity of nutrients delivered to the foetus.

Employment during pregnancy. An increased incidence of low birth weight among women employed outside the home is reported by Räihä (1947), Douglas (1950), Nørregaard (1953), and Steward (1959). Räihä (1956) thinks that the risk of low birth weight due to employment depends on the response of the mother's heart, as judged by its volume. But Rantakallio (1969) could find no effect of work on the birthweight. This factor is difficult to investigate because much will depend on the type of work undertaken and number of hours worked, and some of the disadvantages may be offset by the advantages of an increased income.

Prenatal care. The association of poor prenatal care with an increased incidence of low-weight babies has been shown by Douglas (1950) and Nørregaard (1953). The quality of care is probably more important than the quantity.

Prenatal care is closely associated with other factors, e.g. high parity mothers seek prenatal care latest (Butler and Bonham, 1963) and it is often those at greatest risk (social classes IV and V, young unmarried mothers, etc.) who are least likely to attend for care.

Van der Ahe and Bach (1951) reduced the incidence of low-weight babies in young mothers by giving good prenatal care and Parmelee (1961) did the same with unmarried mothers.

Illegitimacy. The increased incidence of low birth weight among illegitimate births is well known (Räihä, 1947; Maternity in Great

Britain, 1948; Blegen, 1952; Nørregaard, 1953; Butler and Bonham, 1963; Drillien, 1964).

In Edinburgh, during the year October 1953–October 1954, 8·7% of the illegitimate births were low-weight babies compared with 6·4% of the legitimate births. Among mothers aged 15–19, 13% of the illegitimate births were low-weight babies compared with 11·3% of the legitimate births (Drillien and Richmond, 1956). The investigators thought that the high incidence of low birth weight among the illegitimate children might have been partly due to the poor economic status of the mother and partly due to the fact that they were often first babies of young mothers. However, Parmelee (1961) has shown that good prenatal care of unmarried mothers can substantially reduce the number of low-weight babies.

Among the unmarried mothers in the British Perinatal Mortality Survey (Butler and Alberman, 1969), 5·9% of their single-born babies were born before 37 weeks gestation and 10·8% weighed 2,500 g. and less at birth. The corresponding figures for all single-born babies were 4·9% and 6·7%.

Race. Taff and Wilbar (1953) demonstrated the difference between the mean birth weights of the various races living in Hawaii (Filipinos, Chinese, Japanese and Caucasian). Salber and Bradshaw (1951) found 18·5% low-weight babies among Indians as compared with 4·2% among Europeans, in South Africa; while in Rhodesia, Houghton and Fraser-Ross (1953) found 16·6% among Africans and 5·9% among Europeans. In the United States, the coloured population has a higher incidence of low-weight babies than the white population (Peckham, 1938). In all these studies, the close association with poverty and malnutrition has been considered more important than the racial factor.

Millis (1960) found that the mean birth weight among poor Chinese in Singapore was greater than that among poor Indians; but among the higher income groups, the mean birth weights for Chinese and Indians were very similar and close to that of the Caucasians. She felt that race only had a minor effect on the birth weight.

An Expert Committee on Maternity and Child Welfare (W H O Technical Report Series 217, 1961) studied the public health aspects of low birth weight in 18 countries which were at different stages of social development. It found marked differences in the mean birth weights (and therefore in the proportion of babies weighing 2,500 g. and less at birth) in the various countries although the mean gestation rates did not differ significantly. The less well developed countries had lower mean birth weights and higher proportions of low-weight babies than the developed countries, due to a general decrease in birth weight at all stages of maturity. Various biological factors (maternal age and height, birth order, sex, twins, etc.), prenatal complications (especially toxaemia of pregnancy), congenital malformations of the infant, and prenatal care all had their usual influence on birth weight; but after making an allowance for all these factors, the mean birth weights in the various countries still had the same basic relationship to each other. These differences were presumably due to socio-economic conditions or ethnic factors (genetic or racial). The association between low birth weight and poor environment was confirmed by the WHO study but further investigations will be required to separate out the effects of socio-economic conditions (especially nutrition) and ethnic factors.

Maternal nutrition is known to influence the birth weight of a baby, and the differences in nutrition and in the frequencies of various complications of pregnancy, e.g. malaria (Archibald, 1958) probably play a large part in reducing the birth weight among some races.

There is considerable evidence to suggest that the well-to-do classes in any race can produce infants with birth weights very similar to Caucasian birth weights (del Mundo and Cruz-Adiao, 1953; Millis, 1960; Udani, 1963).

Summary of Causes

A *pre-term infant* is associated with:

(1) Certain prenatal complications.
(2) Multiple birth.
(3) A malformed child.
(4) Social class V and illegitimacy.
(5) Mothers aged less than 20 and over 35.
(6) Mothers less than 62 in. (157·48 cm.) tall.
(7) First babies or third onwards.
(8) Mothers who smoke during pregnancy.

A *light-for-dates infant* is associated with:

(1) A history of previous light-for-dates babies.
(2) Certain prenatal complications.
(3) Multiple birth.
(4) A malformed child.
(5) Social classes IV and V and illegitimacy.
(6) Mothers aged less than 20 and over 30.
(7) Mothers less than 62 in. tall.
(8) First babies or third onwards.
(9) Mothers living at a high altitude.
(10) Mothers who smoke during pregnancy.

Distribution of Births by Weight and Gestational Age, with Perinatal Mortality Rates

The following table compiled from figures in the British Perinatal Mortality Survey (Butler and Bonham, 1963) shows the distribution of singleton births in England and Wales in 1958 by birth weight, and the mortality rate in each birthweight group.

Birth weight (g.)	% of total births		Perinatal mortality per 1,000 births in each group	
Up to 1,000 ..	0·3	6·7*	942·6	266·7
1,001–1,500 ..	0·6		724·9	
1,501–2,000 ..	1·0		441·2	
2,001–2,500 ..	4·3		98·8	
Over 2,500	92·9*		16·1	
No information ..	0·4		—	
Total births ..	100·0		33·2†	

* Including estimated.
† Including no information.

The perinatal mortality increases as the birth weight decreases, and is very high among babies weighing 2,500 g. and less at birth.

The following table, compiled from figures in the British Survey (Butler and Alberman, 1969) shows the distribution of single-born births in England and Wales in 1958 by gestational age, and the perinatal mortality rate in each gestational age group.

Gestational age (weeks)	% of total births		Perinatal mortality per 1,000 births in each group
Less than 28 ..	0·2	4·9	897·4
28–36	4·7		267·8
37–38	12·6		37·0
39–41	61·0		15·5
42 and over ..	10·9		27·4
Not known	10·6		36·8
Total births ..	100·0		34·9

The perinatal mortality increases as the gestational age decreases and is very high among babies born before 37 complete weeks gestation.

The figures from the British Perinatal Mortality Survey are based on births which occurred during 1958. Between 1958 and 1969 the incidence of low-weight babies among live births in England and Wales has gone up from 6·8–7·1%; the stillbirth rate among these babies has fallen from 146 to 103·9 per 1,000 total low-weight births; and the neonatal death rate has fallen from 142 to 109 per 1,000 low-weight live births (Report of Ministry of Health for 1958 and Report of Department of Health and Social Security for 1969). The first week deaths are not given in the Report of the Department of Health and Social Security for 1969, so the perinatal death rate cannot be calculated.

Another birth survey has been undertaken by the National Birthday Trust Fund and the Royal College of Obstetricians and Gynaecologists (April 5–11, 1970), and this should show a marked improvement in the perinatal death rate of low weight babies.

In England and Wales 30–40% of all low-weight babies are born after 37 weeks gestation. Their mortality is lower than expected for their birth weight, but higher than expected for their gestational age. Walker (1967) found the perinatal death rate of these babies to be 100, the major component being stillbirth. Usher (1970) found that the perinatal mortality increased as the percentage of underweight for gestational age increased.

Mortality after the first Week of Life

Low-weight infants have a higher mortality rate than babies weighing more than 2,500 g. at birth during the first year of life, as shown in the following table compiled from the City of Birmingham statistics for 1969.

Birth weight (g.)	Age at death	
	1–4 weeks mortality rate (per 1,000 live births)	4 weeks to 1 year mortality rate (per 1,000 live births)
2,500 and less . .	8·5	26·4
Over 2,500	1·7	6·8
All births	2·2	8·3

Several investigators have reported that, compared with babies weighing more than 2,500 g. at birth, low-weight babies continue to have a high mortality rate between the ages of 1 and 4 years (Blegen, 1952; Alm, 1953; Douglas and Mogford, 1953a).

Causes of Mortality

(1) **Primary causes of perinatal death.** The following table shows the perinatal death rate for low-weight babies and babies weighing more than 2,500 g. due to various primary causes of death among babies born in the City of Birmingham during 1969. The primary cause is the condition which started the chain of events which ended in stillbirth or death during the first week of life.

Primary cause of death	Perinatal death rate due to each cause	
	2,500 g. and less	Over 2,500 g.
Prenatal causes		
Toxaemia	26·4	0·6
Non-toxic separation of placenta	32·0	1·4
Haemolytic disease	7·1	0·6
Intranatal cause		
Birth injury or asphyxia	10·2	0·7
Postnatal causes		
Infection	5·1	0·4
Other	30·5	2·2
Congenital abnormalities	26·9	2·7
Atelectasis (including idiopathic respiratory distress)	54·8	2·1
Unknown	17·8	0·9
All causes	210·8	11·6

These primary causes give valuable information in regard to the possibility of preventing some of the deaths.

(2) **Final causes of neonatal death.** The principal causes of neonatal death among pre-term infants are idiopathic respiratory distress (hyaline membrane disease), intraventricular haemorrhage, congenital malformation and infection; while the principal causes among low-weight term babies are birth asphyxia, massive pulmonary haemorrhage, congenital malformation and pneumonia.

Between the ages of 4 weeks and 1 year, low-weight babies die more frequently from congenital malformations and infections than babies weighing more than 2,500 g. at birth (Douglas and Mogford, 1953a).

Factors Influencing Mortality Rates

Complications of pregnancy and labour. It is well known that complications of pregnancy and labour increase the mortality rates (McNeill, 1942; Taylor *et al.*, 1949; Russell and Betts, 1952; Wofinden *et al.*, 1952; Blegen, 1952; Alm, 1953; Butler and Alberman, 1969) and low-weight infants are more often associated with these complications than babies weighing more than 2,500 g. at birth.

The influence of the mode of delivery on the mortality rates of low-weight babies has been studied by various investigators (Beck, 1941; Diddle and Plass, 1942; Dieckmann, 1946; Feeney, 1952; Beck, 1946; Butler and Bonham, 1963; Cavanagh and Talisman, 1969) who have shown that rapid delivery, breech delivery, mid-cavity or high forceps and Caesarean section all increase the risk of death while the suitable use of an episiotomy reduces it.

In the British survey (Butler and Bonham, 1963) the mortality for breech delivery in infants weighing 1,501–2,000 g. was slightly higher than average but for infants weighing 2,001–2,500 g. it was more than treble the average. Unfortunately breech delivery is common among low-weight infants because so many breech presentations only correct themselves during the last few weeks of pregnancy.

In the same survey, Butler and Alberman (1969) found, within groups of similar gestational age, that delivery by Caesarean section increased the risk of hyaline membrane disease, irrespective of the indication for section.

Multiple pregnancy. When *all births* (low-weight and over 2,500 g. at birth) are considered, the multiple-born have higher mortality rates than the single-born; this being due to the smaller average birth weight of the multiple-born (Duffield *et al.*, 1940; Beck, 1941) and their greater risk of association with complications of pregnancy and labour (Beck, 1941; Alm, 1953).

However, when *low-weight infants only* are considered, the multiple-born have lower mortality rates than the single-born due to the greater gestational age which the multiple-born enjoy over the single-born of the same birth weight (Dunham and McAlenny, 1936; Peckham, 1938; Beck, 1941; Tyson, 1946; Record *et al.*, 1952; Butler and Alberman, 1969).

Before 37 weeks gestation the perinatal mortality of twins is lower than that of singletons; but after 37 weeks gestation it is higher than that of singletons; and the smaller one of the pair has the higher mortality (Butler and Alberman, 1969).

Second-born twins have a much higher mortality rate than first-born twins (Corston, 1957; Camilleri, 1963; Keuth *et al.*, 1964; Butler and Alberman, 1969; Kavanagh and Talisman, 1969); and the mortality increases as the interval between the two deliveries increases (MacDonald, 1962; Graves *et al.*, 1962). In the British Survey (Butler and Alberman, 1969) the mortality of first twins was 9·7% and that of second twins 12·1% while the mortality of singletons was 3·3%.

Congenital malformations. The presence of a congenital malformation increases the risk of mortality in any baby, whether low-weight or over 2,500 g. at birth, and there is a higher incidence of malformation among low-weight babies than among babies over 2,500 g. especially among light-for-dates babies.

Sex. A higher stillbirth rate for females under 3 lb. (1,360 g.) due to an excess of anencephalic infants among female stillbirths was reported by Gibson and McKeown (1952a). Above the weight of 3 lb. these workers found that the stillbirth and neonatal death rates were higher among males than females; and this sex difference has been reported also by Tyson (1946), Russell and Betts (1952) and Blegen (1952). When male and female low-weight infants are compared, weight for weight, the females have a slightly higher gestational age than the males and higher survival rates would be expected. When the sexes are compared at similar gestational ages, the male mortality is higher than that of the female at all periods of gestation except between 32–35 weeks, when the slightly greater death rate in females could be due to an excess of anencephaly (Butler and Bonham, 1963).

Other factors. The low-weight baby shares with the baby over 2,500 g. the risk of a higher mortality due to certain biological and socio-economic factors detailed below.

Social Class. Baird (1945) showed that the mortality among infants weighing 2,500 g. and less at birth was highest among the poorest class (Registrar General's social classes III, IV and V).

In the British Perinatal Mortality Survey (Butler and Bonham, 1963) the mortality in each birth weight group rose as the social class fell; and there was a similar, but smaller, rise in mortality among infants of less than 38 weeks maturity, as the social class fell. The Register General's social classes are based entirely on the class of the husband, but the social class of the mother herself is equally important (Drillien, 1964; Butler and Bonham, 1963).

Maternal age. The stillbirth rate is believed to rise with increasing maternal age (Sutherland, 1949; Wofinden *et al.*, 1952; Heady and Morris, 1959). An excess of neonatal deaths is reported among infants of mothers under 23 (Wofinden *et al.*, 1952), while infant mortality is believed to decrease with increasing maternal age (Gibson and McKeown, 1952b), but Heady and Morris (1959) found that it rose again after the age of 30. In the British Perinatal Mortality Survey (Butler and Bonham, 1963) the mortality for infants up to 2,500 g. was lowest when the mother was between 25 and 29 years of age. Peaks in the death rate occurred at each extreme of the child-bearing age. Among infants born before 38 weeks maturity, the mortality was lowest when the mother was between 20 and 24 years of age: the mortality then rose with increasing maternal age.

Maternal height. Baird (1952) has shown marked association between maternal height and perinatal death. Maternal height can be regarded as an index of the mother's social and nutritional experience, and therefore should have as much influence on the outcome of the pregnancy as the social class of the father. The British Perinatal Mortality Survey (Butler and Alberman, 1969) found that the mortality rate increased as the maternal height decreased, in each social class.

Birth order. Birth order is intimately associated with the age of the mother. The stillbirth rate is believed to be highest for first births, lowest for second births and then to rise with increasing parity (Yerushalmy, 1938; Sutherland, 1949; Gibson and McKeown, 1952b; Heady and Morris, 1959). Yerushalmy (1938) and Heady and Morris (1959) report the same pattern for neonatal deaths, but Gibson and McKeown (1952b) only found a higher incidence of neonatal death for fourth and later births. Heady and Morris (1959) found that the death rate after the first 4 weeks of life rose with increasing parity.

In the British Perinatal Mortality Survey there was a similar pattern of mortality among babies weighing 2,500 g. and less, and among babies born before 38 weeks maturity. In both groups the death rate was lowest for second babies with an increased death rate for the first, and for each succeeding baby after the second. This pattern occurred within each social class and in each maternal age group; in fact, maternal age, parity and social class all acted independently of each other (Butler and Bonham, 1963).

Previous obstetric history. It has been stressed in the British Perinatal Mortality Survey that the perinatal mortality is considerably raised if there has been a previous abortion, stillbirth, low-weight baby or a neonatal death; and also if there is a previous history of toxaemia, antepartum haemorrhage or Caesarean section. Unfortunately, a low-weight infant is more likely to have this type of background than an infant weighing more than 2,500 g.

Smoking during pregnancy. Higher mortality rates for infants of smokers have been recorded by Frazier *et al.* (1961), Russell *et al.* (1968) and Butler and Alberman (1969). This is mainly due to an excess of stillbirths. The increase in the neonatal death rate is due to the excess of babies who are light-for-dates.

The increased mortality cannot be explained by parity or social class differences (Butler, 1965).

Overcrowding. In "Maternity in Great Britain" (1948), among first births there was an increase in the combined stillbirth and neonatal death rate as overcrowding increased. Wofinden *et al.* (1952) found no evidence of the influence of overcrowding on the stillbirth or neonatal death rate.

Employment of mother during pregnancy. The effect of employment of the mother outside her home during pregnancy is difficult to gauge because so much depends on the type of work, the benefit due to the extra income, etc., but Wofinden *et al.* (1952) thought it might have some influence on the stillbirth rate, while Woolf (1947) believed that it increased both foetal and infant mortality.

Prenatal care. For all births (low-weight and over 2,500 g.) the British Perinatal Mortality Survey found that the mortality of infants of women who had not had prenatal care was five times the overall mortality, and that the lowest mortality occurred among infants of mothers who had 15–24 prenatal examinations (Butler and Bonham, 1963).

Illegitimacy. It is generally believed that illegitimacy increases both foetal and infant mortalities; and Blegen (1952) showed

(1) higher stillbirth and neonatal death rates, and
(2) higher death rates during the remainder of the first year and the second year of life among illegitimate low-weight babies,

in comparison with legitimate low-weight babies.

Place of care during the neonatal period. In the British Survey the mortality of low-weight babies born to women booked and delivered in hospital was the same as the overall average in spite of "high risk" selection for hospital (Butler and Bonham, 1963). There is no doubt that "high risk" infants should be under expert care during the neonatal period.

Employment of mothers during first year after birth. This could only be expected to influence the death rate after the age of 4 weeks. Again the influence is difficult to assess, because so much depends on where the child is cared for and the possibility of improvement of the financial status.

Method of feeding. Wilcox (1936) drew attention to the fact that low-weight infants receiving little or no human milk after the first 10 days of life showed a relatively greater susceptibility to disease and a higher mortality rate.

Gonzaga and his colleagues (1963) have shown that human milk can act as an effective agent for the prevention of various types of enteric infection provided the mother is immune and excretes the respective antibodies in the milk; and Warren *et al.* (1964) found that human milk contained a polio-virus neutralizing substance in concentrations related to the antibody titre in the mother's serum.

During a special survey in Birmingham, 1,377 low-weight infants were followed up to discover the effects of human milk feeding and cow's milk feeding on the mortality. Of the 1,170 alive after 4 weeks, 88 were excluded (either because of congenital malformation or because they could not be traced), leaving 1,028 who were followed up to the age of 6 months, or death if it occurred before then. These infants were divided into three groups:

(1) 313 fed on human milk from birth until the age of at least 4 months.

(2) 420 fed on cow's milk entirely.

(3) 349 not falling into either of the first two groups.

The death rate between the ages of 1 month and 6 months for the infants fed on human milk was 1·3%, compared with 4·0% for the infants fed on cow's milk.

In order to eliminate other factors which might influence the mortality, groups comparable with regard to birth weight, single or multiple birth, poverty, over-crowding, etc., were examined, but in each case infants fed on human milk had the lowest mortality.

By using human milk, Svirsky Gross (1958) eliminated *E. coli* 0.111 from a premature baby nursery after failure to control a 2-year epidemic of diarrhoea by any other method. Experience in the effect of various diets on the mortality rate has been described on p. 104, and all these results emphasize the fact that every effort should be made to establish and maintain the mother's supply of milk until the infant can be put to the breast.

Long Term Prognosis for Low-weight Babies

Great efforts are being made to save low-weight babies, and more are being saved every year. A programme for saving these babies is expensive and time consuming, but well worth while if the babies develop into normal healthy individuals.

Many reports have now been published on the physical, mental and social development, illnesses, etc., of low-weight babies and results are becoming less conflicting. There is always the difficulty in selecting suitable controls because, as Douglas (1960) has pointed out, the social background of low-weight babies is very different from that of babies weighing more than 2,500 g.

Babies weighing 2,500 g. and less are a very mixed group; some result from a curtailed pregnancy while others are born after 37 weeks gestation but are light-for-dates for many reasons. The only common factor is low birth weight. As a group, low-weight babies include an excess of females, first-born and late-born babies, twins, babies born after a complicated pregnancy, babies born to very young or elderly mothers, illegitimate babies, babies of small light parents, babies of parents living in overcrowded and poor socio-economic conditions, and babies with congenital malformations.

The importance of selecting suitable controls becomes obvious when it is realized how many factors can influence the final development of the infant, i.e.:

(1) *The causes of the low birth weight.* These can influence the subsequent development of the infant. In addition to curtailing pregnancy

and/or retarding intrauterine growth such prenatal conditions as pre-eclamptic toxaemia, placental insufficiency, etc., can also cause birth asphyxia which, in its turn, can result in cerebral palsy, convulsions and mental retardation. Multiple birth (twins, etc.) increases the risk of birth injury and asphyxia, with their possible sequelae. Trans-placental infections which result in low-weight infants can also cause malformations and brain damage. Congenital malformations from other causes which may have led to low-weight infants will obviously influence the later physical and mental development of the child.

First-born babies have an increased risk of birth trauma and asphyxia. Children of very young mothers, illegitimate children, and children from families of low socio-economic status and from large families (high parities) all tend to have less good care and an increased risk of infection, especially if there is overcrowding; and these lead to smaller and lighter children who attend school less regularly. Blegen (1952) drew attention to the correlation between good home care and scholastic achievement.

(2) *Inheritance.* This obviously plays a part in future development, e.g. children of small light parents will probably also be small and light. Intelligence and emotional stability are also inherited.

(3) *Sex.* Girls tend to grow up smaller and lighter than boys.

(4) *The quality of obstetric care during delivery.* Good obstetric care can reduce the extra liability of low-weight babies to birth injury and birth asphyxia, with their possible sequelae.

(5) *The quality of neonatal care.* Good care during the neonatal period can reduce the risk of such complications as anoxia, infections, hypoglycaemia, kernicterus or mental retardation from jaundice, and retrolental fibroplasia from excessive use of oxygen; all of which can affect the prognosis of the low-weight baby.

(6) *Later environmental factors.* These have a tremendous effect on the final development of the child, e.g. the economic, cultural and emotional status of the family; quality of parental care; overcrowding with exposure to infections; quality of diet; quality of paediatric supervision; quality of teaching at school and regularity of attendance; and finally the quality of the parents' educational aspirations for the child (Douglas, 1960).

To discover the true influence of low birth weight *per se* on development it is necessary to exclude the influence of as many of these factors as possible and experience has shown that this is not easy. In addition, for the first 2–3 years of life, it is also necessary to make an allowance for the degree of curtailment of pregnancy by calculating age from the expected date of delivery and not from the date of birth.

Physical development. In comparison with infants born at term, physical development in pre-term infants is retarded for the first 2 years of life, especially among those with the lowest gestational age.

This retardation is eliminated in the majority if an allowance is made for the gestational age by calculating postnatal age from the expected date of delivery.

The malnourished light-for-dates babies seem to do well at first but after 2–3 months they lag behind and generally remain underweight and under height (Warkany *et al.*, 1961; Narbouton *et al.*, 1961; Babson *et al.*, 1964; Drillien, 1964; Illingworth, 1964; Dunn, 1965; Neligan, 1967; MacDonald, 1967; Beargie *et al.*, 1970). Twins tend to grow up smaller and lighter than singletons (Drillien, 1964), especially the smaller of the pair when there is a marked difference between the two birthweights (Babson *et al.*, 1964).

Douglas and Mogford (1953b) matched a national sample of single-born low-weight infants with an equal number of single-born infants weighing more than 2,500 g. at birth born during the same week in March, 1946, in regard to sex, birth order, age of mother, social status and locality; and these workers found:

(1) On the average, the low-weight children had not reduced their weight and height handicaps by the age of 4 years.

(2) The children who had not reduced their height and weight handicaps by the age of 4 years had shorter and lighter mothers than the controls (the shortest and lightest children had the shortest and lightest mothers).

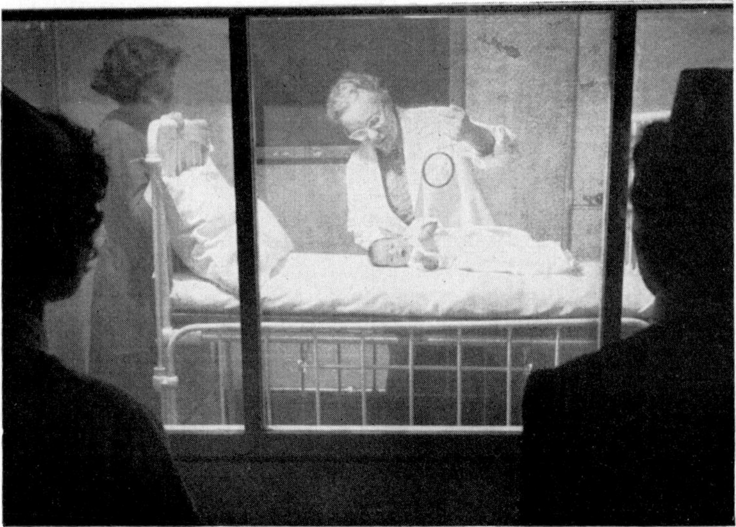

FIG. 49. Follow-up. This photograph was taken in the Follow-up Clinic at Sorrento Special Care Unit, and shows nurses watching an examination from the observation room through a one-way screen.

(3) There was no evidence that either a shorter period of gestation, or complications of pregnancy, retarded growth.

Drillien (1964) has followed up nearly 600 infants (one-third less than $4\frac{1}{2}$ lb. or 2,040 g.; one-third $4\frac{1}{2}$–$5\frac{1}{2}$ lb.; and one-third over $5\frac{1}{2}$ lb. or 2,500 g.) born in two Edinburgh hospitals during 1953 and 1954. She made no attempt to match the low-weight babies with babies over 2,500 g. With the exception of an excess of first-born children among the babies over 2,500 g., each of the three groups of babies had a social class and parity distribution similar to that of all Edinburgh births in these groups; so the low-weight groups had all the usual disadvantages, i.e. more of the lower socio-economic families and more high parities, etc. At the age of 5 years, one-third of the low-weight infants were markedly underweight (i.e. less than the fifth percentile for the groups over 2,500 g.); one-fifth were markedly underheight; and one-sixth were underweight and underheight. The rate of growth varied with:

(a) Maternal efficiency.
(b) Frequency of illness.
(c) Diet and feeding problems.
(d) Parental height.
(e) Maturity at birth.

Genetic and environmental factors were found to be of equal importance in their influence on growth. Generally speaking, the physical development varied inversely with the birth weight: among 72 infants weighing 3 lb. (1,360 g.) or less at birth, one-third were below the fifth percentile in weight; nearly half in height; and over one-quarter in both weight and height. In the group weighing $4\frac{1}{2}$–$5\frac{1}{2}$ lb. at birth, the height and weight were lower among those born *after* 38 weeks gestation, i.e. the low-weight term babies (light-for-dates babies).

In Colorado, Lubchenco and her colleagues (1962) examined 73 infants (birth weight 1,500 g. or less) at the age of 10 years and found 41% below the tenth percentile for weight and 47% below for height. They noticed that light-for-dates infants were particularly likely to remain small.

Warkany *et al.* (1961) and Narbouton *et al.* (1961) also found that light-for-dates infants often remained underweight and underheight.

Robinson and Robinson (1965) followed up 227 infants to 8–10 years of age (33 weighed 1,500 g. or less, 102 weighed 1,501–2,500 g. and 92 over 2,500 g. at birth). The smallest babies were shorter and lighter: they belonged to the lower socio-economic classes and this was considered to have been more important than the birth weight.

It must therefore be accepted that pre-term babies are likely to have a lower average height and weight than term babies of the same age during the first 1 or 2 years of life unless an allowance is made for the

length of gestation; and that a few infants will never reach a normal height and weight due either to genetic causes or socio-economic factors, these factors being the cause of both the curtailed pregnancy and the subsequent small stature. If pre-term babies are compared with controls matched in regard to both these genetic and socio-economic factors, and an allowance is made for their gestational age, there is little difference in their physical development.

Light-for-dates babies weighing less than 2,500 g. at birth are more likely to remain small and light than pre-term babies under this birth weight. Again this may be due to genetic and socio-economic factors.

Mental development. Many investigators have reported mental retardation of varying severity among low-weight babies as a group (Blegen, 1932; Alm, 1953; Knobloch *et al.*, 1956; Harper *et al.*, 1959; Drillien, 1964; Wiener, 1968; Drillien, 1969).

Among pre-term infants, mental development is known to be retarded during the first year or so. They are late in reaching the various milestones, e.g. smiling, sitting without support, standing, walking, talking, bladder control, etc., if the chronological age is used. It is generally found that, in the absence of congenital malformation and of cerebral damage, this early retardation is largely eliminated if age is calculated from the expected date of delivery.

Babies who are light-for-dates are, as a group, liable to be mentally retarded (McDonald, 1964; Neligan, 1967 and 1970) especially if they are more than two standard deviations below the mean birth weight for their gestational age (McDonald, 1965). Twins (usually light-for-dates) have lower I Q levels and verbal reasoning scores than single-born infants (Babson *et al.*, 1964; Dunn, 1965; Barker and Edwards, 1967).

Bazso *et al.* (1964) and Parmelee and Schulte (1970) have shown that light-for-dates babies are more liable to be mentally retarded than pre-term babies. Parmelee and Schulte performed Gesell developmental tests on normal term babies, light-for-dates babies and pre-term babies at the chronological age of 40 weeks. Their developmental quotients (D Q) were respectively: 99, 96 and 88; but when corrected for gestational age the D Q for the pre-term babies was 99, i.e. the same as that of the term babies.

Birth weight and gestational age are influenced by so many factors and many of these factors can affect mental development. As long ago as 1941 Brander showed the effects of poor heredity and complications of childbirth on the intelligence of low-weight babies. Among those with both poor heredity and complications of childbirth, 35% had an I Q less than 70. A similar low I Q was found in 24·1% of babies with poor heredity only, in 13·6% of babies with good heredity but complications of childbirth, and only in 4·3% of babies with good heredity and no birth complications. Various workers have shown that the I Q is highest among low-weight babies coming from the higher social classes (Blegen, 1952; Alm, 1953; Dann *et al.*, 1958; Drillien, 1959); and Drillien (1959) found that the D Q (Developmental Quotient) of the baby was closely related to the I Q of the mother. Also it is generally recognized that certain adverse environmental conditions lead to a failure to realize potential mental capacity, e.g. lack of educational opportunity, or large size of family. An inverse relationship has been shown between family size and intelligence (The Scottish Council for Research in Education, 1949; Barker and Edwards, 1967) and between inadequacy of the home and intelligence (Burt, 1955). Butler (1970) found that the chance of having a backward child was 11 times higher in an unskilled family than in a professional family.

Douglas (1956a) reported on the age at which his matched low-weight infants and controls walked and talked. After eliminating three defective low-weight infants and one defective control, the low-weight infants were not retarded in walking or talking if age was considered from conception and not from birth. Douglas (1956b) gave reading, vocabulary and intelligence tests to the low-weight infants and their controls at the age of 8 years. The low-weight children scored less than their controls in each of the tests, being proportionally the most handicapped in reading. The handicaps of the low-weight children did not increase significantly with either falling birth weight or decreasing length of gestation. In general the handicaps found were small, but there was a small well-defined group with no obstetric or genetic explanation of their low birth weight who were heavily handicapped in all tests: he found that relatively high scores were made by low-weight children with a history of toxaemia or other abnormality during pregnancy (i.e. with a definite cause for the low weight) whereas the absence of such a maternal history was associated with low scores. Further tests were given to the same children when they were 11 years old; and the results of their "eleven-plus" examinations were also known (Douglas, 1960). At this age, the low-weight infants made consistently lower scores than their matched controls in various tests of mental ability and school achievement; and they were less than half as likely as their controls to gain grammar school places in the "eleven-plus" examination. The extent of the handicap was not related to the birth weight or length of gestation. On investigating the home circumstances Douglas found that these handicaps were due to adverse home conditions (in particular to lack of parental care and low educational aspirations) rather than to the effects of low birth weight. Although the low-weight children were of the same birth rank and had originally been in the same broad social group as their controls, there were considerable differences in parental attitudes (noted by health visitors and school teachers). When these further factors were taken into account much of the difference between the low-weight and control children disappeared. This illustrates the extreme difficulty in obtaining suitable controls.

May (1958) investigated the mental development of children weighing less than 5 lb. (2,250 g.) at birth who were born in Birmingham between July 1 and December 31, 1948; and who were legitimate, single-born, free from congenital malformation, born after a normal pregnancy and a spontaneous onset of labour (but the labour itself and the neonatal period were not necessarily normal). Each of these children was matched for sex, age and type of housing and locality, with a control weighing more than $5\frac{1}{2}$ lb. at birth and answering the same criteria as the lower birth weight group. This matching produced samples comparable on all the main points of socio-economic status and family background: the only marked difference between the two groups was the presence of many more low-weight siblings among the families of the low-weight group than among the families of the control group. The ages of the matched pairs ranged between 7 and 8 years and the investigation included various intelligence tests, reading, arithmetic, etc. These tests failed to show any inferiority of the lower birth weight group except in arithmetic where the low-weight boys had slightly lower scores than the rest. It is interesting that these children were matched just before the tests, whereas the matching of babies by Douglas took place 8 and 11 years before the tests, and many social changes could have occurred among the families concerned during this period.

Drillien (1964) found that the mean D Q (Developmental Quotient) fell steadily with decreasing birth weight; twins showed consistently lower scores than singletons of like birth weight at all ages; and that ability was related to social class (social class differences increased with the age of the child). She followed 72 infants, who weighed 3 lb. (1,360 g.) or less at birth, to the age of 5 years or more. Sixty-six were of school age and only six (9%) had an I Q of 100 or more. One-third were likely to be ineducable in normal schools (because of severe mental or physical defects or both); one-third were dull; and one-third were low average, average, or above average as regards mental ability. A marked excess of mental handicaps was found among the babies born during 1953 and 1954, when a very prolonged initial starvation period was being practised (no milk until the 5th to 9th day), and the mean loss of weight was 20·7% of the birth weight. Drillien suggests that this degree of dehydration might have resulted in impairment of the cerebral circulation. In the light of present knowledge, the risk of cerebral damage from hyperbilirubinaemia and hypoglycaemia must also have been greater than at present.

McDonald (1964) followed up 1,066 babies weighing 4 lb. (1,820 g.) and less at birth, to the age of 6–9 years. After excluding 10–15%

disabled children, the remainder had an average I Q of 102·4, no different from that of the general population. The average I Q of twins was 98·3 and of triplets 91·3. The I Q varied with the social class at all birth weights. Among those weighing less than 3 lb. (1,360 g.) at birth, the average I Q was 98·6, compared with 103·4 among those weighing 3–4 lb. at birth: those with a maturity *over* 33 weeks (light-for-dates) had a lower average I Q than those born before this time, in all social classes.

In a Baltimore study (Knobloch *et al.*, 1956; Harper *et al.*, 1959), 500 babies weighing 2,500 g. or less at birth (12% up to 1,500 g., 20% 1,501–2,000 and 68% 2,001–2,500 g.) have been followed up and compared with matched controls (over 2,500 g.). At the age of 3–5 years, most of the low-weight babies were within the normal range of intelligence; and it was only among those weighing less than 1,500 g. at birth that any appreciable handicap was found. Among this group, 24% were mentally handicapped, 37% dull or low average and 39% average or above average (comparable percentages for the matched controls were 5, 26 and 69). Social factors were beginning to influence the D Q by the age of 3 years.

Difficulties in reading and arithmetic have been found among low-weight babies (Wiener, 1968); and among pre-term babies (Davie, 1969), even after making an allowance for social class. However Davie points out that social class *per se* explains little and masks important facets of environment including parental care, parental interest in the child's education, and the quality of ideas, experience and vocabulary in the home.

Barker and Edwards (1967) have shown how the verbal reasoning (V R) scores at the age of 11 years decrease as the birth rank increases, and as the length of gestation decreases; but Record *et al.* (1969) found very small differences in V R scores between sibs with different birthweights and gestational ages. According to McKeown (1970) these investigations suggest that curtailed pregnancy and retarded intrauterine growth have little influence on intelligence as measured at 11 years of age. He considers that the differences in scores were due mainly to a difference *between* families (not *in* families), i.e. that they are due to postnatal rather than prenatal influences.

Record *et al.* (1969) also found that twins whose co-twins did not survive beyond 1 month after birth, performed almost as well as single-born babies, while the V R scores were substantially lower when both twins survived; and this supports McKeown's view that differences in postnatal experience are largely responsible for the differences in mental development.

Unfortunately low-weight babies come more often from large families in poor socio-economic circumstances with a poor heredity and poor postnatal experience. The association of poor mental development with a poor home has been shown by Dann *et al.* (1964), di Toro *et al.* (1964) and Eaves *et al.* (1970). Drillien (1968) and Eaves *et al.* (1970) report an increasing effect as the child grows older. Stock and Smyth (1963) studied cape coloured children and found that the undernourished had a lower I Q.

Certain postnatal complications are known to influence later mental development, e.g. intracranial birth injury or asphyxia, neonatal anoxia, certain infections, hyperbilirubinaemia, hypoglycaemia, etc.

Low gestational age *per se* is probably less important in relation to the mental development of a baby than the influences of heredity, perinatal complications and socio-economic factors.

Low-weight term babies (light-for-dates) are more likely to be mentally retarded than pre-term babies, presumably as the result of intrauterine anoxia.

Social development. Low-weight children are believed to be more restless and irritable, and have less power of concentration, more temper display and behaviour problems than babies born at term (Shirley, 1939; Drillien, 1948; Beskow, 1949; Kahl, 1950; Howard and Worrell, 1952).

Alm (1953) found no significant or probable difference between the social adjustment of low-weight and control infants, based on fitness for active service, military promotion, the receipt of various forms of public assistance (unemployment, poverty or sickness), the net income earned, and convictions for crime and drunkenness.

May (1958) assessed the social development of the Birmingham low-weight babies between the ages of 7 and 8 years, using the Vineland social maturity scale and reports from the mother and school teacher. She found that the degree of social maturity depended on the home conditions and not on whether the child had a low birth weight or not.

Douglas (1960) found that at the age of 11 years the low-weight babies were the subject of more adverse comment (than their controls) by their teachers, in respect of their attitude to work, power of concentration, and discipline in class but, here again, these differences were eliminated when parental attitudes were matched.

Drillien (1964) found that behaviour problems increased as the birth weight decreased (70% of those weighing 3 lb. (1,360 g.) or less at birth had such difficulties). In all birth weight groups, maladjustment at school increased with declining social class and poor maternal care: boys were more often disturbed than girls. A marked excess of disturbed behaviour was found in all birth weight groups, if there was a history of severe complication of pregnancy or labour. Babies with a birth weight of 4½ lb. (2,040 g.) or less, showed more behaviour problems than their siblings over this birth weight. In 1968 Drillien reported that pre-term children were more likely to have behaviour problems than light-for-dates babies. She also found that such problems were less marked at the age of 11 years than they had been at the age of 6–7 years.

A correlation between disturbed behaviour and complications of pregnancy and labour was also demonstrated by Pasamanick *et al.* (1956).

Instability and maladjustment among low-weight babies was also reported by Minkowski (1964), Frisk *et al.* (1964) and Wiener (1968).

Low birth weight *per se* is probably of less importance in relation to social development than the home influence and especially parental attitude. If the parental attitude is good, low birth weight should not delay or alter social development.

Physical and mental handicaps. Infants with very low birth weight are known to have a relatively high incidence of physical handicaps (with or without mental handicaps), especially neurological and sensory defects; and the incidence increases as the birth weight decreases (Illingworth, 1939; Howard and Worrall, 1952; Blegen, 1952; Alm, 1953; Dann *et al.*, 1958; Drillien, 1959; Pasamanick *et al.*, 1959; Grewar *et al.*, 1962; Lubchenco *et al.*, 1962 and 1963; Crosse, 1963; Frisk *et al.*, 1964; Heimer *et al.*, 1964; Robinson and Robinson, 1965; Wiener *et al.*, 1965; McDonald, 1967).

Pre-term infants are liable to suffer from spastic diplegia (McDonald, 1967; Griffiths and Barrett, 1967) and deafness (McDonald, 1967).

Low weight babies who are light-for-dates are more liable to have defects than pre-term infants (Warkany *et al.*, 1961; Lubchenco *et al.*, 1963; Ammann, 1963; Robinson and Robinson, 1965; Wiener *et al.*, 1965; Scott and Usher, 1966; Drillien, 1970), especially those who are retarded in length as well as weight (Warkany *et al.*, 1961), and those who are more than two standard deviations below the mean birth weight for their gestational age (McDonald, 1965). These infants are liable to suffer from cerebral palsy, cataract and fits as well as mental deficiency. Dunn (1965) has reported an increased incidence of defects, including cerebral palsy, among twins.

Causes of handicaps. In an effort to discover the causes of handicaps among low-weight babies, the author followed up 7,283 low-weight babies born in the City of Birmingham during 1951–1957, and every sixth baby weighing more than 2,500 g. born during 1954 (Crosse, 1963). Among the low-weight babies, 4·7% had physical and/or mental handicaps of which 17% were probably acquired during or after birth; while among the larger babies only 0·8% had handicaps of which 22% were probably acquired during or after birth.

Thurston *et al.* (1960) found an increased incidence of neurological defects among low-weight infants who had anoxia, blood incompatibility or obstetric trauma while low-weight infants without these complications had the same incidence as infants weighing more than 2,500 g.

Drillien (1967) thought that 75% of the handicaps among low-weight babies were due to prenatal conditions (50% developmental in origin and 25% due to intrauterine hypoxia from prenatal complications). She found more neurological defects after certain prenatal complications such as toxaemia, antepartum haemorrhage, chronic maternal heart or kidney disease, etc., and she also found complications of labour associated with neurological defects (Drillien, 1968), especially breech delivery in a pre-term infant (Drillien, 1967).

The incidence of infertility is higher among mothers of handicapped children than among mothers of normal children with the same birth weight (Drillien, 1964).

Major congenital malformations may result in low-weight babies, and Drillien (1970) found more neurological and mental defects among children with congenital malformations. Poor socio-economic status is associated with both low birth weight and congenital malformations (Butler and Bonham, 1963).

McDonald (1963) found less diplegia in centres giving oxygen for the longest periods; but Lubchenco *et al.* (1963) could find no association between oxygen administration and the incidence of handicaps at 10 years of age in children who weighed up to 1,500 g. at birth. Bacola *et al.* (1966) found that apnoea, cyanotic attacks and respiratory distress were not associated with defects in babies weighing 1,501–2,500 g. but that there might be some association (not statistically significant) among babies weighing 1,500 g. and less at birth.

An excessive concentration of unconjugated bilirubin can cause kernicterus with brain damage; and McDonald (1967) found spastic diplegia and deafness more commonly among babies who had been jaundiced, especially if their gestational age was less than 31 weeks.

Cox and Dunn (1967) showed more neurological defects among babies with clinical signs associated with hypoglycaemia than among normal babies of the same birth weight. It is not yet known whether asymptomatic hypoglycaemia can also lead to defects.

A marked excess of mental handicaps were found among babies submitted to prolonged initial starvation periods (Drillien, 1964); and the later mental and neurological status is reported to be improved by early feeding with full strength human milk (Davies and Russell, 1968). Davies and Davis (1970) found (among infants weighing 1,500 g. and less) the head circumference increased more rapidly if the early food intake and body temperature were both high.

Health. It has long been recognized that low-weight babies suffer more from respiratory infections than larger babies (Capper, 1928; Hess *et al.*, 1934; Drillien, 1948; Alm, 1953; Knobloch and Pasamanick, 1959).

Douglas and Mogford (1953a) reported a higher incidence of respiratory infection and a higher incidence of hospital admissions among the low-weight children, in comparison with their controls, for the first 2 years of life: after this age they appeared to be as healthy as those born at term.

May (1958) found that the Birmingham low-weight babies required more hospital care during the first 2 years of life than their matched controls. Some of this need for hospital care was for correction of defects, and if this reason for admission was excluded there was little difference between the low-weight babies and their controls. In regard to illnesses not requiring admission to hospital, the two groups were very similar.

Drillien (1964) found that the incidence of illness was markedly increased among babies of all birth weights when maternal care was deficient. There was a peak incidence in the second year of life for babies weighing over 4½ lb. (2,040 g.) at birth, and in the first year for those under this weight. Low-weight infants were twice as likely to be admitted to hospital during their first 2 years of life than the babies over 2,500 g. and this was not entirely due to inferior maternal care. Nine-tenths of all admissions of babies of all birth weights were on account of infective illness. Lowe and McKeown (1954) showed the association between poor social circumstances and the incidence of infection.

Summary. In comparison with babies weighing more than 2,500 g. at birth:

(1) Low-weight babies (especially light-for-dates babies) are more likely to be born with a physical or mental handicap due to a congenital malformation; and some of these handicaps can be modified by early diagnosis and expert surgical treatment of the malformation.

(2) Low-weight babies are more likely to develop physical or mental handicaps as the result of complications of labour or the neonatal period. Some of the complications which have led to such defects in the past are now usually preventable, e.g. retrolental fibroplasia and kernicterus, while others can be greatly reduced by specialized care and management, e.g. birth injury or asphyxia, hypoglycaemia, and infections.

(3) The development of any baby is influenced by hereditary factors, e.g. height, weight, intelligence and social maturity of the parents; and low-weight babies tend to be born to small light parents who are less intelligent and less socially mature.

(4) Socio-economic factors play a very important part in the development of any child; and the proportion of low-weight babies born into

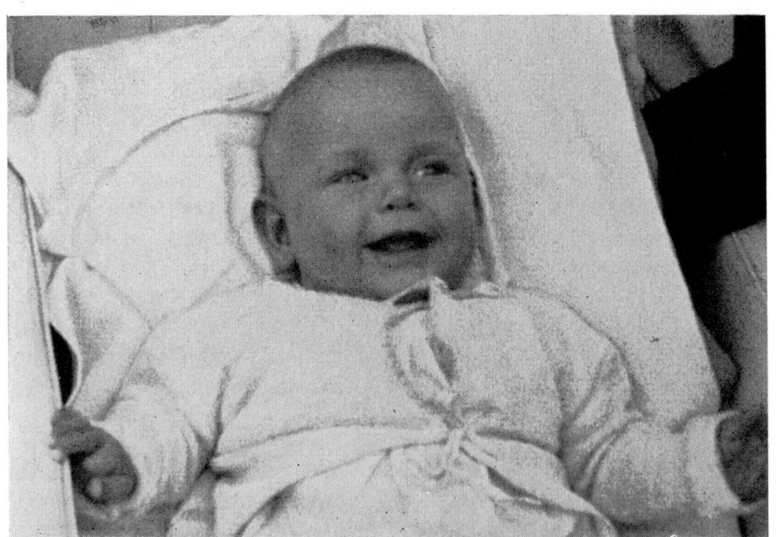

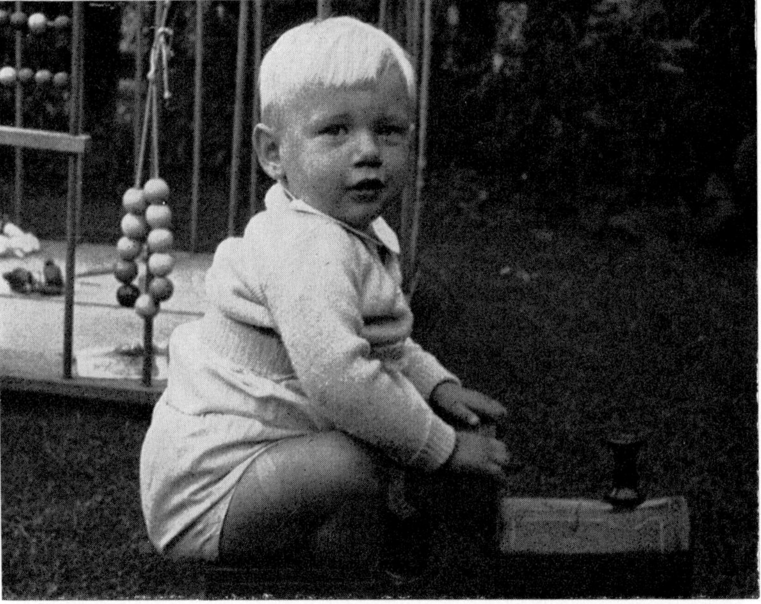

FIG. 50 (*a*) and (*b*). Two ex-pre-term babies: one 4 lb. 6 oz. (2,000 g.) and the other 3 lb. 4 oz. (1,450 g.). These are brothers, and Caesarean section was performed at 34 and 32 weeks respectively because of five previous macerated stillbirths due to Rh-immunization. Both were severely affected and required several replacement transfusions, but both grew up healthy intelligent children.

families of poor socio-economic status is higher than average. In addition, environment is believed to exert a greater influence on low-weight babies than on babies weighing more than 2,500 g. at birth (Grewar *et al.*, 1962; Drillien, 1964; Robinson and Robinson, 1965).

(5) If a baby weighs over 2,000 g. at birth, the physical, social, and mental development shows little difference from that of babies weighing more than 2,500 g. with similar genetic and social status and environment (Harper *et al.*, 1959; Wiener, 1962; Drillien, 1964).

A pre-term baby weighing 1,500–2,000 g. at birth has only a small increased risk of retarded physical and mental development, social maladjustment or neurological defect if other variables are taken into account. Babies of this weight who are light-for-dates are rather more likely to be retarded in all fields.

Babies weighing less than 1,500 g. have a definite excess of gross mental and physical defects; but if this defective group is excluded, the physical, mental and social development again depends more on genetic and environmental factors than on birth weight.

Many of the handicaps are congenital in origin; but others are the result of complications of pregnancy, labour and the neonatal period, and these should be preventable. If a baby is born free from congenital malformation and escapes the hazards of birth and the neonatal period, then low birth weight *per se* should not alter the normal course of physical and mental development if allowances are made for the length of gestation, and the effect of heredity and socio-economic factors.

As a rule babies who are going to be mentally or physically defective show early signs of abnormality. Mentally defective babies tend to twitch, show abnormalities in muscle tone and have feeding difficulties. Later they are slow in developing the usual motor skills; certain responses persist beyond the age at which they usually disappear; and abnormal signs may develop. Holt (1969) has described the neurological responses which can be elicited in the infant and their importance in diagnosing delay in development and abnormalities of the nervous system.

Many famous people are believed to have been very small at birth, for example: Isaac Newton, Charles Darwin, Voltaire, Napoleon Bonaparte, Renoir, Victor Hugo and Winston Churchill. As examples of physical strength after a low birth weight, Hackenschmidt and Lieutenant J. P. Muller can be mentioned.

Programme for the Reduction of Mortality and Morbidity due to Low Birth Weight

It is not sufficient just to save low-weight babies from death: they must be saved in a healthy condition, without physical or mental handicaps.

The reduction of both mortality and morbidity can be achieved in two ways:

(1) By reducing the incidence of low birth weight.
(2) By the provision of adequate perinatal care for all low-weight infants.

Reduction of incidence. The W H O Expert Committee on the Public Health Aspects of Low Birth Weight (1961) stressed the importance of a preventive programme for low-weight babies, whatever the incidence. It believed that preventive measures could be carried out by all countries, regardless of their level of technological development or extent of health services. Where the incidence of low birth weight is high, simple public health measures can be expected in themselves to bring an improvement, not only in reducing the incidence but also in saving many lives.

The content of a preventive programme was discussed in detail by the W H O Expert Group on Prematurity (1950), and it includes:

(a) Improvement of socio-economic conditions, especially nutrition.
(b) An educational programme, stressing the need for early and continuous prenatal care, and the maintenance of good health and nutrition during pregnancy.
(c) Provision of good prenatal care including hospitalization for women with prenatal complications.
(d) Provision of good social services during pregnancy, including domestic help when needed.

The W H O Expert Committee (1961) suggested that health education and prenatal care might sometimes have to be brought to the patient (rather than the other way round) because patients most in need of treatment and advice are the slowest and least likely to seek it. In countries where a considerable number of deliveries are attended by untrained persons, the Committee suggested that these traditional birth-attendants should be given simple instructions in health education and prenatal care. It stressed the need to take local customs and seasonal shortages into account when advising a satisfactory diet; and the importance of recognizing local diseases existing before and during pregnancy. In fact, careful thought must be given to the special problems of the country concerned.

Public Health measures. These can do much to improve the general health, nutrition and socio-economic status of the lower social classes and so reduce the incidence of low-weight births.

Family planning should be included in these measures, to allow parents to have a limited number of children with adequate spacing.

To reduce the incidence of low-weight babies due to congenital malformations all school girls should be vaccinated against rubella; and for families with a history of malformations, genetic counselling should be available.

Care during pregnancy. All mothers with a high risk of having a pre-term or growth-retarded infant should be booked for prenatal care and delivery in a specialist hospital. Mothers should also be transferred to specialist care if they are found to be having twins; if they develop such complications as severe anaemia, pre-eclamptic toxaemia, antepartum haemorrhage, pyuria, etc.; or if foetal growth appears to be retarded.

Mothers should be warned against taking any medicine or drug during pregnancy without medical advice, and they should also be warned against smoking during pregnancy.

Retarded intrauterine growth must be diagnosed as early as possible and suitably treated (see Chapter 2).

Causes of curtailed pregnancy must also be diagnosed and treated as early as possible. Labour should only be induced before 37 weeks if definite indications are present. In some cases it may be possible to prolong pregnancy if the foetal well-being can be monitored (see Chapter 2).

Care during delivery. This has been dealt with fully in Chapter 2.

Neonatal care. The major part of this book discusses neonatal care and the prevention of late sequelae.

The W H O Expert Committee (1961) expected that, before special care was planned for low-weight babies, good infant care would already be available to all infants. This alone saves many low-weight babies, especially those weighing between 2,000 and 2,500 g. at birth. All activities for the care of low-weight babies must be part of the whole programme for child care. Special care for low-weight babies would have little value if the chances of later survival were poor because of deficiencies in other aspects of the public health programme, such as poor sanitation, a high incidence of malaria or other disease, lack of suitable provision for immunization, etc. The Committee warned against undue emphasis being given to the smaller infants before doing all that is possible to save the larger ones; and they stressed the fact that special care does not necessarily mean incubator care, particularly for babies between 2,000 and 2,500 g. who not only form the largest proportion of low-weight babies but also offer the best prospect for healthy development.

Two types of special care were recommended by the Committee:

(1) **Extra care by simple means.** This can be given in the hospital or in the home. It involves less expenditure and less highly trained personnel than are required for the more specialized type of hospital care. All the basic principles of good infant care are required, with additional simple measures suited to the special needs of the

low-weight infant, e.g. the provision of extra heat by hot-water bottles, advice to the mother on artificial feeding if breast feeding is impossible, and all the necessary precautions to protect the infant from infection. In the hospital it is generally necessary to keep the low-weight baby for a longer period than usual. Care in the home involves visits by personnel trained for this purpose. If fully trained midwives and nurses are not available, suitably trained auxiliaries (supervised by more highly trained personnel) can be used. The loan of simple equipment may be necessary.

(2) **Specialized hospital care.** This should only be provided if it can be done without neglecting health services with higher priorities, and if adequately trained personnel is available. This care is only necessary for a small percentage of the babies, and these infants have a high mortality even with skilled care. This type of care is expensive and the saving of very small babies usually leads to an increased need for services for the physically and mentally handicapped who survive.

A centre for specialized care must also provide simple care, in order to allow a smooth transition from specialized hospital care to care at home after discharge. It must be in close relationship with delivery, paediatric and public health services. One of the functions of the centre is the training of all categories of personnel; and it should also provide simple practical teaching for the mothers.

In areas where specialized hospital care is not generally warranted, it may be desirable to establish a pilot centre for demonstration, teaching and research.

A centre for specialized care entails the use of incubators or heated cots, oxygen, catheter feeding, etc. Equipment and accommodation must be good; the medical and nursing personnel must be adequately trained in this very specialized branch of paediatrics if such complications as infections, hypoglycaemia, kernicterus and retrolental fibroplasia are to be avoided; and all necessary ancillary services (especially laboratory services) should be available.

A complete programme for the care of low-weight babies includes:

(1) Preventive programme.
(2) Care programme.
  (a) Assessment of requirements.
  (b) Care during delivery.
  (c) Extra care by simple means { hospital / home.
  (d) Specialized hospital care (special care units and intensive care nurseries).
  (e) Transport.
  (f) Follow-up.
(3) Integration with other health services.

(4) Educational programme.
   (a) Professional personnel.
   (b) Parents.
   (c) General public.
(5) Research programme.
(6) Regular appraisal of results.

The needs of any area can be assessed if the following data are available:

(1) Live birth rate.
(2) Incidence of live-born low-weight infants.
(3) Weight distribution of low-weight infants.
(4) Percentage of low-weight infants born in hospital and at home.

If these data are not available for any particular area, an average incidence of 7% low birth weight may be assumed in England and Wales. Approximately 30% of these babies weigh less than 2,000 g. (4 lb. 6 oz.) at birth (see p. 254) and should have the benefit of specialized hospital care if possible. The average stay in a hospital unit is 5 weeks and one hospital cot should be provided for every 10 babies to be treated annually; while the average duration of domiciliary care (for infants of 2,000 g. and over) is 4 weeks.

The care of the low-weight baby must be integrated with other health services such as:

(a) Maternity and Child Welfare (Maternal and Child Health) Services.
(b) Human milk bank.
(c) Home Help (Home Maker) Service.

In addition to training doctors, midwives, nurses and auxiliaries for hospital care of low-weight infants, centres for specialized hospital care should accept midwives and health visitors (public health nurses) from the local health authorities for training in the care of low-weight babies, both in the home and after discharge from hospital care. Ambulance nurses who will care for the low-weight babies during transport from home to hospital, or from one hospital to another, should also be given a suitable training. The hospital centres should co-operate with those responsible for the home care of low-weight babies, so that all personnel gain experience in home care as well as hospital care.

Mothers (and the families) must be taught how to look after their own infants. This teaching is started in the hospital unit, or by the special nurse in the home, and is continued by the health visitor (public health nurse) when she takes over supervision of the infant. Such education is particularly necessary for young mothers with their first baby, mothers of twins and triplets, and mothers living in poor and overcrowded homes. Correct management should prevent the development of emotional problems and reduce the risk of infection to which low-weight babies are particularly susceptible during the first few years of life.

Regular appraisal of results is important and accurate statistics are required. The W H O Expert Committee (1961) recommended that birth registration should be as complete as possible in all countries, and that the birth weight should be added to the official birth certificate (live birth or stillbirth) used in each country. It also recommended that all countries, hospitals, domiciliary services, etc. should collect all births in 500 g. birth weight groups as follows: 0–1,000 g., 1,001–1,500 g., 1,501–2,000 g., 2,001–2,500 g., 2,501–3,000 g., 3,001–3,500 g., 3,501–4,000 g., 4,001–4,500 g., 4,501–5,000 g., 5,001 g. or more. The group 2,001–2,500 g. can be divided if preferred.

Ideally, the birth weight should also be added to all death certificates of infants who die within the first year of life.

In the light of present knowledge, the length of gestation should also be added to all birth certificates; and if possible to all death certificates of infants who die during the first year of life.

REFERENCES

ABRAMOWICZ, M. and KASS, E. H. (1966). *New Engl. J. Med.*, **275**, 938.

AHVENAINEN, E. (1959). *J. Pediat.*, **55**, 691.

ALM, I. (1953). Suppl. 94. *Acta Paediat. Stockh.*

AMMANN, P. (1963). *Helv. paediat. Acta*, **18**, 438.

ANDERSON, N. A., BROWN, E. W. and LYON, R. A. (1941). *Amer. J. Dis. Child.*, **61**, 72.

ARCHIBALD, H. M. (1958). *Brit. med. J.*, **2**, 1512.

BABSON, S. G., KANGAS, J., YOUNG, N. and BRAMHALL, J. L. (1964). *Pediatrics*, **33**, 327.

BACOLA, E., BEHRLE, F. C., DE SCHWEINITZ, L., MILLER, H. C. and MIRA, M. (1966). *Amer. J. Dis. Child.*, **112**, 359.

BAIRD, D. (1945). *J. Obstet. Gynaec. Brit. Emp.*, **52**, 339.

BAIRD, D. (1952). *New Eng. J. Med.*, **246**, 561.

BARKER, D. J. P. and EDWARDS, J. H. (1967). *Brit. med. J.*, **3**, 695.

BAZSO, J., KARMAZSIN, L. and GELEI, K. (1964). International Copenhagen Congress on the Scientific Study of Mental Retardation, p. 411.

BEARGIE, R. A., JAMES, V. L. and GREENE, J. W. (1970). *Ped. Clin. N. Amer.*, **17**, 159.

BECK, A. C. (1941). *Amer. J. Obstet. Gynec.*, **42**, 355.

BECK, A. C. (1946). *Amer. J. Obstet. Gynec.*, **51**, 173.

BESKOW, B. (1949). *Acta Paediat. Stockh.*, **37**, 125.

BLEGEN, S. D. (1952). Suppl. 88. *Acta Paediat. Stockh.*

BODER, E., quoted by Parmelee, A. H. (1952). "The Management of the Newborn". Year Book Publishers, Chicago.

BRANDER, T. (1941). *Nord. Med.*, **2**, 2380 and 2181.

BUNDESEN, H. N., POTTER, E. L., FISHBEIN, W. I., BAUER, F. C. and PLOTZKE, G. V. (1951). Annual report of Chicago Health Dept.

Burke, B. S., Beale, V. A., Kirkwood, S. B. and Stuart, H. C. (1943a). *Amer. J. Obstet. Gynec.*, **46**, 38.
Burke, B. S., Harding, V. V. and Stuart, H. (1943b). *J. Pediat.*, **23**, 506.
Burt, C. (1955). "The Subnormal Mind". London, p. 123.
Butler, N. R. (1965). *J. Obstet. Gynaec. Brit. Cwlth.*, **72**, 1001.
Butler, N. R. (1970). *World Medicine*, **6**, 71.
Butler, N. R. and Alberman, E. D. (1969). "Perinatal Problems". E. & S. Livingstone, Edinburgh and London.
Butler, N. R. and Bonham, D. G. (1963). "Perinatal Mortality". E. & S. Livingstone, Edinburgh and London.
Camilleri, A. P. (1963). *J. Obstet. gynaec. Brit. Cwlth.*, **70**, 258.
Capper, A. (1928). *Amer. J. Dis. Child.*, **35**, 262.
Cavanagh, D. and Talisman, M. R. (1969). "Prematurity and the Obstetrician". Appleton-Century-Crofts, New York.
Corston, J. McD. (1957). *Obstet. and Gynec.*, **10**, 181.
Cox, M. and Dunn, H. G. (1967). *Devel. Med. Child. Neurol.*, **9**, 430.
Crosse, V. M. (1963). *Med. J. Aust.*, **2**, 1009.
Dann, M., Levine, S. Z. and New, E. V. (1958). *Pediatrics*, **22**, 1037.
Dann, M., Levine, S. Z. and New, E. V. (1964). *Pediatrics*, **33**, 945.
Davie, R. (1969). "Perinatal Problems", p. 321. E. & S. Livingstone, Edinburgh and London.
Davies, P. and Davis, J. P. (1970). *Lancet*, **2**, 1216.
Davies, P. A. and Russell, H. (1968). *Devel. Med. Child. Neurol.*, **10**, 725.
del Mundo, F. and Cruz-Adiao, A. (1953). *J. Philippine Med. Ass.*, **29**, 505.
di Toro, R., Prato, C. and de Cicco, N. (1964). *Pediatria (Napoli)*, **72**, 633.
Diddle, A. W. and Plass, E. D. (1942). *Amer. J. Obstet. Gynec.*, **44**, 279.
Dieckmann, W. J. (1946). *Amer. J. Obstet. Gynec.*, **52**, 349.
Donnelly, J. F., Flowers, C. E., Creadick, R. N., Wells, H. B., Greenberg, B. G. and Surles, K. B. (1964). *Amer. J. Obstet. Gynec.*, **88**, 918.
Douglas, J. W. B. (1950). *J. Obstet. Gynaec. Brit. Emp.*, **57**, 143.
Douglas, J. W. B. (1956a). *Med. Offr.*, **95**, 33.
Douglas, J. W. B. (1956b). *Brit. med. J.*, **1**, 1210.
Douglas, J. W. B. (1960). *Brit. med. J.*, **1**, 1008.
Douglas, J. W. B. and Mogford, C. (1953a). *Brit. med. J.*, **1**, 748.
Douglas, J. W. B. and Mogford, C. (1953b). *Arch. Dis. Childh.*, **28**, 436.
Drillien, C. M. (1947). *J. Obstet. Gynaec. Brit. Emp.*, **54**, 300.
Drillien, C. M. (1948). *Arch. Dis. Childh.*, **23**, 69.
Drillien, C. M. (1957). *J. Obstet. Gynaec. Brit. Emp.*, **64**, 161.
Drillien, C. M. (1959). *J. Obstet. Gynaec. Brit. Emp.*, **66**, 721.
Drillien, C. M. (1964). "The Growth and Development of the Prematurely Born Infant". E. and S. Livingstone, Edinburgh and London.
Drillien, C. M. (1967). *Hosp. Med.*, **1**, 937.
Drillien, C. M. (1968). *Arch. Dis. Childh.*, **43**, 283.
Drillien, C. M. (1969). *Arch. Dis. Childh.*, **44**, 562.
Drillien, C. M. (1970). *Ped. Clin. N. Amer.*, **17**, 9.
Drillien, C. M. and Richmond, F. (1956). *Arch. Dis. Childh.*, **31**, 390.
Duffield, T. J., Parker, S. L. and Baumgartner, L. (1940). *The Child*, **5**, 123.
Dunham, E. C. and McAlenny, P. F. Jr. (1936). *J. Pediat.*, **9**, 717.
Dunn, P. M. (1965). *Devel. Med. Child. Neurol.*, **7**, 121.
Eaves, L. C., Nuttall, J. C., Klonoff, H. and Dunn, H. G. (1970). *Pediatrics*, **45**, 9.
Ebbs, J. H., Tisdall, F. F. and Scott, W. A. (1941). *J. Nutrit.*, **22**, 515.
Feeney, J. K. (1952). *J. Irish Med. Assoc.*, **31**, 252.

FRAZIER, T. M., DAVIS, G. H., GOLDSTEIN, H. and GOLDBERG, I. D. (1961). *Amer. J. Obstet. Gynec.*, **81**, 988.

FRISK, M., TAKKUNEN, R. L. and HOLMSTRÖM, G. (1964). *Ann. Paediat. Finn.*, **10**, 79.

GIBSON, J. R. and MCKEOWN, T. (1952a). *Brit. J. Soc. Med.*, **6**, 152.

GIBSON, J. R. and MCKEOWN, T. (1952b). *Brit. J. Soc. Med.*, **6**, 183.

GONZAGA, A. J., WARREN, R. L. and ROBBINS, F. C. (1963). *Pediatrics*, **32**, 1039.

GRAHN, D. and KRATCHMAN, J. (1963). *Amer. J. Human Genet.*, **15**, 329.

GRAVES, L. R., ADAMS, J. O. and SCHREIER, P. C. (1962). *Obstet. and Gynec.*, **19**, 246.

GREWAR, D. A. I., MEDOVY, H., WYLIE, K. O. (1962). *Canad. med. Ass. J.*, **84**, 822.

GRIFFITHS, M. I. and BARRETT, N. M. (1967). *Devel. Med. Child. Neurol.*, **9**, 33.

HARPER, P. A., FISCHER, L. K. and RIDER, R. V. (1959). *J. Pediat.*, **55**, 679.

HEADY, J. A. and MORRIS, J. N. (1959). *J. Obstet. Gynaec. Brit. Emp.*, **66**, 577.

HEIMER, C. B., CUTLER, R. and FREEDMAN, A. M. (1964). *Amer. J. Dis. Child.*, **108**, 122.

HERRIOT, A., BILLEWICZ, W. Z. and HYTTEN, F. E. (1962). *Lancet*, **1**, 771.

HESS, J. H., MOHR, G. J. and BARTELME, P. F. (1934). "The Physical and Mental Growth of Prematurely Born Children". Univ. of Chicago Press.

HOLT, K. S. (1969). *Proc. roy. Soc. Med.*, **62**, 997.

HOUGHTON, J. W. and FRASER ROSS, W. (1953). *Trans. roy. Soc. trop. Med. Hyg.*, **47**, 62.

HOWARD, P. J. and WORRELL, C. H. (1952). *Pediatrics*, **9**, 577.

HOWARD, R. C., LICHTY, J. A. and BRUNS, P. D. (1957). *Amer. J. Dis. Child.*, **93**, 670.

ILLESLEY, R. (1955). *Brit. med. J.*, **2**, 1520.

ILLINGWORTH, R. S. (1964). "The Normal Child". J. & A. Churchill, London.

ILLINGWORTH, R. S. (1939). *Arch. Dis. Childh.*, **14**, 121.

KAHL, M. (1950). *Arch. Kinderh.*, **138**, 138.

KEUTH, U. E., SCHMIDT, G., TZIEPLY, G. and WEIDTMAN, V. (1964). *Z. Kinderheilk.*, **91**, 265.

KNOBLOCH, H. and PASAMANICK, B. (1959). *J. Obstet. Gynaec. Brit. Emp.*, **66**, 729.

KNOBLOCH, H., RIDER, R., HARPER, P. and PASAMANICK, B. (1956). *J. Amer. med. Assoc.*, **161**, 581.

LICHTY, J. A., TING, R. Y., BRUNS, P. D. and DYAR, E. (1957). *Amer. J. Dis. Child.*, **93**, 666.

LOWE, C. R. (1959). *Brit. med. J.*, **2**, 673.

LOWE, C. R. and MCKEOWN, T. (1954). *Brit. J. Soc. Med.*, **8**, 24.

LUBCHENCO, L. O., HORNER, F. A., HIX, I. E., METCALF, D., HASSEL, L., COHIG, R. and ELLIOTT, H. C. (1962). *Amer. J. Dis. Child.*, **102**, 752.

LUBCHENCO, L. O., HORNER, F. A., HIX, I. E., METCALF, D., COHIG, R., ELLIOTT, H. C. and BOURG, M. (1963). *Amer. J. Dis. Child.*, **106**, 101.

MACMAHON, B., ALPERT, M. and SALBER, E. J. (1965). *Amer. J. Epidem.*, **82**, 247.

MATERNITY IN GREAT BRITAIN. JOINT COMMITTEE OF THE ROYAL COLLEGE OF OBSTETRICIANS AND GYNAECOLOGISTS AND THE POPULATION INVESTIGATION COMMITTEE (1948). Oxford University Press, London.

MAY, E. F. (1958). Thesis for Ph.D. Univ. Birmingham.

MCDONALD, A. D. (1963). *Arch. Dis. Childh.*, **38**, 579.

MCDONALD, A. D. (1964). *Brit. J. prev. Soc. Med.*, **18**, 59.

MCDONALD, A. D. (1965). *Clin. devel. Med. No.* 19, p. 28. Ed. Dawkins and MacGregor.

McDonald, A. D. (1967). "Children of Very Low Birth Weight". Spastics Society in association with W. Heinemann, London.
McDonald, R. R. (1962). *Brit. med. J.*, **1,** 518.
McKeown, T. (1970). *Brit. med. J.*, **2,** 63.
McKeown, T. and Gibson, J. R. (1951). *Brit. med. J.*, **2,** 513.
McKeown, T. and Record, R. G. (1952). *J. Endocrin.*, **8,** 386.
McNeill, C. (1942). *Glasg. Med. J.*, **137,** 87.
Millis, J. (Working Paper No. 6). W.H.O. Expert Committee on Maternal and Child Health, Geneva, 21–26 Nov. 1960.
Minkowski, A. (1964). *Maternité*, **13,** 356.
Murphy, D. P. (1947). "Congenital Malformations". Lippincott, Philadelphia.
Naeye, R. L., Benirschke, K., Hagstrom, J. W. C. and Marcus, C. C. (1966). *Pediatrics*, **37,** 409.
Narbouton, R., Michelin, J. M., Alison, F. and Rossier, A. (1961). *Ann. pédiat.*, **37,** 197.
Neligan, G. A. (1967). *Proc. roy. Soc. Med.*, **60,** 881.
Neligan, G. A. (1970). *Brit. J. hosp. Med.*, **3,** 587.
Nørregaard, S. (1953). "Causes of Prematurity; a Clinical Study", Arne Frost-Hansens Forlag, Copenhagen.
Ounsted, M. (1965). *Develop. Med. Child. Neurol.*, **7,** 479.
Palmelee, A. H. (1961). *Amer. J. Obstet. Gynec.*, **81,** 81.
Parmelee, A. H. Jr. and Schulte, F. J. (1970). *Pediatrics*, **45,** 21.
Pasamanick, B., Rogers, M. E. and Lilienfeld, A. M. (1956). *Amer. J. Psychiat.*, **112,** 613.
Peckham, C. H. (1938). *J. Pediat.*, **13,** 474.
People's League of Health (1942). *Lancet*, **2,** 10.
Räihä, C. E. (1947). *Ann. med. int. Fenniae*, **36,** 619.
Räihä, C. E. (1956). *Neonatal Studies*, **5,** 87.
Rantakallio, P. (1969). *Act. Paed. Scand.*, Suppl. 193.
Ravenholt, R. T. and Levinski, M. J. (1965). *Lancet*, **1,** 961.
Record, R. G., Gibson, J. R. and McKeown, T. (1952). *J. Obstet. Gynaec., Brit. Emp.*, **59,** 471.
Record, R. G., McKeown, T. and Edwards, J. H. (1969). *Ann. Human Genet.*, **33,** 71.
Report of the Ministry of Health for 1958. Part II. H.M. Stationery Office, London.
Robinson, M. R. and Robinson, H. B. (1965). *Pediatrics*, **35,** 425.
Russell, C. S., Taylor, R. and Law, C. E. (1968). *Brit. J. Soc. Med.*, **22,** 119.
Russell, G. R. and Betts, W. A. (1952). *J. Pediat.*, **40,** 722.
Salber, E. J. and Bradshaw, E. S. (1951). *Brit. J. Soc. Med.*, **5,** 113.
Scott, K. E. and Usher, R. (1966). *Amer. J. Obstet. Gynec.*, **94,** 951.
Scottish Council for Research in Education (1949). The Trend of Scottish Intelligence, London, p. 101.
Shirley, M. (1939). *Child. Dev.*, **10,** 115.
Shutt, W. (1965). Little Club Clin. devel. Med. No. 19. W. Heinemann, London.
Simpson, A. S. (1964). *Med. Offr.*, **112,** 155.
Simpson, W. J. (1957). *Amer. J. Obstet. Gynec.*, **73,** 807.
Smith, C. A. (1947). *Amer. J. Obstet. Gynec.*, **53,** 599.
Stewart, A. M. (1959). *J. Obstet. Gynaec. Brit. Emp.*, **66,** 739.
Stock, M. B. and Smyth, P. M. (1963). *Arch. Dis. Childh.*, **38,** 546.
Sutherland, I. (1949). "Stillbirths: their Epidemiology and Social Significance". Oxford University Press, London.

SVIRSKY-GROSS, S. (1958). *Ann. Paediat. (Basel)*, **190,** 109.

TAFF, M. A. and WILBAR, C. L. (1953). *Amer. J. Dis. Child.*, **85,** 279.

TAYLOR, E. S., PHALEN, J. R. and DYER, H. L. (1949). *J. Amer. med. Assoc.*, **141,** 904.

TERRIS, M. and GOLD, E. M. (1969). *Amer. J. Obstet. Gynec.*, **103,** 371.

THOMPSON, A. M. (1951). *Brit. J. Nutrit.*, **5,** 158.

THOMSON, F. A. (1962). *J. Trop. Paediat.*, **8,** 3.

THURSTON, D., GRAHAM, F. K., ERNHART, C. B., EICHMAN, P. L. and CRAFT, M. (1960). *Neurol.*, **10,** 680.

TOVERUD, K. (1939). *Acta Paediat. Stockh.*, **24,** 116.

TYSON, R. M. (1946). *J. Pediat.*, **28,** 648.

UDANI, P. M. (1963). *Ind. J. Child. Hlth.*, **12,** 593.

USHER, R. H. (1970). *Ped. Clin. N. Amer.*, **17,** 199.

VAN DEN BERG, B. and YERUSHALMY, J. (1966). *J. Pediat.*, **69,** 531.

VON DER AHE, C. V. and BACH, J. L. (1951). *West J. Surg.*, **59,** 235.

WALKER, J. (1967). *Proc. roy. Soc. Med.*, **60,** 877.

WARKANY, J., MUNROE, B. B. and SUTHERLAND, B. S. (1961). *Amer. J. Dis. Child.*, **102,** 127.

WARREN, R. J., LEPOW, M. L., BARTSCH, G. E. and ROBBINS, F. C. (1964). *Pediatrics*, **34,** 4.

WHO (1950). Expert Group on Prematurity. Technical Report Series No. 27.

WHO (1961). Expert Committee on Maternal and Child Health. "Public Health Aspects of Low Birth Weight". Technical Report Series No. 217.

WIENER, G. (1962). *J. Nerv. ment. Dis.*, **134,** 129.

WIENER, G. (1968). *J. spec. Educ.*, **2,** 237.

WIENER, G., RIDER, R. V., OPPEL, W. C., FISCHER, L. K. and HARPER, P. A. (1965). *Pediatrics*, **35,** 434.

WILCOX, D. A. (1936). *Amer. J. Dis. Child.*, **52,** 848.

WOFINDEN, R. C., ROSS, A. I., AIDEN, R. and HARTLEY, G. (1952). "An Enquiry into Stillbirths and Neonatal Deaths in Bristol (1948–50)", Southmead General Hospital Group Management Committee.

WOODBURY, R. M. (1925). U.S. Children's Bureau, Pub. 142. Washington, D.C.

WOOLF, B. (1947). *Brit. J. Soc. Med.*, **1,** 73.

YERUSHALMY, J. (1938). *Amer. J. Hyg.*, **28,** 244.

YERUSHALMY, J. (1964). *Amer. J. Obstet. Gynec.*, **88,** 505.

INDEX